Nurses' Handbook of Health Assessment

THIRD EDITION

Nurses' Handbook of Health Assessment

Janet Weber, R.N., Ed.D.
Associate Professor
Department of Nursing
Southeast Missouri State University
Cape Girardeau, Missouri

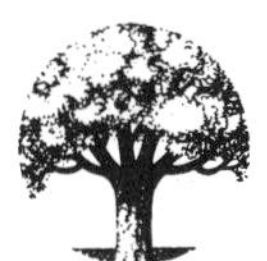

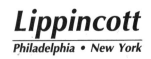

Lippincott
Philadelphia • New York

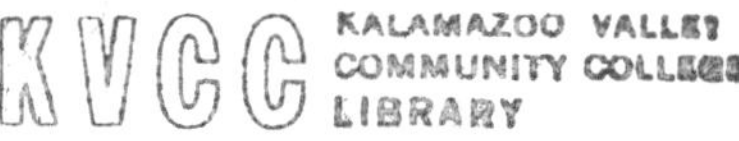

Acquisitions Editor: Mary P. Gyetvan, RN, MSN
Assistant Editor: Susan M. Keneally
Production Editor: Virginia Barishek
Production Manager: Janet Greenwood
Production: Caslon, Inc.
Cover Design: Lou Fuiano
Compositor: Maryland Composition Company
Cover Printer: Lehigh Press
Printer/Binder: R.R. Donnelley & Sons Company/Crawfordsville

Third Edition

Library of Congress Cataloging-in-Publication Data

Weber, Janet.
Nurses' handbook of health assessment / Janet Weber. — 3rd ed.
p. cm.
Includes bibliographical references and index.
ISBN 0-397-55326-9
1. Nursing assessment—Handbooks, manuals, etc. I. Title.
[DNLM: 1. Nursing Assessment—handbooks. 2. Physical Examination—handbooks. WY 39 W374n 1997]
RT48.N863 1997
610.73—dc20
DNLM/DLC
for Library of Congress 96-21001
CIP

The material contained in this volume was submitted as previously unpublished material, except in the instances in which credit has been given to the source from which some of the illustrative material was derived.

Any procedure or practice described in this book should be applied by the health-care practitioner under appropriate supervision in accordance with professional standards of care used with regard to the unique circumstances that apply in each practice situation. Care has been taken to confirm the accuracy of information presented and to describe generally accepted practices. However, the authors, editors, and publisher cannot accept any responsibility for errors or omissions or for any consequences from application of the information in this book and make no warranty, express or implied, with respect to the contents of the book.

The authors and publisher have exerted every effort to ensure that drug selection and dosage set forth in this text are in accordance with current recommendations and practice at the time of publication. However, in view of ongoing research, changes in government regulations, and the constant flow of information relating to drug therapy and drug reactions, the reader is urged to check the package insert for each drug for any change in indications and dosage and for added warnings and precautions. This is particularly important when the recommended agent is a new or infrequently employed drug.

9 8 7 6 5 4 3 2 1

To Bill, my husband,
for all your encouragement, patience, & good humor

To my sons, Joey and Wesley,
for your endless enthusiasm and joy.

To my mother for all your support

To all my students for those special
insights you gave me

To the nursing staff at Southeast Missouri Hospital
for your encouragement

To Donna Hilton and Mary Gyetvan, my editors,
who affirm my efforts & encourage new ideas.

Contributors

Jill Cash, RN, MSN
Instructor
Southeast Missouri State University
Cape Girardeau, Missouri

Jane Kelley, R.N., Ph.D.
Professor of Nursing
Southeast Missouri State University
Cape Girardeau, Missouri

Contributors to Previous Editions

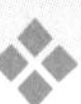

Peggy Ellis, R.N., M.S.N.
Assistant Professor of Nursing
University of Alabama—Birmingham
Birmingham, Alabama

Jane Kelley, R.N., Ph.D.
Professor of Nursing
Southeast Missouri State University
Cape Girardeau, Missouri

Kathy Lancaster, R.N.
Former Student Nurse
Southeast Missouri State University
Cape Girardeau, Missouri

Priscilla LeMone, R.N., D.S.N.
Assistant Professor of Nursing
University of Missouri—Columbia
Columbia, Missouri

Glenda McGaha, R.N., Ph.D.
Dean, School of Nursing
Troy State University
Troy, Alabama

Melissa Spezia, R.N.C., D.S.N.
Assistant Professor, College of Nursing
University of Tennessee
Memphis, Tennessee

Joy Wayman, C.N.M., M.S.N.
Clinical Midwifery Practice
Murphysboro, Illinois

Terri Woods, R.N., M.S.N.
Certified Adult Nurse Practitioner
Assistant Professor of Nursing
Southeast Missouri State University
Cape Girardeau, Missouri

Reviewers

Jane Kelley, RN, PhD.
Professor
Department of Nursing
International Coordinator
College of Health and Human Services
Southeast Missouri State University
Cape Girardeau, Missouri

Margaret G. Marks, RN, BSNE
Former Instructor
Juniata-Mifflin Area Vocational Technical School
Lewistown, Pennsylvania

Reviewers to Previous Editions

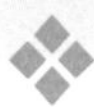

Mary Brown, R.N.
Adult Nurse Practitioner
University of Missouri—St. Louis
St. Louis, Missouri

Eileen Riviello Giardino, R.N., Ph.D.
Assistant Professor
Department of Nursing
LaSalle University
Philadelphia, Pennsylvania

Kathy Lancaster, R.N.
Returning Student
Department of Nursing
Southeast Missouri State University
Cape Girardeau, Missouri

Jacquelyn D. Reid, R.N., C., Ed.D.
Associate Professor
School of Nursing
University of Louisville
Louisville, Kentucky

Melissa Spezia, R.N.C., D.S.N.
Assistant Professor, College of Nursing
University of Tennessee
Memphis, Tennessee

Preface

The purpose of *Nurses' Handbook of Health Assessment,* a pocket-size nursing history and physical assessment guide, is to provide the student or practicing nurse with a ready reference to assist with collection of subjective and objective client data. This handbook is not intended to contain detailed anatomy and physiology or an in-depth explanation of how to do the health history and physical assessment. Many textbooks are available with specific in-depth information. Instead, this guide is intended to remind the student or nurse of information needed when assessing the client, including normal and abnormal findings. Illustrations highlight parts of the physical assessment that are easily forgotten.

The guide is divided into 20 chapters. Chapter 1 gives an overview of the nursing history. Chapter 2 consists of guideline questions necessary to elicit subjective data for a complete nursing health history. The chapter begins with questions for a client profile and developmental history, followed by health history questions organized according to Gordon's 11 functional health patterns (Gordon, 1987). The reader is referred to specific physical assessment chapters for related objective data as appropriate. A list of associated nursing diagnoses that may be identified by client responses follows each section. The nursing diagnoses used are based on the North American Nursing Diagnoses Association's (NANDA's) currently accepted list of diagnostic categories. This functional health pattern format focuses the health history within the independent domain of professional nursing.

Chapter 3 consists of guidelines for performing the physical assessment. This is followed by 17 chapters consisting of procedures for assessment of each body system. Focus questions related to each body system are listed at the beginning of each of these chapters. The physical assessment guide is followed by pediatric, geriatric, and cultural variations. Chapters 4 through 17 end with a list of possible related collaborative problems and teaching tips for selected nursing diagnoses. Chapter 18 describes the procedure for nutritional assessment. Chapter 19 explains maternal health assessment, a normal variation. A new chapter (Chapter 20) on newborn assessment has been added to this third edition.

The appendices contain tables and charts of interest in health assessment. These include common laboratory values, developmental norms, growth charts, immunization tables, recommended dietary allowances, a calorie and protein counter, sample history and physical assessment, height and weight charts, and an eye chart. In addition to the nursing diagnoses and collaborative problems appendices, a new appendix has been developed to describe possible wellness diagnoses. These are grouped according to functional health patterns. Additionally, a new appendix that focuses on family assessment has also been added.

Janet Weber, R.N., Ed.D.

Contents

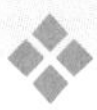

Appendices

CHAPTER 1

The Nursing Health History

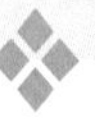

Definition and Purpose

A nursing health history can be defined as the systematic collection of subjective data (stated by the client) and objective data (observed by the nurse) used to determine a client's functional health pattern status. The nurse collects physiological, psychological, sociocultural, developmental, and spiritual client data. These data assist the nurse in identifying nursing diagnoses and/or collaborative problems.

The North American Nursing Diagnoses Association (NANDA, 1994) defines a nursing diagnosis as a clinical judgment about individual, family, or community responses to actual and potential health problems and life processes. A nursing diagnosis provides the basis for selection of nursing interventions to achieve outcomes for which the nurse is accountable. Nursing diagnoses fall into three categories: (1) Wellness diagnoses (opportunity to enhance health status), (2) Risk diagnoses, and/or (3) Actual nursing diagnoses.

Wellness diagnoses may be described as opportunities for enhancement of a healthy state (Kelley, Avant, & Frisch, 1995). There are occasions when clients are ready to improve an already healthy level of function. When such an opportunity exists, the nurse can support the client's movement toward greater health and wellness by identifying "Opportunities for Enhancement." If a client does not have a diagnosis but data reveal a risk for its development, the nurse can focus on reducing factors for a Risk diagnosis (see Table 1-1). Actual diagnoses present a current client problem.

Carpenito (1995) defines collaborative problems as certain "physiological complications that nurses monitor to detect their onset or changes in status. Nurses manage collaborative problems by implementing both physician-prescribed and nurse-prescribed interventions in order to reduce further complications (p. 30). The definitive treatment for a nursing diagnosis is developed by the nurse; the definitive treatment for a collaborative problem is developed by both the nurse and the physician. Nursing diagnoses, wellness nursing diag-

Table 1-1. Comparison of Wellness, Risk, and Actual Nursing Diagnoses

	Wellness Diagnoses	*Risk Diagnoses*	*Actual Diagnoses*
Client Status	State of harmony and balance	State of risk for identified problem	State of health problems
Format for Stating	"Opportunity for enhanced . . . or to enhance"	"Risk for . . ."	"Nursing diagnoses and related to clause."
Examples	Opportunity to enhance body image	Risk for Altered Body Image	Altered Body Image related to wound on hand that is not healing.
	Opportunity to enhance family processes	Risk for Altered Family Processes	Altered Family Processes related to hospitalization of patient
	Opportunity to enhance effective breastfeeding	Risk for Ineffective Breastfeeding	Ineffective Breastfeeding related to poor mother–infant attachment
	Opportunity to enhance skin integrity	Risk for Impaired Skin Integrity	Impaired Skin Integrity related to immobility

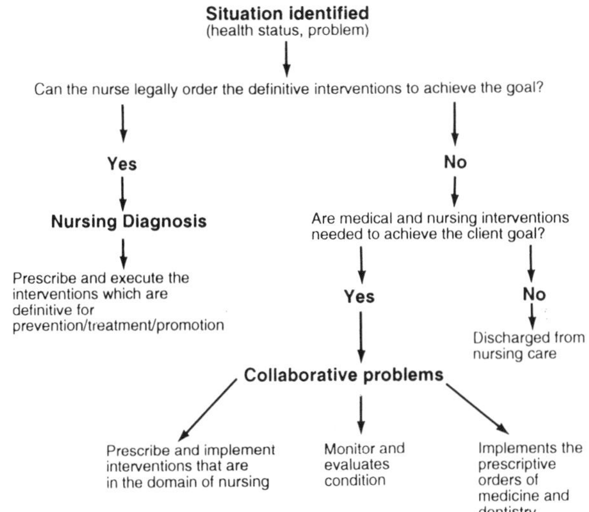

Figure 1-1. Differentiation of nursing diagnoses from collaborative problems. (© 1995, 1988, 1985, Lynda Juall Carpenito) (Carpenito, LJ: Nursing Diagnoses: Application to Clinical Practice, 4th ed. Philadelphia, JB Lippincott, 1992).

noses, and collaborative problems are listed in Appendices XIII, XIV, & XV.

Collaborative problems are equivalent in importance to nursing diagnoses but represent the interdependent or collaborative role of nursing, whereas nursing diagnoses represent the independent role of the nurse (Carpenito, 1995). Figure 1-1 illustrates the decision-making process involved in distinguishing a nursing diagnosis from a collaborative health problem. The nurse can use this model to decide whether the identified problem can be treated independently as a nursing diagnosis, or whether the nurse will monitor and use both medical and nursing interventions to treat or prevent the problem. If medical and nursing interventions are not needed, the problem is discharged from nursing care and referred to medicine and/or dentistry. The difference between a medical diagnosis, a collaborative problem, and a nursing diagnosis is explained with the following examples:

Medical Diagnosis	*Collaborative Problem*	*Nursing Diagnoses*
Fractured jaw	Potential complication: Aspiration	Altered Oral Mucous Membrane related to difficulty with hygiene secondary to fixation devices Chronic Pain related to tissue trauma
Diabetes mellitus	Potential complication: Hyperglycemia Potential complication: Hypoglycemia	Impaired Skin Integrity related to poor circulation to lower extremities Knowledge Deficit: Effects of exercise on need for insulin
Pneumonia	Potential complication: Hypoxemia	Ineffective Airway Clearance related to presence of excessive mucus Fluid Volume Deficit related to poor fluid intake

Guidelines for formulating nursing diagnoses and collaborative problems can be found in Table 1-2.

A nursing health history usually precedes the physical assessment and guides the nurse as to which body systems must be assessed. It also assists the nurse in establishing a nurse-client relationship and allows client participation in identifying problems and goals. The primary source of data is the client. Valuable information may also be obtained from the family, other health team members, and the client record.

Nursing Model versus Medical Model

There are several models of nursing that may be used to guide the nurse in data collection. However, Marjory Gordon's Functional Health Pattern assessment framework (1987) is very useful in collecting health data to formulate nursing diagnoses. Gordon has defined 11 functional health patterns that provide for a holistic client data base. A pattern is a sequence of related behaviors that assists the nurse in collecting and categorizing data. These 11 functional health patterns can be used for nursing assessment in all practice areas for clients of all ages and in the assessment of families and communities. For the purpose of this handbook, assessment is focused on the individual. However, guideline questions for families organized according to functional health patterns are included in appendix XIII. The NANDA list of accepted nursing diagnoses has been grouped according to the appropriate functional health patterns. These diagnoses

Table 1-2. Comparison of Nursing Diagnoses and Collaborative Problems

Identifying Criteria of a Nursing Diagnosis	*Identifying Criteria of a Collaborative Problem*
1. The client problem is physiological, psychosocial, or spiritual.	1. The client problem is a physiological complication.
2. The nurse monitors and treats.	2. The nurse monitors for signs and symptoms of the complication and notifies the physician if a change occurs. (In some cases the nurse may initiate interventions.)
3. The nurse independently orders and implements the primary nursing interventions.	3. The physician orders the primary treatment, and the nurse collaborates to implement those treatments he or she is licensed to implement.
Format for Stating Nursing Diagnoses	*Format for Stating Collaborative Problems*
1. Use problem + "related to" + etiology.	1. Use "Potential" complication: ________."
2. Write specific client goals.	2. Write nursing goals.
3. Write specific nursing orders (interventions), including assessments, teaching, counseling, referrals, and direct client care.	3. Write which parameters the nurse must monitor, including how often. Indicate when the physician should be notified. Identify nursing interventions to prevent the complication and those to be initiated if a change occurs.

are listed at the end of each of the functional health pattern sections in Chapter 2. Following is a brief overview of the subjective and objective assessment focus for each functional health pattern.*

1. Health Perception–Health Management Pattern
   Subjective data: Perception of health status and health practices used by client to maintain health

*Adapted from Gordon M. Nursing Diagnosis: Process and Application, 2d ed. New York, McGraw-Hill, 1987.

Objective data: Appearance, grooming, posture, expression, vital signs, height, weight

2. Nutrition–Metabolic Pattern
   Subjective data: Dietary habits, including food and fluid intake
   Objective data: General physical survey, including examination of skin, mouth, abdomen, and cranial nerves (CN V, IX, X, and XII)
3. Elimination Pattern
   Subjective data: Regularity and control of bowel and bladder habits
   Objective data: Skin examination, rectal examination
4. Activity–Exercise Pattern
   Subjective data: Activities of daily living that require expenditure of energy
   Objective data: Examination of musculoskeletal system, including gait, posture, range of motion (ROM) of joints, muscle tone, and strength; cardiovascular examination, peripheral vascular examination, and thoracic examination
5. Sexuality–Reproduction Pattern
   Subjective data: Sexual identity, activities, and relationships; expression of sexuality and level of satisfaction with sexual patterns; reproduction patterns
   Objective data: Male and female genitalia examination, breast examination
6. Sleep–Rest Pattern
   Subjective data: Perception of effectiveness of sleep and rest habits
   Objective data: Appearance and attention span
7. Cognitive–Perceptual Pattern
   For the purpose of this handbook the cognitive-perceptual pattern has been divided into two parts: (a) the sensory-perceptual pattern, to include the senses of hearing, vision, smell, taste, and touch and (b) the cognitive pattern, to include knowledge, thought perception, and language.
   a. Sensory-Perceptual Pattern
      Subjective data: Perception of ability to hear, see, smell, taste, and feel (including light touch, pain, and vibratory sensation)
      Objective data: Visual and hearing examinations, pain perception, cranial nerve examination; testing for taste, smell, and touch
   b. Cognitive Pattern
      Subjective data: Perception of messages, decision making, thought processes
      Objective data: Mental status examination
8. Role-Relationship Pattern
   Subjective data: Perception and level of satisfaction with family, work, and social roles

Objective data: Communication with significant others and visits from significant others and family; family genogram

9. Self-Perception—Self-Concept Pattern

Subjective data: Perception of self-worth, personal identity, feelings

Objective data: Body posture, movement, eye contact, voice and speech pattern, emotions, moods, and thought content

10. Coping-Stress Tolerance Pattern

Subjective data: Perception of stressful life events and ability to cope

Objective data: Behavior, thought processes

11. Value–Belief Pattern

Subjective data: Perception of what is good, correct, proper, and meaningful; philosophical beliefs; values and beliefs that guide choices

Objective data: Presence of religious articles, religious actions and routines, and visits from clergy

Using a nursing functional pattern framework assists the nurse with collecting data necessary to identify and validate nursing diagnoses. This approach eliminates repetition of medical data already obtained by physicians and other members of the health care team. The medical systems history model (biographical data, chief complaint, present health history, past health history, family history, psychosocial history, and review of systems) is more useful for the physician in making medical diagnoses. Patients often complain that the same information is asked by both nurses and physicians. A nursing history, based on functional health patterns, will help eliminate this problem by assisting the nurse to assess client responses associated with nursing diagnoses and collaborative problems.

It is important for the nurse to assess each of the functional health patterns with clients because alterations in health can affect functioning in any of these areas, and alterations in functional health patterns can in turn affect health. See Appendix I for a sample nursing assessment form based on functional health patterns.

Guidelines for Obtaining a Nursing Health History

Professional interpersonal and interviewing skills are necessary to obtain a valid nursing health history. The nursing interview is a communication process that focuses on the client's developmental, psychological, physiological, sociocultural, and spiritual responses that can be treated with nursing and collaborative interventions. The nursing interview has three basic phases; these phases are briefly explained below by describing the roles of the nurse and the client during each phase.

1. *Introductory Phase.* The nurse introduces self and explains the purpose of the interview to the client. An explanation of note taking,

confidentiality, and type of questions to be asked should be given. Comfort, privacy, and confidentiality are provided.
2. *Working Phase.* The nurse facilitates the client's comments about major biographical data, reason for seeking health care, and functional health pattern responses. The nurse must listen and observe cues in addition to using critical thinking skills to interpret and validate information received from the client. The nurse and client collaborate to identify client problems and goals. The approach used for facilitation may be either free flowing or more structured with specific questions, depending on time available and the type of data needed.
3. *Summary and Closure Phase.* The nurse summarizes information obtained during the working phase and validates problems and goals with the client. Possible plans to resolve the problem (nursing diagnoses and collaborative problems) are identified and discussed with the client.

There are specific communication techniques used to facilitate the interview. Following are some specific guidelines for phrasing statements and questions to promote an effective and productive interview.

1. Types of Questions to Use

a. Use open-ended questions to elecit the client's feelings and perceptions. These questions begin with "what," "how," or "which," because they require more than a one-word response.
b. Use closed-ended questions to obtain facts and to zero in on specific information. The client can respond with one or two words. These questions begin with "how," "when," or "did"; they help to avoid rambling by the client.
c. Use a "laundry list" (scrambled words) approach to obtain specific answers. For example, "Is pain severe, dull, sharp, mild, cutting, piercing? Does pain occur once every year, day, month, hour?" This reduces the likelihood of the client's perceiving and providing an expected answer.
d. Explore all data that deviate from normal with the following questions: What alleviates or aggravates the problem? How long has it occurred? How severe is it? Does it radiate? When does it occur? Is its onset gradual or sudden?

2. Types of Statements to Use

a. Rephrase or repeat your perception of client's response in order to reflect or clarify information shared. For example, "You feel you have a serious illness?"
b. Encourage verbalization of client by "um hum," "yes," "I agree," or nodding.
c. Describe what you observe in the client. For example, "It seems you have difficulty on the right side."

3. Additional Helpful Hints

a. Accept the client; display a nonjudgmental attitude.
b. Use silence to help the client and yourself reflect and reorganize thoughts.

c. Provide the client with information during the interview as questions and concerns arise.

4. Communication Styles to Avoid

a. Excessive or not enough eye contact (varies with cultures).
b. Doing other things while getting the history and being mentally distant or physically far away from client (more than 2–3 feet).
c. Biased or leading questions. For example, "You don't feel bad, do you?"
d. Relying on memory to recall all the information or recording all the details.
e. Rushing the patient.
f. Reading questions from the history form, distracting attention from the client.

5. Specific Age Variations

a. Interviewing the pediatric client: Birth–early adolescence (through age 14). All information from the history should be validated for reliability with the responsible significant other (i.e., parent, grandparent).
b. Interviewing the geriatric patient
   (1) Use simple, straightforward questions in lay terms.
   (2) Establish and maintain privacy (especially important).
   (3) Assess hearing acuity; with loss, speak slowly, face the client, and speak on the side on which hearing is more adequate.
   (4) *Remember:* Age affects and often slows all body systems within an individual to varying degress.

6. Emotional Variations

a. *Angry client:* Approach in a calm, reassuring, in-control manner. Allow ventilation of feelings. Avoid arguing, and provide personal space.
b. *Anxious client:* Approach with simple, organized information. Explain your role and purpose.
c. *Manipulative client:* Provide structure and set limits.
d. *Depressed client:* Express interest and understanding in a neutral manner.
e. *Sensitive issues* (e.g., sexuality, dying, spirituality): Be aware of your own thoughts and feelings regarding dying, spirituality, and sexuality. These factors may affect the client's health and need to be discussed with someone. Such personal, sensitive topics may be referred when the nurse does not feel comfortable discussing these topics.

7. Cultural Variations: Ethnic variations in communication and self-disclosure styles may seriously affect the information obtained. Be aware of possible variations in the communication styles of self and patient. If misunderstanding or difficulty in communicating is evident, seek help from a culture broker who is skilled at crosscultural communication. Frequently noted variations are:

a. Reluctance to reveal personal information to strangers for various culturally based reasons.
b. Variation in willingness to openly express emotional distress or pain.
c. Variation in ability to receive information/listen.
d. Variation in meaning conveyed by use of language (e.g., by nonnative speakers; by use of slang).
e. Variation in use and meaning of nonverbal communication: eye contact, stance, gestures, demeanor (e.g., eye contact may be perceived as rude, aggressive, or immodest by some cultures, but lack of eye contact may be perceived as evasive, insecure, or inattentive by other cultures; slightly bowed stance may indicate respect in some groups; size of personal space affects one's comfortable interpersonal distance; touch may be perceived as comforting or threatening).
f. Variation in disease/illness perception; culture-specific syndromes or disorders are accepted by some groups (e.g., *susto* in Latin America).
g. Variation in past, present, or future time orientation (e.g., U.S. dominant culture is future-oriented; others vary).
h. Variation in family decision making process: person other than client or client's parent may be the major decision maker re: appointments, treatments, or follow-up care for client.

8. Assessing non-English-speaking clients

a. Use a bilingual interpreter familiar with the client's culture and with health care when possible (i.e., a nurse culture broker).
b. Consider the relationship of the interpreter to the client. If the interpreter is a child or of a different sex, age, or social status, interpretation may be impaired.
c. Not all clients can read. Basic care terms can be communicated best by pictures.

CHAPTER 2

Components of the Nursing Health History

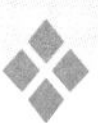

Following are the components of a nursing health history incorporating a functional health pattern approach (Gordon, 1987). Prior to data collection for each functional health pattern, a client profile and developmental history are obtained.

1. Client Profile
2. Developmental History
3. Health Perception–Health Management Pattern
4. Nutritional—Metabolic Pattern
5. Elimination Pattern
6. Activity—Exercise Pattern
7. Sexuality—Reproduction Pattern
8. Sleep—Rest Pattern
9. Sensory—Perceptual Pattern
10. Cognitive Pattern
11. Role—Relationship Pattern
12. Self-Perception–Self-Concept Pattern
13. Coping–Stress Tolerance Pattern
14. Value—Belief Pattern

The purpose of each nursing health history component will be explained, followed by guideline statements and questions to elicit subjective data from the client. Guideline questions should be preceded by open-ended statements to encourage the client to verbalize freely. Then specific questions are asked to obtain specific information. It is important to remember that not every question will apply to every client. Common sense and professional judgment must be used to determine which questions are a priority and are appropriate for each individual client.

Certain factors such as comfort level, level of anxiety, age, and current health status influence the client's ability to participate fully in the interview and must be considered. When appropriate, an objective data outline follows the subjective data questions and refers the examiner to the section where the specific examination technique, normal findings, and deviations from normal are located. At the end of each section is a list of corresponding nursing diagnostic categories for that specific nursing health history component. This list is divided into wellness nursing diagnoses, risk nursing diagnoses, and actual (problem) nursing diagnoses. Although clients can be at risk for most problem diagnoses, only NANDA-approved and a few selected other risk diagnoses are listed. Appendix I provides a documentation form for collection of subjective and objective data for each of the functional health patterns.

Client Profile

Purpose

The purpose of the client profile is to determine biographical client data and to obtain an overview of past and present medical diagnoses and treatment that may alter a client's response. This section also helps the interviewer elicit collaborative health problems.

Subjective Data: Guideline Questions

Biographical Data

What is your name?
Tell me about your background.
When were you born?
What is your ethnic origin?
How old are you?
What level of education have you completed?
Have you ever served in the military?
Do you have a religious preference? Specify.
Where do you live
What form of transportation do you use to come here or go other places?
Where is the closest health care facility to you that you would go to if ill or in an emergency?

Reason for Seeking Health Care and Current Understanding of Health

Explain your major reason for seeking health care.
What has the doctor told you regarding your health?
Do you feel you understand your medical diagnosis?

Treatments/Medications

Describe the treatments and medications you have received.
How has your illness been treated in the past?
What is being planned for your treatment now?
Do you understand the purpose of your treatment?
Have you been satisfied with your past treatments?
What prescribed medications are you taking?
What over-the-counter medications are you taking?
Do you have any difficulties with these medications?

How do they make you feel?
What is the purpose of these medications?

Past Illnesses/Hospitalizations
Tell me about any past illnesses/surgeries you have had.
Have you had other illnesses in the past? Specify.
How were the past illnesses treated?
Have you ever been in the hospital before?
How did you feel about your past hospital stays?
How can we help to improve this hospital stay for you?
Have you received any home health care? Explain.
How satisfied were you with this care?

Allergies
Are you allergic to any drugs, foods, or other environmental substances (e.g., dust, molds, pollens)?
Describe the reaction you have when exposed to the allergic substance.
What do you do for your allergies?

Developmental History

Purpose

The purpose of the developmental history is to determine the physical, cognitive, and psychosocial development of the client, in order to assess any developmental delays. Subjective data obtained from Assessment of the Functional Health Patterns (Role Relationship, Cognitive, Value-Belief, and Coping–Stress Tolerance) will assist you in determining cognitive and psychosocial development. Appendix II provides a comparison developmental table for the child. Psychosocial development of the adult and aging adult is provided in Appendix IV. Objective data obtained from the physical examination regarding height, weight, and musculoskeletal function provide a basis for determining physical development (see Developmental Information, Appendix II, and growth charts, Appendix V.)

Subjective Data: Guideline Questions

Do you have any physical handicaps?
Tell me about your health and growth as a child.
Tell me about your accomplishments in life.
What are your lifelong goals?
Has your illness interfered with these goals?

Objective Data

Appendixes II, III, V, and VI provide normal developmental charts based on age to provide a baseline by which to compare your client's physical, psychosocial, and cognitive development.

1. Does this client have obvious developmental lags that need further assessment?

2. Does this client's illness interfere with ability to accomplish the necessary developmental, physical, psychosocial, and cognitive tasks required at each age level for normal development?
3. Does this client have any physical, psychosocial, or cognitive developmental lags that aggravate his or her illness or inhibit self-care?

Health Perception–Health Management Pattern

Purpose

The purpose of assessing the client's health perception–health maintenance pattern is to determine how the client perceives and manages his or her health. Compliance with current and past nursing and medical recommendations is assessed. The client's ability to perceive the relationship between activities of daily living and health is also determined.

Subjective Data: Guideline Questions

Client's Perception of Health

Describe your health.

How would you rate your health on a scale of 1 to 10 (10 is excellent) now, 5 years ago, and 5 years ahead?

Client's Perception of Illness

Describe your illness or current health problem.

How has this affected your normal daily activities?

How do you feel your current daily activities have affected your health?

What do you feel caused your illness?

What course do you predict your illness will take?

How do you feel your illness should be treated?

Do you have or anticipate any difficulties in caring for yourself or others at home? If yes, explain.

Health Management and Habits

Tell me what you do when you have a health problem.

When do you seek nursing or medical advice?

How often do you go for professional exams (dental, Pap smears, breast, BP)?

What activities do you feel keep you healthy? contribute to illness?

Do you perform self-exams (blood pressure, breast, testicular)?

When were your last immunizations? Are they up to date? (See Immunization Tables, Appendix III.)

Do you use alcohol, tobacco, drugs? Describe the amount and length of time used.

Are you exposed to pollutants or toxins?

Compliance with Prescribed Medications and Treatments

Have you been able to take your prescribed medications? If not, what caused your inability to do so?

Have you been able to follow through with your prescribed nursing and medical treatment (e.g., diet, exercise)? If not, what caused your inability to do so?

Objective Data

Refer to Chapter 4, General Physical Survey.

Associated Nursing Diagnoses Categories to Consider

Wellness Diagnoses

Health Seeking Behaviors
Effective Management of Therapeutic Regimen

Risk Diagnoses

Risk for Injury
Risk for Suffocation
Risk for Poisoning
Risk for Trauma
Risk for Perioperative Positioning Injury

Actual Diagnoses

Energy Field Disturbance
Altered Growth and Development
Altered Health Maintenance
Ineffective Management of Therapeutic Regimen: Individual
Ineffective Management of Therapeutic Regimen: Family
Ineffective Management of Therapeutic Regimen: Community
Noncompliance

Nutritional-Metabolic Pattern

Purpose

The purpose of assessing the client's nutritional–metabolic pattern is to determine the client's dietary habits and metabolic needs. The conditions of hair, skin, nails, teeth and mucous membranes are assessed.

Subjective Data: Guideline Questions

Dietary and Fluid Intake

Describe the type and amount of food you eat at breakfast, lunch, and supper on an average day.

Do you attempt to follow any certain type of diet? Explain.

What time do you usually eat your meals?

Do you find it difficult to eat meals on time? Explain.

What types of snacks do you eat? How often?

Do you take any vitamin supplements? Describe.

Do you consider your diet high in fat? sugar? salt?

Do you find it difficult to tolerate certain foods? Specify.
What kind of fluids do you usually drink? How much per day?
Do you have difficulty chewing or swallowing food?
When was your last dental exam? What were the results?
Do you ever experience sore throats, sore tongue, or sore gums? Describe.
Do you ever experience nausea and vomiting? Describe.
Do you ever experience abdominal pains? Describe.
Do you use antacids? How often? What kind?

Condition of Skin
Describe the condition of your skin.
How well and how quickly does your skin heal?
Do you have any skin lesions? Describe.
Do you have excessively oily or dry skin?
Do you have any itching? What do you do for relief?

Condition of Hair and Nails
Describe the condition of your hair and nails.
Do you have excessively oily or dry hair?
Have you had difficulty with scalp itching or sores?
Do you use any special hair or scalp care products?
Have you noticed any changes in your nails? color? cracking? shape? lines?

Metabolism
What would you consider to be your "ideal weight"?
Have you had any recent weight gains or losses?
Have you used any measures to gain or lose weight? Describe.
Do you have any intolerances to heat or cold?
Have you noted any changes in your eating or drinking habits? Explain.
Have you noticed any voice changes?
Have you had difficulty with nervousness?

Objective Data

Assess the client's temperature, pulse, respirations, and height and weight. Refer to Chapter 5, Skin, Hair, and Nail Assessment; Chapter 6, Head, Neck, and Cervical Lymph Node Assessment; and Chapter 7, Mouth, Oropharynx, Nose, and Sinus Assessment

Associated Nursing Diagnoses Categories to Consider

Wellness Diagnoses
*Opportunity to enhance nutritional metabolic pattern
Opportunity to enhance effective breastfeeding
*Opportunity to enhance skin integrity

(* not on current NANDA list)

Risk Diagnoses

Risk for Altered Body Temperature
Hypothermia
Hyperthermia
Risk for Infection
*Risk for altered nutrition: more than body requirements
*Risk for altered nutrition: less than body requirements
Risk for Aspiration

Actual Diagnoses

Decreased Adaptive Capacity: Intracranial
Ineffective Thermoregulation
Fluid Volume Deficit
Fluid Volume Excess
Altered Nutrition: Less than body requirements
Altered Nutrition: More than body requirements
Ineffective Breastfeeding
Interrupted Breastfeeding
Ineffective Infant Feeding Pattern
Impaired Swallowing
Altered Protection
Impaired Tissue Integrity
Altered Oral Mucous Membrane
Impaired Skin Integrity

Elimination Pattern

Purpose

The purpose of assessing the client's elimination pattern is to determine the adequacy of function of the client's bowel and bladder for elimination. The client's bowel and urinary routines and habits are assessed. In addition, any bowel or urinary problems and use of urinary or bowel elimination devices are examined.

Subjective Data: Guideline Questions

Bowel Habits

Describe your bowel pattern. Have there been any recent changes?
How frequent are your bowel movements?
What is the color and consistency of your stools?
Do you use laxatives? What kind and how often do you use them?
Do you use enemas? How often and what kind?
Do you use suppositories? How often and what kind?
Do you have any discomfort with your bowel movements? Describe.

(* not on current NANDA list)

Have you ever had bowel surgery? What type? Ileostomy? Colostomy?

Bladder Habits

Describe your urinary habits.
How frequently do you urinate?
What is the amount and color of your urine?
Do you have any of the following problems with urinating:
- Pain?
- Blood in urine?
- Difficulty starting a stream?
- Incontinence?
- Voiding frequently at night?
- Voiding frequently during day?
- Bladder infections?

Have you ever had bladder surgery? Describe.
Have you ever had a urinary catheter? Describe. When? How long?

Objective Data

Refer to Chapter 14, Abdominal Assessment, and the rectal assessment section in Chapter 15.

Associated Nursing Diagnoses Categories to Consider

Wellness Diagnoses

*Opportunity to enhance adequate bowel elimination pattern
*Opportunity to enhance adequate urinary elimination pattern

Risk Diagnoses

*Risk for constipation
*Risk for altered urinary elimination

Actual Diagnoses

Altered Bowel Elimination
- Constipation
- Colonic constipation
- Perceived constipation
- Diarrhea
- Bowel Incontinence

Altered Urinary Elimination Patterns of Urinary Retention
- Total Incontinence
- Functional Incontinence
- Reflex Incontinence

(* not on current NANDA list)

Urge Incontinence
Stress Incontinence

Activity-Exercise Pattern

Purpose

The purpose of assessing the client's activity–exercise pattern is to determine the client's activities of daily living, including routines of exercise, leisure, and recreation. This includes activities necessary for personal hygiene, cooking, shopping, eating, maintaining the home, and working. An assessment is made of any factors that affect or interfere with the client's routine activities of daily living. Activities are evaluated in reference to the client's perception of their significance in his or her life.

Subjective Data: Guideline Questions

Activities of Daily Living

Describe your activities on a normal day. (Including hygiene activities, cooking activities, shopping activities, eating activities, house and yard activities, other self-care activities.)
How satisfied are you with these activities?
Do you have difficulty with any of these self-care activities? Explain.
Does anyone help you with these activities? How?
Do you use any special devices to help you with your activities?
Does your current physical health affect any of these activities (e.g., dyspnea, shortness of breath, palpations, chest pain, pain, stiffness, weakness)? Explain.

Leisure Activities

Describe the leisure activities you enjoy.
Has your health affected your ability to enjoy your leisure? Explain.
Do you have time for leisure activities?
Describe any hobbies you have.

Exercise Routine

Describe those activities that you feel give you exercise.
How often are you able to do this type of exercise?
Has your health interfered with your exercise routine?

Occupational Activities

Describe what you do to make a living.
How satisfied are you with this job?
Do you feel it has affected your health?
How has your health affected your ability to work?

Objective Data

Refer to Chapter 10, Thoracic and Lung Assessment; Chapter 11, Cardiac Assessment; Chapter 12, Peripheral Vascular Assessment; and Chapter 16, Musculoskeletal Assessment.

Associated Nursing Diagnoses Categories to Consider

Wellness Diagnoses

Potential for enhanced organized infant behavior
*Opportunity to enhance effective cardiac output
*Opportunity to enhance effective diversional activity pattern
*Opportunity to enhance effective activity-exercise pattern
*Opportunity to enhance effective home maintenance management
*Opportunity to enhance effective self-care activities
*Opportunity to enhance adequate tissue perfusion
*Opportunity to enhance effective breathing pattern

Risk Diagnoses

Risk for Disorganized Infant Behavior
Risk for Peripheral Neurovascular Dysfunction
*Risk for altered respiratory function

Actual Diagnoses

Activity Intolerance
Impaired Gas Exchange
Ineffective Airway Clearance
Ineffective Breathing Pattern
Decreased Adaptive Intracranial Capacity
Decreased Cardiac Output
*Disuse syndrome
Diversional Activity Deficit
Impaired Home Maintenance Management
Impaired Physical Mobility
Dysfunctional Ventilatory Weaning Response
Inability to Sustain Spontaneous Ventilation
Self-Care Deficit: (Feeding, Bathing/Hygiene, Dressing/Grooming, Toileting)
Altered Tissue Perfusion: (Specify type: Cardiac, Cerebral, Cardiopulmonary, Renal, Gastrointestinal, Peripheral)
Disorganized Infant Behavior

Sexuality–Reproduction Pattern

Purpose

The purpose of assessing the client's sexuality–reproduction pattern is to determine the client's fulfillment of sexual needs and perceived level of satisfaction. The reproductive pattern and developmental level of the client is determined, and perceived problems related to sexual activities, relationships, or self-concept are elicited. The physical and psychological effects of the client's current health status on his or her sexuality or sexual expression are examined.

(* not on current NANDA list)

Subjective Data: Guideline Questions

1. Female

a. Menstrual history

How old were you when you began menstruating?
On what date did your last cycle begin?
How many days does your cycle normally last?
How many days elapse from the beginning of one cycle until the beginning of another?
Have you noticed any change in your menstrual cycle?
Have you noticed any bleeding between your menstrual cycles?
Do you experience episodes of flushing, chilling, or intolerance to temperature changes?
Describe any mood changes or discomfort before, during, or after your cycle.

b. Obstetric history

How many times have you been pregnant?
Describe the outcome of each of your pregnancies.
If you have children, what are the ages and sex of each?
Describe your feelings with each pregnancy.
Explain any health problems or concerns you had with each pregnancy.
If pregnant now,

Was this a planned or unexpected pregnancy?
Describe your feelings about this pregnancy.
What changes in your life-style do you anticipate with this pregnancy?
Describe any difficulties or discomfort you have had with this pregnancy.
How can I help you meet your needs during this pregnancy?

2. Male/female

a. Contraception

What do you or your partner do to prevent pregnancy?
How acceptable is this method to both of you?
Does this means of birth control affect your enjoyment of sexual relations?
Describe any discomfort or undesirable effects this method produces.
Have you had any difficulty with fertility? Explain.
Has infertility affected your relationship with your partner? Explain.

b. Perception of sexual activities

Describe you sexual feelings. How comfortable are you with your feelings of femininity/masculinity?
Describe your level of satisfaction from your sexual relationship(s) on scale of 1 to 10 (with 10 being very satisfying).
Explain any changes in your sexual relationship(s) that you would like to make.
Describe any pain or discomfort you have during intercourse.

Have you (has your partner) experienced any difficulty achieving an orgasm or maintaining an erection? If so, how has this affected your relationship?

c. Concerns related to illness
   How has your illness affected your sexual relationship(s)?
   How comfortable are you discussing sexual problems with your partner?
   Who would you seek help from for sexual concerns?
d. Special problems
   Do you have or have you ever had a sexually transmitted disease? Describe.
   What method do you use to prevent contracting a sexually transmitted disease?
   Describe any pain, burning, or discomfort you have while voiding.
   Describe any discharge or unusual odor you have from your penis/vagina.
   What is the date of your last Pap smear?
e. History of sexual abuse
   Describe the time and place the incident occurred.
   Explain the type of sexual contact that occurred.
   Describe the person who assaulted you.
   Identify any witnesses present.
   Describe your feelings about this incident.
   Have you had any difficulty sleeping, eating, or working since the incident occurred?

Objective Data

Refer to Chapter 13, Breast Assessment; Chapter 14, Abdominal Assessment; and Chapter 15, Genitourinary-Reproductive Assessment.

Associated Nursing Diagnoses Categories to Consider

Wellness Diagnosis
*Opportunity to enhance sexuality patterns

Risk Diagnosis
*Risk for altered sexuality pattern

Actual Diagnoses
Sexual Dysfunction
Altered Sexuality Patterns

Sleep–Rest Pattern

Purpose

The purpose of assessing the client's sleep–rest pattern is to determine the client's perception of the quality of his or her sleep, relaxation,

(* not on current NANDA list)

and energy levels. Methods used to promote relaxation and sleep are also assessed.

Subjective Data: Guideline Questions

Sleep Habits

Describe your usual sleeping time at home.
How would you rate the quality of your sleep?

Special Problems

Do you ever experience difficulty with falling asleep? remaining asleep? Do you ever feel fatigued after a sleep period?
Has your current health altered your normal sleep habits? Explain.
Do you feel your sleep habits have contributed to your current illness? Explain.

Sleep Aids

What helps you to fall asleep? medications? reading? relaxation technique? watching TV? listening to music?

Objective Data

1. Observe appearance
  a. Pale
  b. Puffy eyes with dark circles

2. Observe behavior
  a. Yawning
  b. Dozing during day
  c. Irritability
  d. Short attention span

Associated Nursing Diagnoses Category to Consider

Wellness Diagnosis

*Opportunity to enhance sleep

Risk Diagnosis

*Risk for sleep pattern disturbance

Actual Diagnosis

Sleep Pattern Disturbance

Sensory–Perceptual Pattern

Purpose

The purpose of assessing the client's sensory–perceptual pattern is to determine the functioning status of the five senses: vision, hearing, touch (including pain perception), taste, and smell. Devices and

(* not on current NANDA List)

methods used to assist the client with deficits in any of these five senses are assessed.

Subjective Data Guideline Questions

Perception of Senses

Describe your ability to see, hear, feel, taste, and smell.

Describe any difficulty you have with your vision, hearing, ability to feel (e.g., touch, pain, heat, cold), taste (salty, sweet, bitter, sour), or smell.

Pain Assessment

Describe any pain you have now.

What brings it on? What relieves it?

When does it occur? How often? How long does it last?

What else do you feel when you have this pain?

Show me where on this drawing [of a figure] you have pain.

Rate your pain on a scale of 1 to 10, with 10 being the most severe pain. (Have a child use the Oucher Scale, with faces ranging from frowning to crying.)

How has your pain affected your activities of daily living?

Special Aids

What devices (e.g., glasses, contact lenses, hearing aids) or methods do you use to help you with any of the above problems?

Describe any medications you take to help you with these problems.

Objective Data

Refer to the section on Nose and Sinus Assessment in Chapter 7; Chapter 8, Eye Assessment; Chapter 9, Ear Assessment; and the section on Cranial Nerve Assessment in Chapter 17.

Associated Nursing Diagnoses Categories to Consider

Wellness Diagnosis

*Opportunity to enhance comfort level

Risk Diagnoses

*Risk for pain

Risk for Aspiration

Actual Diagnoses

Pain

Chronic Pain

Dysreflexia

Sensory/Perceptual

(* not on current NANDA list)

Alterations: (Specify: visual, auditory, kinesthetic, gustatory, tactile, olfactory)
Unilateral Neglect

Cognitive Pattern

Purpose

The purpose of assessing the client's cognitive pattern is to determine the client's ability to understand, communicate, remember, and make decisions.

Subjective Data: Guideline Questions

Ability to Understand
Explain what your doctor has told you about your health.
Do you feel you understand your illness and prescribed care?
What is the best way for you to learn something new (read, watch TV, etc.)?

Ability to Communicate
Can you tell me how you feel about your current state of health?
Are you able to ask questions about your treatments, medications, and so forth?
Do you ever have difficulty expressing yourself or explaining things to others?

Ability to Remember
Are you able to remember recent events and events of long ago? Explain.

Ability to Make Decisions
Describe how you feel when faced with a decision.
What assists you in making decisions?
Do you find decision making difficult, fairly easy, or variable?

Objective Data

Refer to the Mental Status Assessment section of Chapter 17.

Associated Nursing Diagnoses Categories to Consider

Wellness Diagnosis
*Opportunity to enhance cognition

Risk Diagnosis
*Risk for altered thought processes

Actual Diagnoses
Acute Confusion
Chronic Confusion

(* not on current NANDA list)

Decisional Conflict
Impaired Environmental Interpretation Syndrome
Knowledge Deficit (Specify)
Altered Thought Processes
Impaired Memory

Role–Relationship Pattern

Purpose

The purpose of assessing the client's role–relationship pattern is to determine the client's perceptions of responsibilities and roles in the family, at work, and in social life. The client's level of satisfaction with these is assessed. In addition, any difficulties in the client's relationships and interactions with others are examined.

Subjective Data: Guideline Questions

Perception of Major Roles and Responsibilities in Family
Describe your family.
Do you live with your family? alone?
How does your family get along?
Who makes the major decisions in your family?
Who is the main financial supporter of your family?
How do you feel about your family?
What is your role in your family? Is this an important role?
What is your major responsibility in your family? How do you feel about this responsibility?
How does your family deal with problems?
Are there any major problems now?
Who is the person you feel closest to in your family? Explain.
How is your family coping with your current state of health?

Perception of Major Roles and Responsibilities at Work
Describe your occupation.
What is your major responsibility at work?
How do you feel about those you work with?
What would you change if you could about your work?
Are there any major problems you have at work?

Perception of Major Social Roles and Responsibilities
Who is the most important person in your life? Explain.
Describe your neighborhood and the community in which you live.
How do you feel about the people in your community?
Do you participate in any social groups or neighborhood activities?
What do you see as your contribution to society?
What about your community would you change if you could?

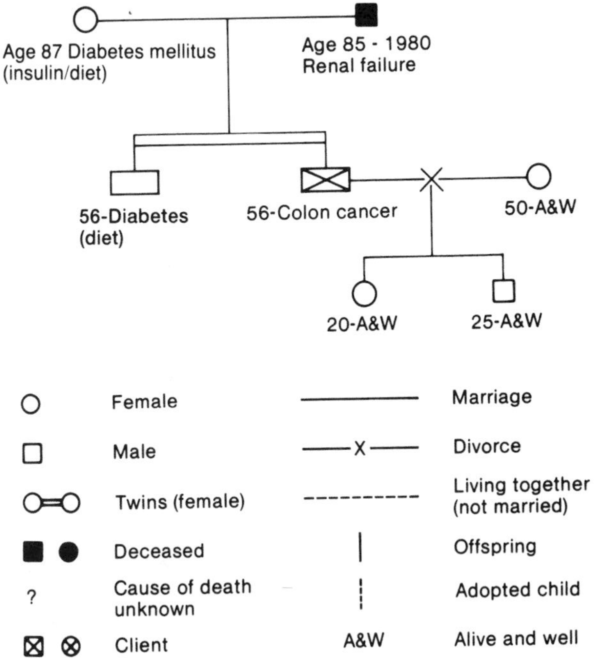

Age 87 Diabetes mellitus (insulin/diet)

Age 85 - 1980 Renal failure

56-Diabetes (diet)

56-Colon cancer

50-A&W

20-A&W

25-A&W

○	Female	———	Marriage
□	Male	—X—	Divorce
○=○	Twins (female)	- - - - -	Living together (not married)
■ ●	Deceased	|	Offspring
?	Cause of death unknown	¦	Adopted child
⊠ ⊗	Client	A&W	Alive and well

Figure 2-1. A family genogram.

Objective Data

1. **Outline a family genogram for your client. See Figure 2-1 for an example.**
2. **Observe your client's family members.**
   a. How do they communicate with each other?
   b. How do they respond to the client?
   c. Do they visit, and how long do they stay with the client?

Associated Nursing Diagnoses Categories to Consider

Wellness Diagnoses

*Opportunity to enhance effective relationships
*Opportunity to enhance effective parenting
*Opportunity to enhance effective role performance
*Opportunity to enhance effective communication
*Opportunity to enhance effective social interaction

(* not on current NANDA list)

*Opportunity to enhance effective caregiver role
*Opportunity to enhance effective grieving

Risk Diagnoses
*Risk for dysfunctional grieving
High risk for Loneliness
Risk for Altered Parent/Infant/Child Attachment

Actual Diagnoses
Impaired Verbal Communication
Altered Family Processes
Altered Family Process: Alcoholism
Anticipatory Grieving
Dysfunctional Grieving
Altered Parenting
Parental Role Conflict
Altered Role Performance
Impaired Social Interaction
Social Isolation

Self-Perception–Self-Concept Pattern

Purpose

The purpose of assessing the client's self-perception–self-concept pattern is to determine the client's perception of his or her identity, abilities, body image, and self-worth. The client's behavior, attitude, and emotional patterns are also assessed.

Subjective Data: Guideline Questions

Perception of Identity
Describe yourself.
Has your illness affected how you describe yourself?

Perception of Abilities and Self-Worth
What do you consider to be your strengths? weaknesses?
How do you feel about yourself?
How does your family feel about you and your illness?

Body Image
How do you feel about your appearance?
Has this changed since your illness? Explain.
How would you change your appearance if you could?
How do you feel about other people with disabilities?

Objective Data

Refer to the procedures for observing appearance, behavior and mood under the Mental Status Assessment section Chapter 17.

(* not on current NANDA list)

Associated Nursing Diagnoses Categories to Consider

Wellness Diagnoses
*Opportunity to enhance self-perception
*Opportunity to enhance self-concept

Risk Diagnoses
*Risk for hopelessness
*Risk for body image disturbance
*Risk for low self esteem

Actual Diagnoses
Anxiety
Fatigue
Fear
Hopelessness
Powerlessness
Personal Identity Disturbance
Body Image Disturbance
Self Esteem Disturbance
Chronic Low Self Esteem
Situational Low Self Esteem

Coping–Stress Tolerance Pattern

Purpose

The purpose of assessing the client's coping–stress tolerance pattern is to determine the areas and amount of stress in a client's life and the effectiveness of coping methods used to deal with it. Availability and use of support systems such as family, friends, and religious beliefs are assessed.

Subjective Data: Guideline Questions

Perception of Stress and Problems in Life
Describe what you believe to be the most stressful situation in your life.
How has your illness affected the stress you feel? *or* How do you feel stress has affected your illness?
Has there been a personal loss or major change in your life over the last year? Explain.
What has helped you to cope with this change or loss?

Coping Methods and Support Systems
What do you usually do first when faced with a problem?
What helps you to relieve stress and tension?

(* not on current NANDA List)

To whom do you usually turn when you have a problem or feel under pressure?
How do you usually deal with problems?
Do you use medication, drugs, or alcohol to help relieve stress? Explain.

Objective Data

Refer to the Mental Status Assessment section of Chapter 17.

Associated Nursing Diagnoses Categories to Consider

Wellness Diagnoses
*Opportunity to enhance effective individual coping
*Opportunity to enhance family coping
Potential for Enhanced Spiritual Well Being
Potential for Enhanced Community coping

Risk Diagnoses
*Risk for ineffective coping (individual, family, or community)
*Risk for self-harm
*Risk for self-abuse
Risk for Self-Mutilation
*Risk for suicide
Risk for Violence: Self-directed or directed at others

Actual Diagnoses
Impaired Adjustment
Caregiver Role Strain
Ineffective Individual Coping:
Defensive Coping I
Ineffective Denial
Ineffective Family Coping: Disabling
Ineffective Family Coping: Compromised
Ineffective Community Coping
Post-Trauma Response
Rape-Trauma Syndrome
Relocation Stress Syndrome

Value–Belief Pattern

Purpose

The purpose of assessing the client's value–belief pattern is to determine the client's life values and goals, philosophical beliefs, religious beliefs, and spiritual beliefs that influence his or her choices and decisions. Conflicts between these values, goals, beliefs, and expectations that are related to health are assessed.

(* not on current NANDA list)

Subjective Data: Guideline Questions

Values, Goals, and Philosophical Beliefs

What is most important to you in life?
What do you hope to accomplish in your life?
What is the major influencing factor that helps you make decisions?
What is your major source of hope and strength in life?

Religious and Spiritual Beliefs

Do you have a religious affiliation?
Is this important to you?
Are there certain health practices or restrictions that are important for you to follow while you are ill or hospitalized? Explain.
Is there a significant person (e.g., minister, priest) from your religious denomination whom you want to be contacted?
Would you like the hospital chaplain to visit?
Are there certain practices (e.g., prayer, reading scripture) that are important to you?
Is a relationship with God an important part of your life? Explain.
Do you have another source of strength that is important to you?
How can I help you continue with this source of spiritual strength while you are ill in the hospital?

Objective Data

1. **Observe religious practices**
   a. Presence of religious articles in room (e.g., Bible, cards, medals, statues)
   b. Visits from clergy
   c. Religious actions of client: prayer, visit to chapel, request for clergy, watching of religious TV programs or listening to religious radio stations
2. **Observe client's behavior for signs of spiritual distress**
   a. Anxiety
   b. Anger
   c. Depression
   d. Doubt
   e. Hopelessness
   f. Powerlessness

Associated Nursing Diagnoses Category to Consider

Wellness Diagnosis

Potential for Enhanced Spiritual Well-Being

Risk Diagnosis

*Risk for spiritual distress

Actual Diagnosis

Spiritual Distress (distress of the human spirit)

(* not on current NANDA list)

CHAPTER 3

Physical Assessment

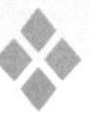

I. Physical Assessment Skills

There are four basic techniques to use in performing a physical assessment: inspection, palpation, percussion, and auscultation. The definition and proper technique for each of these is described below.

A. *Inspection*

Definition: To use the senses of vision, smell, and hearing to observe the normal condition or any deviations from normal of various body parts.

Technique:

1. Expose body parts being observed while keeping the rest of the client properly draped.
2. *Always* look before touching.
3. Use good lighting. Tangential sunlight is best. Be alert for the effect of bluish-red tinted or fluorescent lights that interfere with observing bruises, cyanosis, and erythema.
4. Provide a warm room for examination of the client. (A cold or hot environment may alter skin color and appearance.)
5. Observe for color, size, location, texture, symmetry, odors, and sounds.

B. *Palpation*

Definition: To touch and feel body parts with hands in order to determine the following characteristics:

1. Texture (roughness/smoothness)
2. Temperature (warm/hot/cold)
3. Moisture (dry, wet, or moist)
4. Motion (stillness/vibration)
5. Consistency of structures (solid/fluid filled)

Technique:

1. Examiner's fingernails should be short.
2. The most sensitive part of the hand should be used to detect various sensations. See Table 3-1.
3. Light palpation precedes deep palpation.
4. Tender areas are palpated last.

Table 3-1. Sensitivity of Parts of the Hand

Hand Part Used	*Type of Sensation Felt*
Fingertips	Fine discriminations; pulsations
Palmar/ulnar surface	Vibratory sensations (e.g., thrills, fremitus)
Dorsal surface (back of hand)	Temperature

5. Three different types of palpation may be used depending on the purpose of the exam. The purpose and technique for each are described in Table 3-2.

C. *Percussion*

Definition: To tap a portion of the body to elicit tenderness or sounds that vary with the density of underlying structures.

Technique:

Two types of percussion may be used depending on purpose. These are explained in Table 3-3. Percussion notes elicited through indirect percussion vary with density of underlying structures. Five percussion notes are described in Table 3-4.

D. *Auscultation*

Definition: To listen for various breath, heart, and bowel sounds, using a stethoscope.

Technique:

1. Use a good stethoscope that has
   - Snug-fitting ear plugs
   - Tubing not longer than 15 inches and internal diameter not greater than inch
   - Diaphragm and bell
2. The diaphragm and bell are used differently to detect various sounds, as shown in Table 3-5.

II. Basic Guidelines for Physical Assessment

A. Obtain a nursing history and survey the client's general physical status for an overall impression prior to physical assessment. This is done to determine which specific body systems should be examined (e.g., if the client complains of chest pain, a thoracic and cardiac physical exam should be performed). A complete examination of all body systems may be done only on admission.

B. Maintain privacy and proper draping.

C. Explain the procedure and purpose of each part of the exam to the client.

D. Follow a planned order of examination for each body system, using the four techniques described. Specific history questions related to each body part being examined may be integrated with the physical exam. (For example, when examining vision,

Table 3-2. Palpation

Type	*Purpose*	*Technique*
Light palpation	Used to feel for surface abnormalities (i.e., texture, tenderness, temperature, moisture, elasticity, pulsations, superficial organs and masses)	Depress skin ½" to ¾" with finger pads.
Deep palpation	Used to feel internal organs and masses for size, shape, tenderness, symmetry, mobility	Depress skin 1½" to 2" with firm, deep pressure. May use one hand on top of the other to exert firmer pressure.
Bimanual palpation (use this with caution as it may provoke internal injury)	Used to assess organs deep in abdomen	Use two hands, one on each side of body part or organs being felt. The upper hand is used to apply pressure while the lower hand is used to detect deep structures. Use one hand to push deeply on abdominal wall to move internal structure to the flank. Use the other hand to feel the structure.

ask the date of the client's last eye exam if he or she has a history of blurring, double vision.)

E. Always inspect, palpate, percuss, then auscultate, *except* in the abdominal exam. Auscultate bowel sounds and percuss the abdomen prior to palpation to avoid alterations in bowel sounds.

F. Use each technique to compare symmetrical sides of the body and organs.

Table 3-3. Percussion

Type	*Purpose*	*Technique*
Direct percussion	To elicit tenderness or pain	Directly tap body part with 1 or 2 fingertips.
Indirect percussion	To elicit one of the following sounds over the chest or abdomen: tympany, resonance, hyperresonance, dullness, flatness (see Table 3-4)	Press middle finger of hand firmly on body part. Keep other fingers off body part. Strike the finger on the body part with the middle finger (with short nail) of the dominant hand. Flex wrist quickly (not forearm). Listen to sound. Use quick wrist movement, as if you are giving an IM injection.

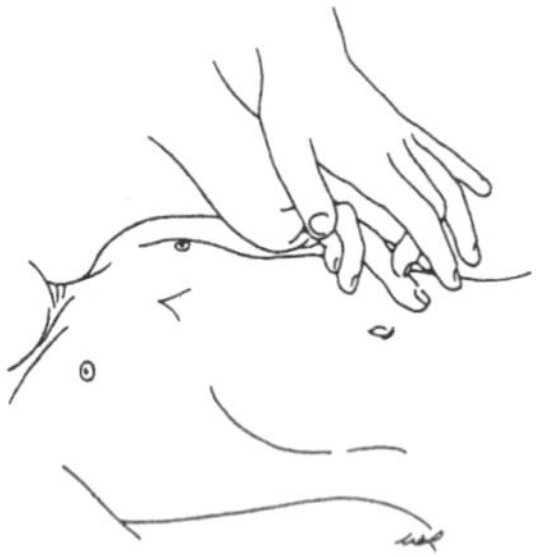

Table 3-4. Percussion

Percussion Note	*Origin*	*Sound*	*Example*
Tympany	Enclosed air	Drumlike	Puffed-out cheek; air in bowel
Resonance	Part air and part solid tissue	Hollow	Normal lung
Hyperresonance	More air	Booming	Lung with emphysema
Dullness	More solid tissue	Thud sound	Liver, spleen, heart
Flatness	Very dense tissue	Flat	Muscle, bone

Table 3-5. Uses for Diaphragm and Bell on Stethoscope

	Purpose	*Technique*
Diaphragm	To detect high-pitched sounds (i.e., breath sounds, normal heart sounds, and bowel sounds)	Press *firmly* on body part.
Bell	To detect low-pitched sounds (i.e., abnormal heart sounds and bruits)	Press *lightly* over body part.

G. Assess both the structure and function of each body part and organ (e.g., the appearance and condition of the ear as well as its hearing function).

H. When you identify an abnormality, assess for further data on the extent of the abnormality and the client's responses to the abnormality. Is there radiation of pain to other areas? Is there an effect on eating? bowels? activities of daily living? (For example, left upper quadrant abdominal pain: Is there radiation of the pain?)

I. Integrate patient teaching with the physical assessment (e.g., self-exam of breast, testicular exam, foot care for the diabetic).

J. Allow time for client questions.

Remember: The most important guideline for adequate physical assessment is conscious, continuous practice of physical assessment skills.

III. Variations in Physical Assessment of the Pediatric Client

A. Sequence of the physical assessment is dependent upon the development level of the client. (See Appendix II, Developmental Information, for detailed discussion.)

B. Establishment of rapport with the child and significant others is the most essential step in obtaining meaningful physical assessment data.

C. Allowing time for interaction with the child prior to beginning the examination helps to reduce fears.

D. In certain age groups, portions of the assessment will require physical restraint of the client with the help of another adult.

E. Distraction and play should be intermingled throughout the examination to assist in maintaining rapport with the pediatric client.

F. Involving assistance from the child's significant caregiver may facilitate a more meaningful examination of the younger client.

G. The examiner should be prepared to alter the order of the assessment and approach to the child based on the child's response.

H. Protest or an uncooperative attitude toward the examiner is a normal finding in children from birth to early adolescence, throughout parts or even all of the assessment process. Appendix II describes normal behavior at various developmental levels for the pediatric patient.

IV. Variations for Physical Assessment of the Geriatric Client

A. *Remember:* Normal variations related to aging may be observed in all parts of the physical exam.

B. Divide the physical assessment into parts in order to avoid fatigue in the older client.

C. Provide room with comfortable temperature and no drafts.

D. Allow sufficient time for client to respond to directions.

E. If possible, assess the elderly clients in a setting where they have an opportunity to perform normal activities of daily living in order to determine the client's optimum potential.

CHAPTER 4

General Physical Survey

Equipment Needed

- Beam balance scale
- Tape measure
- Thermometer
- Sphygmomanometer
- Stethoscope

I. Subjective Data: Focus Questions

Reason for seeking health care and major concern about current health? Current age, height, and weight? Recent weight changes? Fever? History of hypertension/hypotension? Difficulty breathing? Changes in pulse or heart rate?

II. Objective Data: Assessment Techniques

When you meet the client, observe the client from head to toe to note any gross abnormalities in appearance or behaviors. Assess vital signs (temperature, pulse, respirations, and blood pressure) to detect any severe deviations and to acquire baseline data. Then weigh the client and measure for height with shoes and heavy clothing removed.

Procedure	*Normal Findings*	*Deviations from Normal*
A. Observe the following:		
Behavior	Cooperative attitude and behavior	Uncooperative or bizarre, unpredictable behavior
Mood	Mild anxiety or tenseness	Moderate to severe anxiety and tenseness
Appearance	Dressed for occasion	Dress bizarre and inappropriate for occasion
Body movements	Coordinated; smooth and steady	Uncoordinated; shaky and unsteady
B. Assess vital signs by doing the following:		
1. Monitor temperature		
Temperature is usually lowest in early A.M. and highest in early P.M.		
Oral		
Place clean thermometer under tongue near vascular bed with lips closed for 5 minutes.	97°F-100°F (36°C–37.8°C) Strenuous exercise may elevate temperature to 101°F (38.4°C). Hot fluids, smoking, and gum chewing may elevate temperature, while cold fluids may lower it.	<97°F or >100°F (<36°C or >38°C); fever, chills, shivering, restlessness

Procedure	*Normal Findings*	*Deviations from Normal*
Rectal Lubricate clean thermometer with water-soluble lubricant and insert 1–2 inches into rectum for 3 minutes	1°F higher than oral temperature. Strenuous exercise may elevate temperature to 104°F (40°C).	
Axillary Insert under axilla with arm down and across chest for 5-10 minutes	1°F lower than oral temperature. Environmental temperature may alter body temperature, and stress may raise body temperature.	
2. Monitor pulse Radial: Use middle three fingers to palpate radial pulse for 15 seconds and multiply times four. Palpate for the following:		
Rate	60–100 beats/min	>100 beats/min = tachycardia <60 beats/min = bradycardia
Rhythm (if irregular, feel for full minute)	Regular	Irregular
Equality of strength	Equal bilaterally in strength	Asymmetrical in strength

Apical: Auscultate heart sounds for 1 minute with stethoscope.		
Rate	60–100 beats/min	>100 beats/min = tachycardia <60 beats/min = bradycardia
Rhythm	Regular	Irregular
3. Monitor respirations Monitor 1 full minute for the following:		
Rate	12–20/min	<12/min >20/min
Rhythm	Regular	Irregular
Depth	Equal bilateral chest expansion of 1 to 2 inches	Unequal, shallow, or extremely deep chest expansion
See Table 4-1.		
4. Monitor blood pressure Monitor after client is seated or supine quietly for 10 minutes. Repeat after 2 minutes. Repeat with client standing. Verify BP in the contralateral arm. Refer to Table 4-2.	Systolic: 100–140 mm Hg Diastolic: 60–90 mm Hg; varies with individuals	Higher or lower than normal systolic and diastolic readings (Tables 4-2 and 4-3)

C. Weigh client with light clothing and no shoes. Measure height of client. (See Appendix VI for normal and abnormal values.)

Table 4-1. Types of Respirations

	Description	*Pattern*
Normal	12–20/min and regular	
Apnea	Absence of respiration	
Bradypnea	<12/min and regular	
Tachypnea	>20/min and regular	
Hyperventilation	Increased rate and increased depth	
Hypoventilation	Decreased rate and decreased depth	
Cheyne-Stokes	Periods of apnea and hyperventilation	
Kussmaul	Very deep with normal rhythm	

Table 4-2. Classification of Blood Pressure for Adults Age 18 Years and Older*

Category	*Systolic (mm Hg)*	*Diastolic (mm Hg)*
Normal†	<130	<85
High normal	130–139	85–89
Hypertension**		
STAGE 1 (Mild)	140–159	90–99
STAGE 2 (Moderate)	160–179	100–109
STAGE 3 (Severe)	180–209	110–119
STAGE 4 (Very severe)	≥210	≥120

*Not taking antihypertensive and not acutely ill. When systolic and diastolic pressures fall into different categories, the higher category should be selected to classify the individual's blood pressure status. For instance, 160/92 mm Hg should be classified as Stage 2, and 180/120 mm Hg should be classified as Stage 4. Isolated systolic hypertension (ISH) is defined as SBP ≥140 mm Hg and DBP <90 mm Hg and staged appropriately (e.g., 170/85 mm Hg is defined as Stage 2 ISH).

†Optimal blood pressure with respect to cardiovascular risk is SBP <120 mm Hg and DBP <80 mm Hg. However, unusually low readings should be evaluated for clinical significance.

**Based on the average of two or more readings taken at each of two or more visits following an initial screening.

Note: In addition to classifying stages of hypertension based on average blood pressure levels, the clinician should specify presence or absence of target-organ disease and additional risk factors. For example, a patient with diabetes and a blood pressure of 142/94 mm Hg plus left ventricular hypertrophy should be classified as "Stage 1 hypertension with target-organ disease (left ventricular hypertrophy) and with another major risk factor (diabetes)." This specificity is important for risk classification and management.

Source: The 5th Report of the Joint National Committee on Detection, Evaluation, and Treatment of High Blood Pressure, U.S. Dept. Health & Human Services. *Arch Intern Med* (1993) 153:154–183.

Table 4-3. Recommendations for Follow-up Based on Initial Set of Blood Pressure Measurements for Adults Age 18 and Older

Initial Screening Blood Pressure (mm Hg)*		
Systolic	Diastolic	Follow-up Recommended†
<130	<85	Recheck in 2 years
130–139	85–89	Recheck in 1 year**
140–159	90–99	Confirm within 2 months
160–179	100–109	Evaluate or refer to source of care within 1 month
180–209	110–119	Evaluate or refer to source of care within 1 week
≥210	≥120	Evaluate or refer to source of care immediately

*If the systolic and diastolic categories are different, follow recommendation for the shorter time follow-up (e.g., 160/85 mm Hg should be evaluated or referred to source of care within 1 month).

†The scheduling of follow-up should be modified by reliable information about past blood pressure measurements, other cardiovascular risk factors, or target-organ disease.

**Consider providing advice about lifestyle modifications.

Source: The 5th Report of the Joint National Committee on Detection, Evaluation, and Treatment of High Blood Pressure, U.S. Dept. Health & Human Services. *Arch Intern Med* (1993) 153:154–183.

Pediatric Variations

Equipment Needed

- Tape measure
- Growth charts for specific age comparisons (see Appendix V)

I. Subjective Data: Focus Questions

- Inquire about child's development milestones (see Appendix II).
- Inquire about immunizations (see Appendix III).
- Inquire about parent-child relationships (see Appendix II).

II. Objective Data: Assessment Techniques

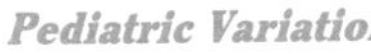

Procedure	***Normal Variations***
A. Observe physical level of development and compare to chronological age.	See Appendix II, Developmental Information.
B. Monitor temperature: *Oral:* Caution against biting glass. *Note:* Take axillary or rectal temperature in children under 6 years if they are uncooperative or unconscious.	Temperature fluctuates markedly in infants and young children.

Procedure	***Normal Variations***
Rectal: Position child prone, supine, or side-lying (may use parent's lap). Insert thermometer no more than 1 inch into rectum.	
C. Monitor pulse: Take apical pulse in children under 3 years. Count pulse for 1 full minute.	See Table 11-2 for average heart rates.
D. Monitor respirations.	Abdominal movement in infants and young children. See Table 10-1 for normal respiratory rates in children. See Figure 4-1 for average blood pressure values.
E. Monitor blood pressure *Size of cuff:* Width of cuff should cover two-thirds of upper arm or be 20% greater than diameter of the extremity. Length of bladder should encircle without overlapping.	
F. Measure height, weight, head circumference, and chest circumference	

Figure 4-1. Blood Pressure percentiles (right arm, seated) of children in Western industrialized countries.

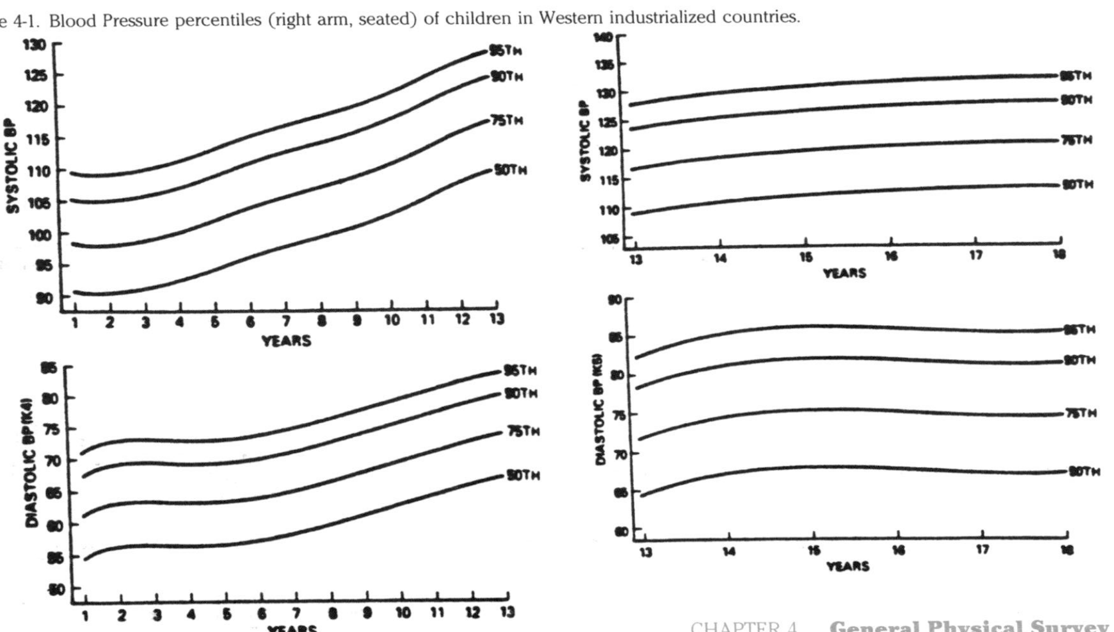

II. Objective Data: Assessment Techniques *(continued)*

Procedure	***Normal Variations***
1. *Height* *Children under 36 months:* Measure length from vertex of head to heels in recumbent position (see Fig. 4-2). *Children over 36 months:* Standing height in bare feet. Plot on growth chart.	See Appendix V for normal height ranges.
2. *Weight* For infants and young children, use platform scale.	See Appendix V. At 1 year the child's weight is three times his or her birth weight.
3. *Head circumference* *Children under 36 months:* Measure slightly above eyebrows, pinna of ears over occipital prominence of skull (see Fig. 4-2). Compare with chest circumference (Appendix V).	*At birth:* Head circumference exceeds chest circumference by 1 inch. *1–2 years:* Head circumference equals chest circumference. *Childhood:* Head circumference 2–4 inches smaller than chest circumference.
4. *Chest circumference* Measure chest diameter at nipple line (see Fig. 4-2).	

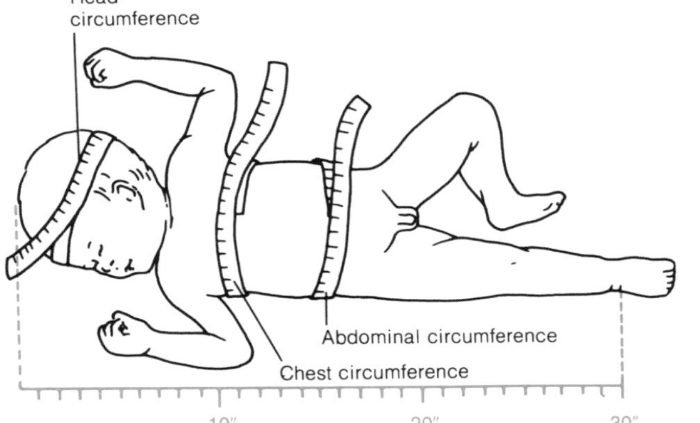

Figure 4-2. Measuring children under 36 months of age.

Geriatric Variations

- Temperature may decrease to 95°F (35°C) in cold weather.
- Temperature may normally be lowered.
- Temperature is not always elevated with an infection.
- Pulse may be increased.
- Systolic blood pressure may be increased.
- Systolic murmurs may be present.
- Height may decrease due to development of kyphosis and osteoporosis.

Cultural Variations

- Caucasian-American men tend to be .5 inches taller than African-American men.
- African-American women consistently weigh more than Caucasian-American women (Overfield, 1985).
- Blood pressure percentiles of prepubertal children in nonindustrialized countries may fall well below Western percentiles.

Possible Related Collaborative Problems

Potential complications:
Hypertension
Hypotension
Infection
Dysrhythmias

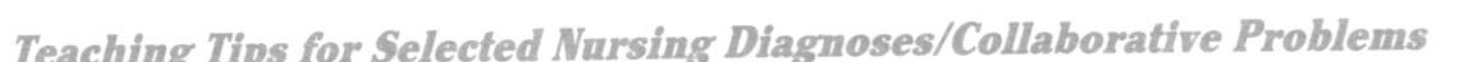

Teaching Tips for Selected Nursing Diagnoses/Collaborative Problems

Nursing Diagnoses/ Collaborative Problems	Teaching Tips
Adult Client	
NURSING DIAGNOSIS: Opportunity to enhance health seeking behaviors (desire to learn more about health promotion)	Teach client self assessment procedures (i.e., breast exam, testicular exam) and the importance of regular medical checkups. Refer to wellness resources in community and support groups as they relate to client.
COLLABORATIVE PROBLEM: Potential complication: Hypertension	Explain the relation of body weight, diet, exercise, stress, and blood pressure. Explain the possible effects of a low-fat and low-cholesterol diet along with vigorous exercise in reducing the atherosclerotic process. Explain methods of preparing food low in sodium, low in fat, and high in potassium. Teach clients who drink alcohol to limit their intake. Refer to Table 4-2 for follow-up and referral.
Pediatric Client	
NURSING DIAGNOSIS: Hyperthermia	Instruct parents on proper method to assess temperature and detect fever. Teach proper method of giving tepid sponge baths and using antipyretics to reduce fever. Explain the use of quiet play and increasing fluids during this time. Instruct parent to notify physician in case of high fever.

Teaching Tips for Selected Nursing Diagnoses/Collaborative Problems *(continued)*

Nursing Diagnoses/ Collaborative Problems	Teaching Tips
NURSING DIAGNOSIS: Altered Protection related to loss of passive immunity of placenta (age 6–12 months)	Instruct parents to clothe infant well and decrease exposure to others with illnesses. Encourage use of good hand-washing techniques and complete immunizations throughout childhood.
Geriatric Client	
COLLABORATIVE PROBLEM: Potential complication: Postural hypotension	Identify postural hypotension in elderly (difference of 20 mm Hg systolic and 10 mm Hg diastolic from a lying to standing position). Instruct client to reduce risk of falls by moving from a lying to sitting position slowly, then to stand for 2–3 minutes before proceeding.
NURSING DIAGNOSIS: Risk for hypothermia related to decreased tactile sensations, decreased cardiac output, and decreased subcutaneous tissue secondary to aging processes	Encourage good heating in homes and added clothing in cold weather. Teach family to observe for signs of hypothermia, including facial edema, pallor, clouding of vision, decreased blood pressure, and decreased heart rate. Refer to community agencies that may provide shelter, clothing, and food when needed.

CHAPTER 5

Skin, Hair, and Nail Assessment

Equipment Needed

- Adequate lighting
- Comfortable room temperature

I. Subjective Data: Focus Questions

Skin infection, rashes, lesions, itching? Precipitating factors: stress, weather, drugs, exposure to allergens? Methods of relief (e.g., medications, lotions, soaks)? Changes in skin color, lesions, bruising? Amount of sun exposure (type of lotions used)? Scalp lesions, itching, infections? Changes in texture and amount of hair? Changes in nails and cuticles? Nail breaking, splitting? Cuticle inflammation?

II. Objective Data: Assessment Techniques

Procedure	Normal Findings	Deviations from Normal
A. Inspection and Palpation		
1. General Inspection		
Expose the body part to be inspected. (Cleanse skin if not clean.)		
a. Inspect skin for generalized color.	*In white skin:* Light to dark pink *In dark skin:* Light to dark brown, olive	*In white skin:* Extreme pallor, flushed, yellow (jaundice) *In dark skin:* Loss of red tones in pallor; ashen gray in cyanosis. • Bluish-colored palms, soles, lips, nails, earlobes with cyanosis • Yellow-colored palms, soles, sclera, oral mucosa with jaundice
b. Inspect skin for color variations in patches of body	*In white skin:* Suntanned areas, white patches (vitiligo) *In dark skin:* Lighter-colored palms, soles, nail beds, and lips; black/blue area over lower lumbar area (mongolian spot); freckle-like pigmentation of nail beds and sclera	Increased pigmented areas • Erythema Decreased pigmented areas; reddened, warm areas (erythemia); black and blue marks (ecchymosis); tiny red spots (petechiae)

II. Objective Data: Assessment Techniques *(continued)*

Procedure	Normal Findings	Deviations from Normal
2. General Palpation Palpate for the following:		
Texture	Smooth and soft	Rough, thick
Temperature and moisture (feel with back of hand)	Warm, dry	Extremely cool or warm; wet, oily
Turgor (pinch up skin on sternum or under clavicle)	Pinched-up skin returns immediately to original position.	Pinched-up skin takes 30 seconds or longer to return to original position.
Edema (press firmly for 5–10 seconds over tibia and ankles)	No swelling, pitting, or edema	Swollen; shallow to deep pitting; ascites
3. Skin Inspection and Palpation *Procedure:* If a skin lesion is detected, inspect and palpate it for size, location, mobility, consistency, and pattern (circular, clustered, or straight-lined).		
	Silver-pink stretch marks (striae), moles (nevi), freckles, birthmarks	Primary lesions (Fig. 5-1), secondary lesions (Fig. 5-2), vascular lesions (Fig. 5-3)

Nonpalpable Lesion

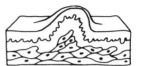

Macule: Flat and colored
(Example: Freckle, petechiae)

Palpable Lesions with Fluid

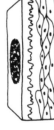

Vesicle: Elevated and
filled with fluid
(Example: Blister)

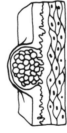

Nodules: Elevated and firm
has dimension of depth
(Example: Wart)

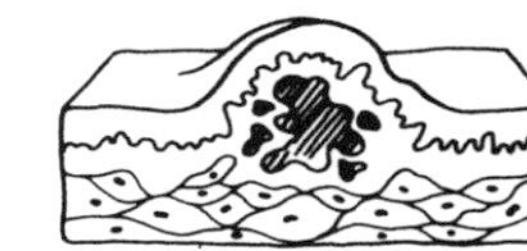

Pustule: Elevated and
filed with pus
(Example: Acne)

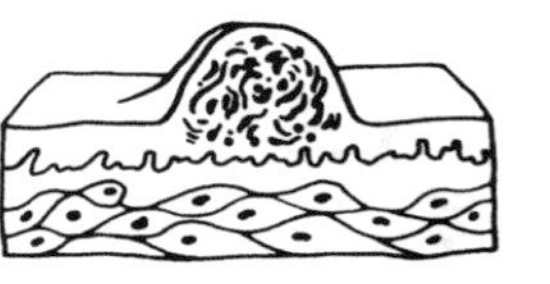

Palpable Lesion

Papule: Elevated, superficial
(Example: Mole)

Tumor: Elevated and deep;
has dimension of depth
(Example: Epithelioma)

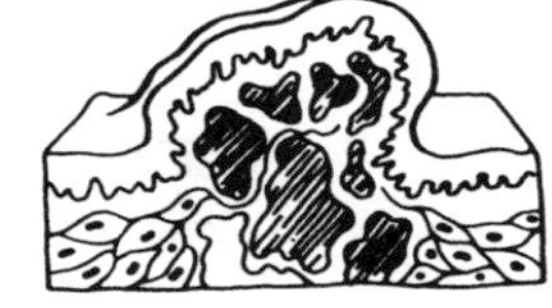

Wheal: Localized edema
(Example: Insect bite)

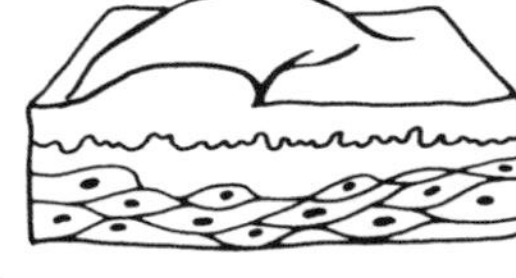

Figure 5-1. Primary skin lesions.

Ulcer: Skin surface loss, often bleeds

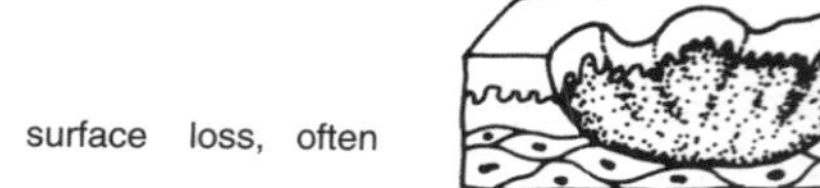

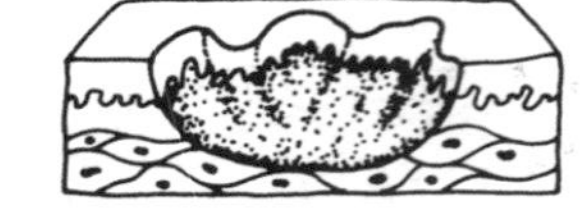

Atrophy: Thin, skinny, taut skin

Crust: Dried pus or blood

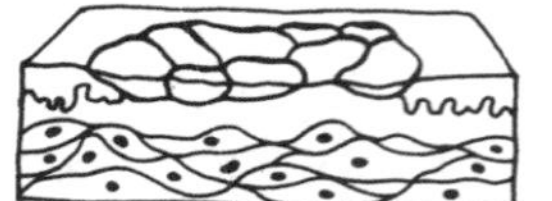

Scar: Fibrous tissue

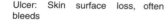

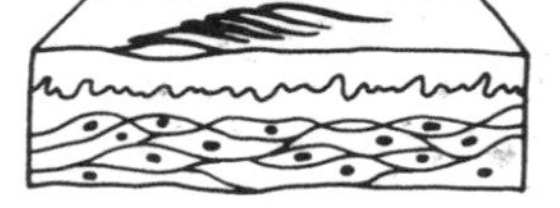

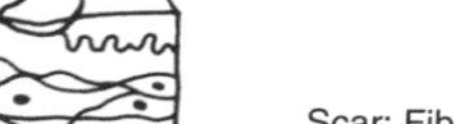

Scale: Thin, flaky skin

Keloid: Hypertrophied scar

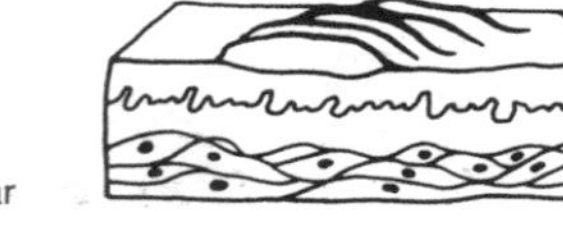

Figure 5-2. Secondary skin lesions. (changes in primary lesions).

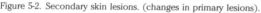

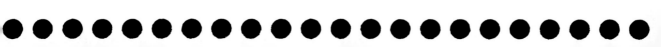

Cherry angioma: Ruby red; flat or raised

Spider angioma: Bright red with radiating legs; pulsating seen on center legs, arms, and upper trunk; blanches when pressure is applied to center

Venous star: Bluish; may have radiating legs; seen mostly on legs

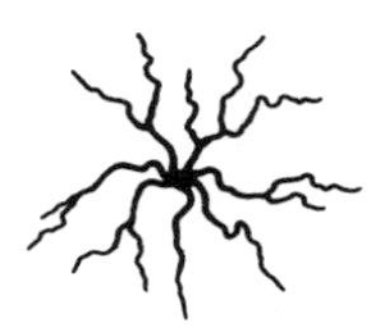

Figure 5-3. Vascular lesions.

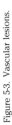

Procedure	Normal Findings	Deviations from Normal
4. Hair Inspection and Palpation Inspect and palpate hair for the following:		
Color	Varies	Copper-red hair in black child may indicate severe malnutrition
Amount and distribution	Varies	Sudden loss of hair (alopecia) or increase in area and growth of hair (hirsutism)
Texture	Fine to coarse; pliant	Change in texture; brittle
Presence of parasites	None	Lice (body or head)
5. Scalp Inspection and Palpation Inspect and palpate scalp for the following:		
Symmetry	Symmetrical	Asymmetrical
Texture	Smooth and firm	Scaly, dry flakes
Lesions	None	Open or closed lesions
6. Nail Inspection and Palpation Inspect and palpate nails for the following:		
Color	Pink nail *In dark skin:* may have small or large pigmented deposits, streaks, freckles	Pale, cyanotic nails, splinter hemorrhages (vertical lines); Beau's lines (horizontal)

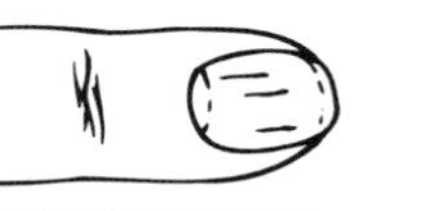

Splinter hemorrhages

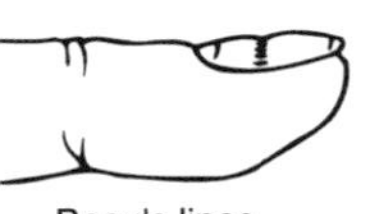

Beau's lines

Shape

Round nail with 160° nail base

160°

Normal angle

Clubbing: 180° or more nail base

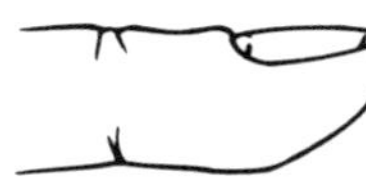

Early clubbing

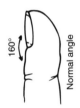

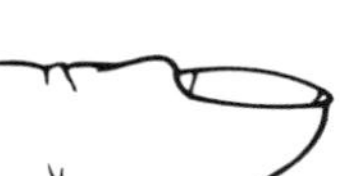

Late clubbing

II. Objective Data: Assessment Techniques *(continued)*

Procedure	**Normal Findings**	**Deviations from Normal**
Texture	Nail round and hard *In dark skin:* may be thick	Nail jagged, soft, and spooned Spoon nails
Condition of nail bed	Smooth, firm and pink	Paronychia: inflamed nail head 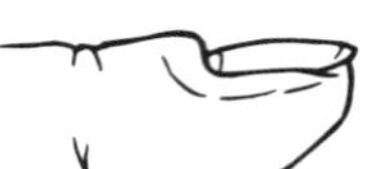 Paronychia

Pediatric Variations

I. Subjective Data: Focus Questions

- Skin eruptions or rashes (and relationship to any allergies)?
- Acne (especially during adolescence)?
- Excessive nail biting?
- History of communicable diseases?
- Immunization history (see Appendix III)

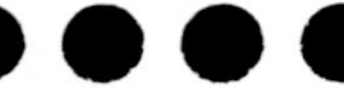
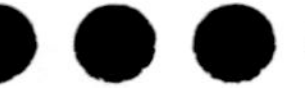
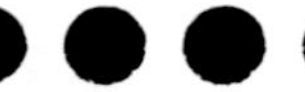
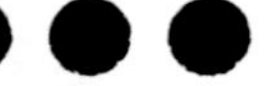

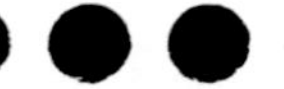

II. Objective Data: Assessment Techniques

Procedure	*Normal Findings*	*Deviations from Normal*
Assess dermatoglyphics by inspecting flexion creases in palm.	Three flexion creases present in palm	More or less than three flexion creases with varied pattern in palm, e.g., one horizontal crease in palm (simian crease)

Normal creases

Simian creases

Geriatric Variations

Skin

- Thinning epithelium
- Wrinkles, decreased turgor and elasticity
- Dry, itchy skin due to decrease in activity of ecrine and sebaceous glands
- Seborrheic or senile keratosis (tantoblack macular-elevated lesions found on neck, chest, or back)
- Senile lentigines ("liver spots" or "age spots"—flat brown macules on hands, arms, neck, face)
- Cherry angiomas (small, round, red elevated spots)
- Senile purpura (vivid purple patches)
- Acrochordons (soft, light pink to brown skin tags)
- Prominent veins due to thinning epithelium

Hair

- Loss of pigment; fine, brittle texture
- Alopecia, especially in men; sparse body hair
- Coarse facial hair, especially in women
- Decreased axillary, pubic, and extremity hair

Nails

- Thickened, yellow, brittle nails
- Ingrown toenails

Cultural Variations

- Infants and newborns of African, Native-American or Asian descent often have Mongolian spots, a blue-black or purple macular area on buttocks and sacrum; sometimes this pattern appears on the abdomen, thighs, or upper extremities.

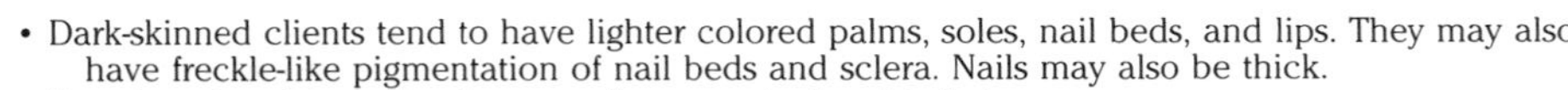

- Dark-skinned clients tend to have lighter colored palms, soles, nail beds, and lips. They may also have freckle-like pigmentation of nail beds and sclera. Nails may also be thick.
- Females of certain cultural groups shave or pluck pubic hair.
- Pallor is assessed in the dark-skinned client by observing the absence of underlying red tones. (Brown skin appears yellow-brown; black skin appears ashen-gray.)
- Erythema is detected by palpation of increased warmth of skin in dark-skinned clients.
- Cyanosis is detected in dark-skinned clients by observing the lips and tongue which become ashen-gray when the client is cyanotic.
- Inspect for petechiae in the oral mucosa or conjunctiva of the dark-skinned client, since it is difficult to see in dark pigment; also observe the sclera, hard palate, palms, and soles for jaundice.

Possible Related Collaborative Problems

Potential complications:

Skin infections	Burns
Skin rashes	Graft rejection
Skin lesions	

Teaching Tips for Selected Nursing Diagnoses/Collaborative Problems

Nursing Diagnoses/ Collaborative Problems	***Teaching Tips***
Adult Client NURSING DIAGNOSIS: Opportunity to enhance skin integrity	Teach client that regular exercise improves circulation and oxygenation of skin. Encourage protective clothing and boots when walking in wooded areas.

Nursing Diagnoses/ Collaborative Problems	***Teaching Tips***
Altered Health Maintenance related to lack of hygienic care of skin, hair, and nails	Assess hair, nail, and skin care, and instruct client on appropriate hygiene measures as necessary (i.e., use of mild soap, lotion for dry skin, wash oily areas with warm soap and water three times a day)
NURSING DIAGNOSIS: Risk for Impaired Skin Integrity related to prolonged sun exposure	Caution client against prolonged sun exposure, and instruct that proper use of sunscreen agents can decrease the risk of skin pathologies. Teach client to report a change in the size or appearance of a mole, nodule, or pigmented area, and/or the appearance of a new growth on the skin; avoid sun exposure between 10 A.M. and 3 P.M., when the sun's ultraviolet rays are strongest; avoid sunlamps and tanning parlors; use a sunscreen with a sun protection factor (SPF) of at least 15; wear protective clothing and hats (American Cancer Society, 1996).
NURSING DIAGNOSIS: Risk for Impaired Nail Integrity related to prolonged use of nail polish	Caution client of nail damage caused by prolonged use of nail polish.
Pediatric Client NURSING DIAGNOSIS: Risk for Impaired Skin Integrity: "Diaper rash" related to parental knowledge deficit of skin care for diapered infant or child.	Inform parents of products available for treatment of rash and the importance of frequent diaper changes and cleansing of skin with mild soap (Ivory or Dove).

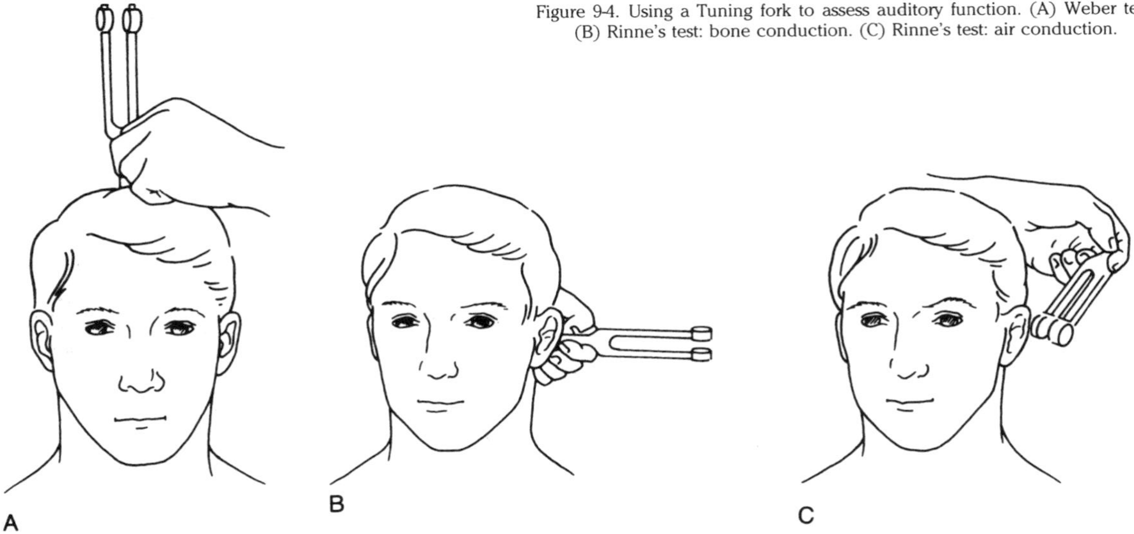

Figure 9-4. Using a Tuning fork to assess auditory function. (A) Weber test. (B) Rinne's test: bone conduction. (C) Rinne's test: air conduction.

A

B

C

II. Objective Data: Assessment Techniques *(continued)*

Procedure	Normal Findings	Deviations from Normal
G. Palpate mastoid process for the following:		
Tenderness	No tenderness or pain when palpated	Painful on palpation of mastoid process
Temperature	Warm	Erythema
Edema	Mastoid process easily palpated	Actual process difficult to palpate; ear displaced outward due to edema

Pediatric Variations

Procedure	Normal Findings	Deviations from Normal
A. Observe for placement and alignment of pinna	Pinna slightly crosses the horizontal line (Fig. 9-5); extends slightly forward from skull symmetrically	Pina falls below horizontal line (Fig. 9-5); ears asymmetrical, protruding, or flattened masses

B. Note on otoscopic exam:
For examination of infants and young children, restraint may be necessary to accomplish a safe, effective assessment (Figs. 9-6 and 9-7). In infants and young children, examination with the otoscope should be postposed until last in the assessment since this part of the examination is often distressing to clients of this age group.

NURSING DIAGNOSIS: Impaired Skin Integrity: Acne related to developmental changes	Teach adolescents proper skin cleansing and the significance of adequate rest, moderate exercise, and balanced diet.
Geriatric Client	
NURSING DIAGNOSIS: Risk for Impaired Skin Integrity related to immobility and decreased production of natural oils and to thinning skin.	Teach client and family the benefits of turning, range-of-movement exercises, massage, and cleaning of skin in reducing skin breakdown. Teach family and client how to observe for reddened pressure areas. Encourage the use of lotions to replace skin oils. Massage skin with lotions. Instruct client to decrease the number of baths and use a humidifier during the cold seasons. Explain the effects of proper nutrition and adequate fluids on skin integrity.
NURSING DIAGNOSIS: Risk for impaired tissue integrity related to thickened, dried toenails	Instruct client to soak nails 15 minutes in warm water prior to cutting. Use good scissors and lighting. Refer to podiatrist as necessary. Ascertain whether shoes fit correctly.

CHAPTER 6

Head, Neck, and Cervical Lymph Node Assessment

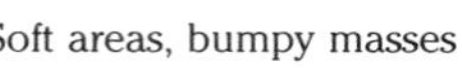

Equipment Needed

None

I. Subjective Data: Focus Questions

Prior neck injury? Swelling? Recent infection? Pain on movement? Prior head injury? Prior thyroid surgery?

II. Objective Data: Assessment Techniques

Procedure	***Normal Findings***	***Deviations from Normal***
A. Inspection and Palpation of Scalp		
Inspect and palpate scalp for the following:		
Size	Varies	Very small, very large
Shape	Symmetrical and round	Asymmetrical
Consistency	Hard and smooth	Soft areas, bumpy masses

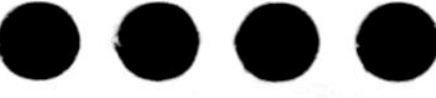
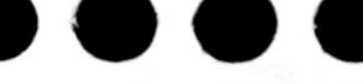

B. Inspection of Face and Neck

1. Observe face for the following:

Symmetry	Symmetrical	Asymmetrical
Facial features	Features vary	Extremely distorted features, lesions, masses

2. Observe neck for the following:

Appearance	Symmetrical, centered head position	Asymmetrical head position, masses or scars present
Movement	Smooth, controlled movements; from upright position: Flexion = 45° Extension = 55° Lateral abduction = 40° Rotation = 70°	Rigid, jerky movement; range of movement less than values given under Normal Findings; pain on movement

Procedure	Normal Findings	Deviations from Normal
C. Palpation of Thyroid, Trachea, and Lymph Nodes First palpate the trachea, then the thyroid using the guidelines described in Figure 6-1. After the thyroid, palpate the cervical lymph nodes.		
1. Palpate trachea for position and landmarks (tracheal rings, cricoid and thyroid cartilage) (Fig. 6-2)	Midline position; symmetrical; landmarks identifiable	Asymmetrical; deviates from the midline
2. Palpate thyroid for the following:		
Position	Midline	Deviates from the midline
Characteristics, landmarks	Smooth, firm, nontender	Enlarged lobes, irregular consistency, tender on palpation

(Note: Ability to see or palpate the thyroid varies considerably with thyroid size and client body build.)

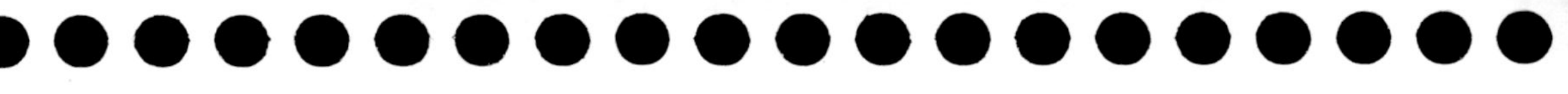

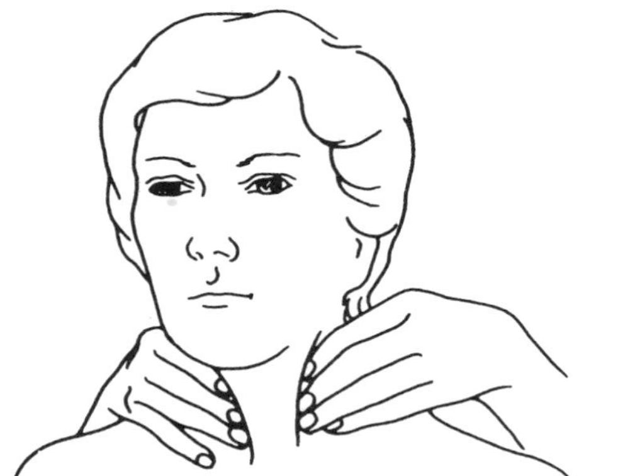

1. Stand behind client and position your hands with thumbs on nape of client's neck.
2. Ask client to flex neck forward and to the right, and use fingers of your left hand to displace thyroid to the right.
3. Palpate the right lobe using your right fingers while client swallows.
4. Repeat procedure to examine the left lobe.

(Note: Ability to see or palpate the thyroid varies considerably with thyroid size and client body build.)

Figure 6-1. Guidelines for palpating thyroid.

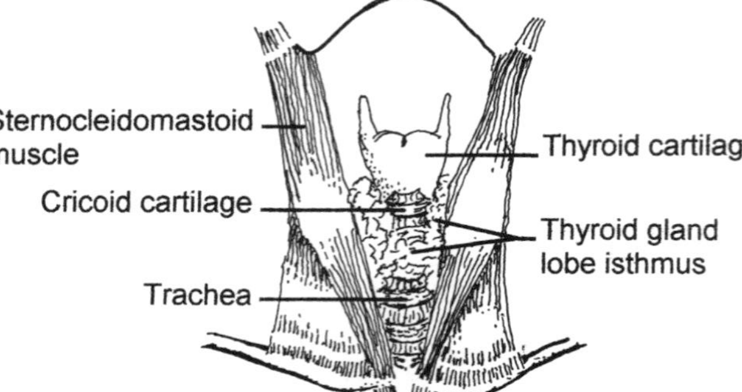

Figure 6-2. Landmarks to palpate thyroid.

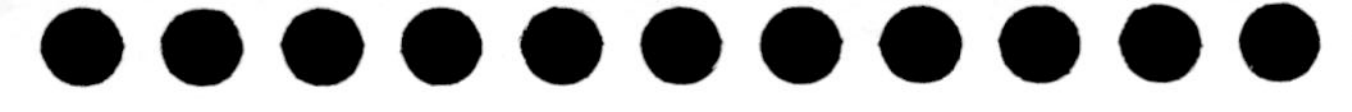

II. Objective Data: Assessment Techniques *(continued)*

Procedure	***Normal Findings***	***Deviations from Normal***
3. Palpate cervical lymph nodes (Fig. 6-3) for the following:		
Size/shape	Cervical lymph nodes are usually not palpable. If palpable, they should be 1 cm or less and round	Enlarged nodes with irregular borders
Delineation	Discrete	Confluent
Mobility	Mobile	Fixed to tissue
Consistency	Soft	Hard, firm
Tenderness	Nontender	Verbalizes pain on palpation

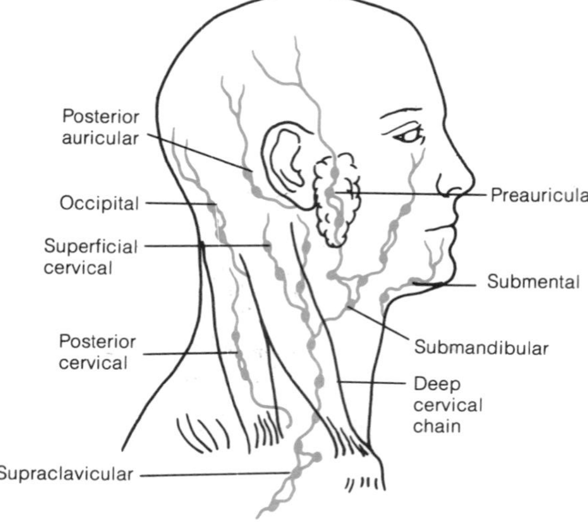

Figure 6-3. Lymph nodes of the head and neck.

Pediatric Variations

Procedure	Normal Findings	Deviations from Normal
Head:		
Observe shape, size, and symmetry	Occipital prominence; features appropriate for size	Uneven molding; asymmetrical masses; enlarged head (hydrocephalus)
Observe head control	Well established by 6 months; moves head up and down, side to side	Resistance to movement; head lag
Palpate skull and fontanels (Fig. 6-4)	Smooth, fused except for fontanels	Ecchymotic areas on scalp; loss of hair in spots; posterior fontanel open after 2 months of age, anterior fontanel after 18 months of age
Lymph Nodes:		
Palpate neck for lymph nodes.	Moderate number of small, firm lymph nodes	Diffuse large lymph nodes, asymmetrical placement

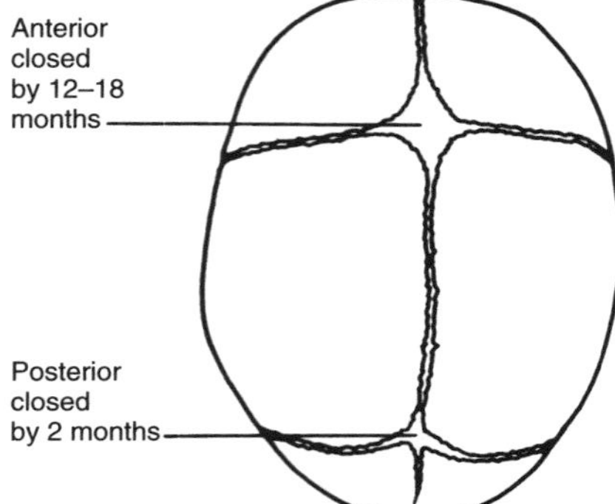

Figure 6-4. Fontanels.

Geriatric Variations

- Bones of face and nose more angular in appearance.
- Muscle atrophy and loss of fat causes shortening of neck.

Possible Related Collaborative Problems

Potential complications:
Lymphedema
Hypercalcemia
Hypocalcemia

Teaching Tips for Pediatric and Adolescent Clients

Nursing Diagnoses	***Teaching Tips***
NURSING DIAGNOSIS: Risk for Injury related to open fontanels	Teach parents normal development of fontanels and how to protect infants from pressure and injury.
NURSING DIAGNOSIS: Altered Health Maintenance management related to a knowledge deficit on the effects of smokeless tobacco	Teach that "dipping snuff" is highly addictive and increases the risk of cheek and gum cancer fifty fold. Explain that this is *not* a healthy substitute for smoking cigarettes (*Cancer Facts and Figures*, 1996).

CHAPTER 7

Mouth, Oropharynx, Nose, and Sinus Assessment

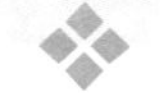

Mouth and Oropharynx Assessment

Equipment Needed

- Penlight
- Tongue blade
- Small gauze (2 × 2)
- Clean gloves

I. Subjective Data: Focus Questions

Prior dental problems? Dentures? Previous oral surgery? Prior lip or oral lesions? Sore throat? Dysphagia? Hoarseness?

II. Objective Data: Assessment Techniques

Procedure	*Normal Findings*	*Deviations from Normal*
A. Observe closed mouth for alignment	Upper teeth resting on top of lower teeth with upper incisors slightly overriding lower ones	Malocclusion of teeth, separation of individual teeth, or protusion of upper or lower incisors
B. Wearing gloves, observe and palpate lips for the following:		
Color	*In white skin:* Pink *In dark skin:* may have bluish hue or freckle-like pigmentation	Cyanotic, pale
Consistency	Moist, smooth with no lesions	Dry, cracked; nodules, fissures, or lesions present
Ask client to remove any dentures or dental appliances prior to continuing examination.		
C. Wearing gloves, observe and palpate buccal mucosa for the following:		
Color	Pink (increased pigmentation often noted in dark-skinned clients)	Pale, cyanotic, or reddened mucosa
Consistency	Smooth, moist, without lesions	Ulcers, dry mucosa, bleeding, or white patches present

II. Objective Data: Assessment Techniques *(continued)*

Procedure	*Normal Findings*	*Deviations from Normal*
Landmarks	Small papilla (parotid duct openings) located near upper second molar	Elevated, markedly reddened area near upper second molar
D. Wearing gloves, inspect and palpate gums, by retracting lips, for the following:		
Color	Pink	Pale, markedly reddened
Consistency	Moist, clearly defined margins	Dry, edema, ulcers, bleeding, white patches, tenderness
E. Wearing gloves, inspect and palpate teeth for the following:		
Number (See Fig. 7-1)	32 teeth	Missing teeth
Position/condition	Stable fixation, smooth surfaces and edges	Loose or broken teeth, jagged edges, dental caries
Color	Pearly white and shiny	Darkened, brown discoloration

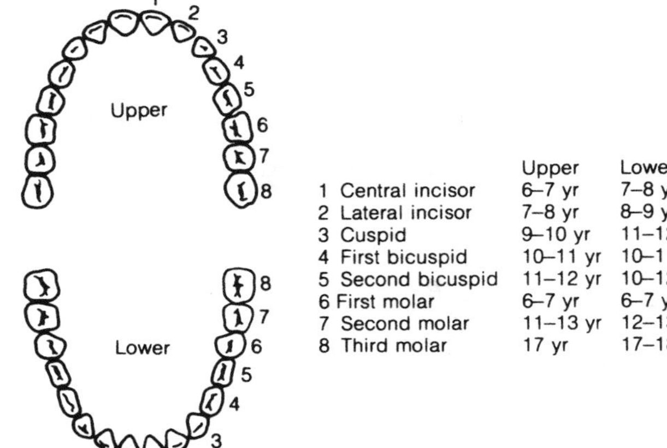

	Upper	Lower
1 Central incisor	6–7 yr	7–8 yr
2 Lateral incisor	7–8 yr	8–9 yr
3 Cuspid	9–10 yr	11–12 yr
4 First bicuspid	10–11 yr	10–11 yr
5 Second bicuspid	11–12 yr	10–12 yr
6 First molar	6–7 yr	6–7 yr
7 Second molar	11–13 yr	12–13
8 Third molar	17 yr	17–18 yr

Figure 7-1. Time Table for eruption of permanent teeth.

II. Objective Data: Assessment Techniques *(continued)*

Procedure	*Normal Findings*	*Deviations from Normal*
F. Inspect protruded tongue for the following:		
Symmetry/texture	Moist; papillae present; symmetrical appearance; midline fissures present Common variations: fissured, geographic tongue	Dry; nodules, ulcers present; papillae or fissures absent; asymmetrical
Movement	Smooth	Jerky or unilateral movement
Color	Pink	Markedly reddened; white patches; pale
G. Inspect ventral surface of the tongue and the mouth floor for the following:		
Color	Pink, slightly pale	Markedly reddened, cyanotic, or extreme pallor
Landmarks	Submaxillary duct openings (located on both sides of the frenulum) free of lesions or increased redness; frenulum centered (Fig. 7-2)	Lesions, ulcers, nodules, or hypertrophied duct openings present on either side of the frenulum
H. Inspect and palpate sides of tongue for color/lesions	Pink, smooth, moist; no lesions	White or reddened areas, ulcerations, or indurations present

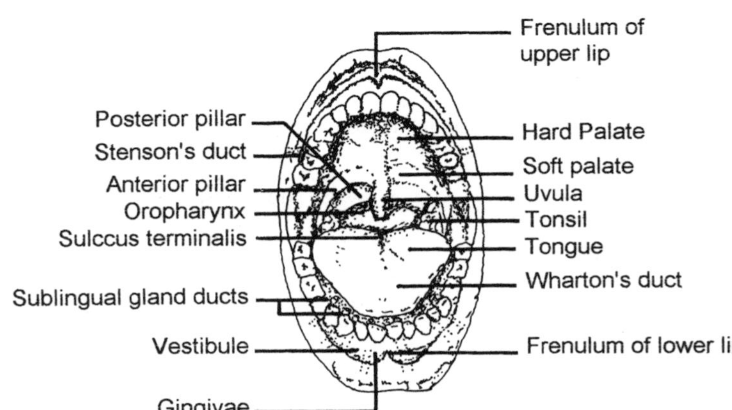

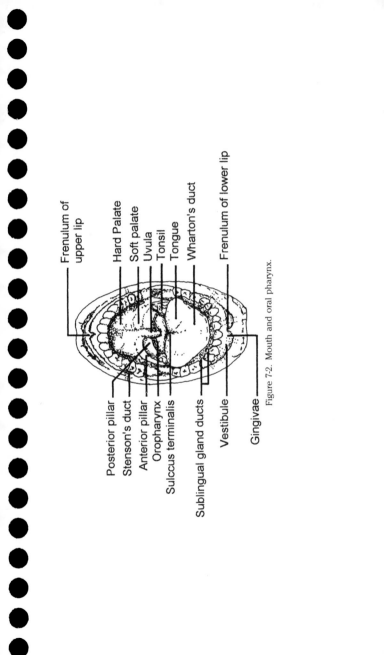

Figure 7-2. Mouth and oral pharynx.

Procedure	Normal Findings	Deviations from Normal
I. Inspect hard and soft palate (Fig. 7-2) for the following:		
Color	Hard palate: pale Soft palate: pink	Extreme pallor, white patches, or markedly reddened areas present
Consistency	Hard palate: firm with irregular transverse rugae Common variation: palatine torus (lump) on hard palate Soft palate: spongy texture with symmetrical elevation or phonation	Softened tissue over hard palate; lesions present; absence of elevation; asymmetrical elevation with phonation
J. Inspect oropharynx (Fig. 7-2) for the following:		
Landmarks	Tonsillar pillars symmetrical; tonsils present (unless surgically removed) and without exudate; uvula at midline and rises on phonation	Enlarged tonsils, with exudate; asymmetrical; uvula deviates from midline; edema, ulcers, lesions
Color	Pink	Markedly reddened; gray membranes

Pediatric Variations

- Eruption of deciduous teeth (Fig. 7-3)
- Eruption of permanent teeth (Fig. 7-1)

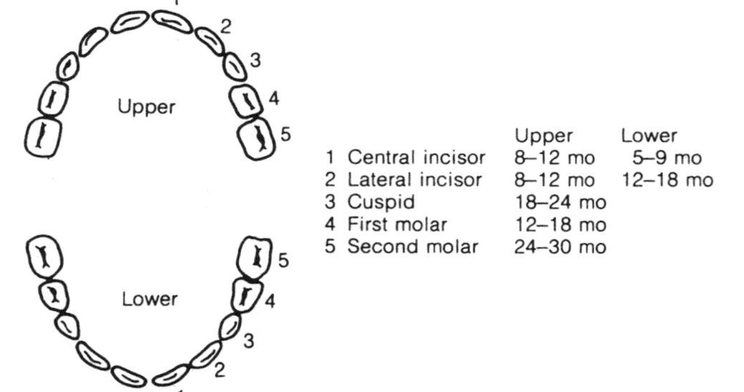

	Upper	Lower
1 Central incisor	8–12 mo	5–9 mo
2 Lateral incisor	8–12 mo	12–18 mo
3 Cuspid	18–24 mo	
4 First molar	12–18 mo	
5 Second molar	24–30 mo	

Figure 7-3. Time table for eruption of deciduous teeth.

Geriatric Variations

- Worn teeth, abraded enamel, and yellowing teeth
- Decreased production of saliva
- Decreased taste sensations due to a decrease in the number of taste buds
- Gums recede
- Poor-fitting dentures may cause facial asymmetry
- Progressive atrophy of olfactory bulbs causes a decreased sense of smell

Cultural Variations

- Dark-skinned clients may have lips with bluish hue or freckle-like pigmentation.
- Some groups have reduced teeth number; Australian aborigines have four extra molars.
- Dark-skinned clients may have dark pigment or freckling on side or ventral surface of tongue and floor of mouth; hard and soft palate may also be darkly pigmented.
- Some groups (especially Asians) may have mandibular torus (lump) on inner mandible near second premolar.
- Native Americans and Asians may have a split uvula.

Possible Related Collaborative Problems

Potential complications:
Stomatitis
Gingivitis
Oral lesions
Periodontal (gum) disease

Teaching Tips for Selected Nursing Diagnoses/Collaborative Problems

Nursing Diagnoses/ Collaborative Problems	Teaching Tips
Adult Client	
NURSING DIAGNOSIS: Altered Oral Mucous Membrane related to inadequate mouth care	Instruct client on proper brushing and flossing. (Client should brush teeth at least twice a day, and floss once a day to remove plaque from under gum line and sides of teeth.) Recommend a toothbrush with soft rounded end or polished bristles, to be replaced every 2–3 months when frayed, in addition to an ADA accepted fluoride toothpaste and mouth rinses. Explain the role of fluoride in decreasing tooth decay. Refer to dentist for fluoride protection advice if client's water supply is not fluoridated. Explain the significance of a well-balanced diet in decreasing tooth decay and periodontal (gum) disease. Dry mouth can cause problems with oral health. Refer to dentist or physician for possible recommendation of artificial saliva or fluoride mouth rinse.

Nursing Diagnoses/ Collaborative Problems	Teaching Tips
COLLABORATIVE PROBLEM: Potential complication: periodontal (gum) disease	*Teach client warning signs:* • Gums that bleed with brushing • Red, swollen, tender gums or gums that pull away from teeth • Presence of pus between teeth or loose teeth • Change in position of teeth or denture fit • Bad breath or bad taste that lasts • Teach prevention: Brush and floss every day Eat balanced diet Schedule regular dental visits (American Dental Association, 1991)
COLLABORATIVE PROBLEM: Potential complication: oral cancer	*Teach client warning signs:* • Sore in mouth that does not heal • White scaly patches in mouth • Swelling or lumps in mouth/throat/on lips • Numbness or pain in mouth/throat/on lips • Repeated bleeding in mouth • Difficulty chewing, swallowing, speaking, or moving tongue or jaw • Change in bite

Pediatric Client

NURSING DIAGNOSIS: Altered Health Maintenance related to lack of proper mouth care	Instruct parents not to put child to bed with a bottle filled with formula, milk, juices, or sugar water, because these liquids pool around teeth and promote decay. Use only water in bottles when putting child to bed, to prevent so-called "baby bottle tooth decay." Teach the importance of fluoride in drinking water and proper nutrition to prevent decay. Fluoride drops are recommended for infants and fluoride tablets for children up through age 14 if adequate fluoride is not in water. Refer child who sucks thumb past age 4 years. Explain the benefits of using a small, cool spoon rubbed over gums or using teething rings during teething period. Instruct parents to start brushing child's teeth with eruption of first tooth. Begin flossing when primary teeth have erupted (2–2 1/2 yrs.) Parents should be taught to brush and floss child's teeth until child can be taught to do this alone (approximately age 5 for brushing and age 8 for flossing). Encourage a dental exam by a dentist between 6 and 12 months of age.
NURSING DIAGNOSIS: Risk for Injury to teeth related to developmental age and play activities	In case of broken or knocked-out tooth, instruct parent to rinse the tooth in cool water (don't scrub it); when possible, insert back in socket and hold in place 5 minutes. If this cannot be done, put tooth in cup of milk or water or wrap it in wet cloth and take child to dentist at once for possible replacement. Recommend use of mouth guards to prevent injuries in contact sports.

Teaching Tips for Selected Nursing Diagnoses/Collaborative Problems *(continued)*

Nursing Diagnoses/ Collaborative Problems	Teaching Tips
Geriatric Client	
NURSING DIAGNOSIS: Altered Nutrition: Less than body requirements related to decreased appetite secondary to decreased sense of taste and smell	Explore food preferences with client and use visual appeal of food to enhance appetite.

Nose and Sinus Assessment

Equipment Needed

- Penlight
- Nasal speculum or otoscope with broad-tipped speculum

I. Subjective Data: Focus Questions

Prior nasal surgery? Trauma? Obstructed nares? Epistaxis? Use of nasal sprays? Frequent infections? Allergies? Headaches located in sinus areas? Postnasal drip?

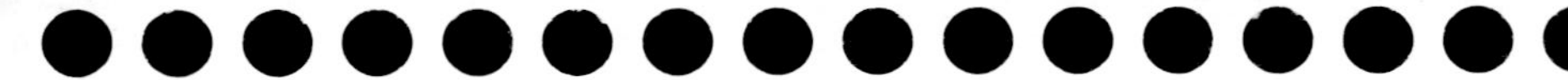

Procedure	Normal Findings	Deviations from Normal

A. Inspection

The external nose is inspected; then the internal nose is inspected, using the following guidelines:

Guidelines for Using Nasal Speculum

- Tilt client's head back to facilitate speculum insertion and visualization.
- Hold speculum in hand and brace with your index finger against the client's nose.
- Insert the speculum tip approximately 1 cm and dilate the naris as much as possible.
- Use the other hand to position client's head and hold penlight.

Procedure	Normal Findings	Deviations from Normal
1. Observe external nose for the following:		
Skin appearance	*Color:* Same as face *Consistency:* Smooth	Nodules, lesions, erythema, visible vasculature
Shape	Symmetrical appearance	Asymmetry
Nares	Symmetrical appearance; no changes in nares with respiration; dry with no crusting; septum midline	Asymmetry; flaring nares; discharge, crusting, displaced septum

II. Objective Data: Assessment Techniques *(continued)*

Procedure	***Normal Findings***	***Deviations from Normal***
2. Inspect internal nose for the following:		
Appearance	Mucosa pink and moist with uniform color and no lesions	Markedly red mucosa, dry or cracked; areas of discoloration; polyps, masses
Landmarks: Turbinates, septum (Fig. 7-4)	Turbinates and middle meatus visible and same color as mucosa, moist and free of lesions; septum symmetrical and uniform without lesions	Turbinates not visible due to edema or occlusion; turbinate pale or markedly reddened; polyps, lesions, copious discharge, bleeding, perforation, deviation present
3. Assess function of nose for patency (with mouth closed and one naris occluded, feel for air).	Air is felt being exhaled through opposite naris; noiseless	Noisy or obstructed exhalation when mouth is closed and one naris is occluded

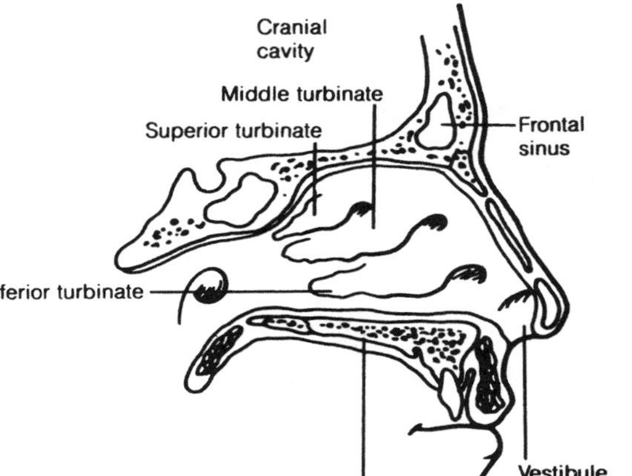

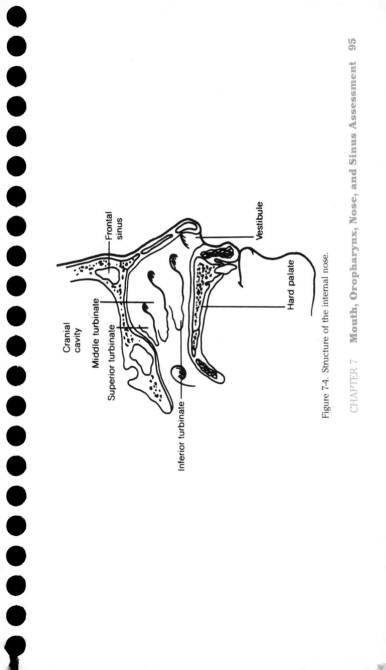

Figure 7-4. Structure of the internal nose.

II. Objective Data: Assessment Techniques *(continued)*

Procedure	*Normal Findings*	*Deviations from Normal*
B. Palpation		
1. Palpate external nose for firmness.	Solid placement; no pain reported on palpation	Unstable placement; no nodules or masses present; verbalizes pain on palpation
2. Palpate sinuses (both frontal and maxillary; Fig. 7-5) for tenderness.	Nontender on palpation	Verbalizes pain or discomfort on palpation
C. Percussion		
Percuss sinuses for resonance.	Hollow tone elicited.	Flat, dull tone elicited; expresses pain on percussion

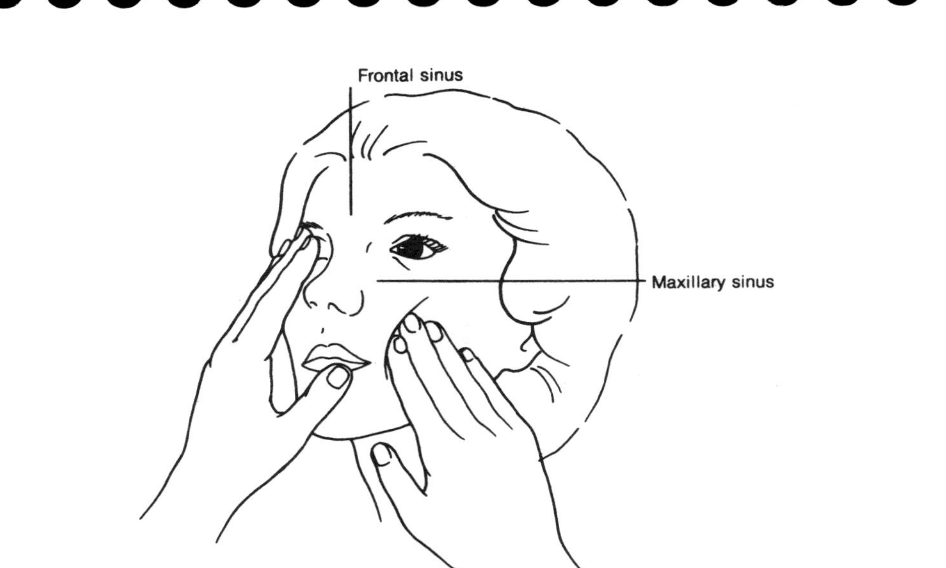

Figure 7-5. Palpation of frontal and maxillary sinuses.

Geriatric Variation
Decreased sense of taste and smell due to the aging process.

Possible Related Collaborative Problem
Potential complication: Nosebleed

Teaching Tips for Selected Nursing Diagnoses/Collaborative Problems

Nursing Diagnoses/ Collaborative Problems	***Teaching Tips***
Adult Client	
NURSING DIAGNOSIS: Altered Health Maintenance related to a lack of information regarding over-the-counter nasal medications	Instruct client on use, proper dosage, and effects of overuse of nasal sprays.
COLLABORATIVE PROBLEM: Potential complication: Nosebleed	Instruct client to apply pressure for 5 minutes while breathing through mouth and leaning forward. Caution against blowing nose for several hours afterward. Refer as necessary.
Pediatric Client	
NURSING DIAGNOSIS: Risk For Injury related to insertion of foreign bodies into nasal cavity	Caution and give instructions to parents.

CHAPTER 8

Eye Assessment

Equipment Needed

- Eye chart (Snellen or hand-held Rosenbaum; see Appendix VII)
- Near-vision chart or newsprint
- Cover card
- Penlight
- Ophthalmoscope
- Ruler

I. Subjective Data: Focus Questions

History of prior eye surgery? Trauma? Use of corrective glasses or contact lenses? Blurred vision? Dyplopia? Strabismus? Recent changes in vision? Allergies? Eye redness? Frequent watering? Discharge? Date of previous vision test?

II. Objective Data: Assessment Techniques

Client should be seated comfortably in a well-lighted room that can be darkened for ophthalmic examination. First, the external eye structures are examined. Then eye function is tested, followed by the ophthalmic examination, using the following guidelines:

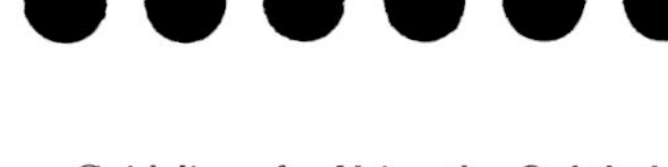

Guidelines for Using the Ophthalmoscope

1. Position dial so that the small, round white light can be used.
2. Client and examiner shoud remove glasses.
3. Darken room.
4. Ask client to fix gaze on object straight ahead and slightly upward.
5. For examination of the client's right eye, place opthalmoscope in your right hand with index finger on the lens wheel and place instrument to your right eye.
6. With diopter setting at 0, stand slightly to the client's right (about 15 degrees).
7. Holding ophthalmoscope firmly against your head, approach client while shining the instrument beam toward the pupil.
8. After viewing the red reflex, continue approach until 3 to 5 cm from the client's eye; retinal structures should come into view.
9. Focus on retinal structures by rotating the lens wheel if refractory errors are present.
10. After completing retinal inspection, rotate the lens wheel slowly to +5, +10, +15, and +20 to assess the anterior structures of the eye.

Procedure	*Normal Findings*	*Deviations from Normal*
External Eye Examination		
A. Inspect eyelids and lashes (Fig. 8-1) for the following:		
1. Position and appearance	Lid margins moist and pink; lashes short, evenly spaced, and curled outward; lower margins at bottom edge of iris; upper margins of lid cover approximately 2 mm of iris	Crusting, scales; lashes absent or curled inward; edema, ptosis, or xanthelasma present; asymmetry of lids Ectropion: lower lids turn outward Entropion: lower lids turn inward Chalazion: inflammation of meibomian glands Hordeolum: stye or inflammation of glands in lid Blepharitis: waxy white scales (seborrheic) or inflammation of hair follicles (staphylococci) Itching Ulcerative lesions
2. Blinking	Blinking symmetrical, involuntary, at approximately 15 blinks/min	Asymmetrical blink, incomplete closure, rapid blinking

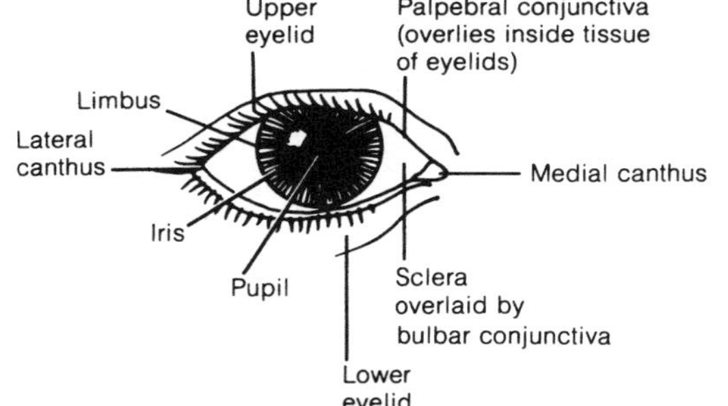

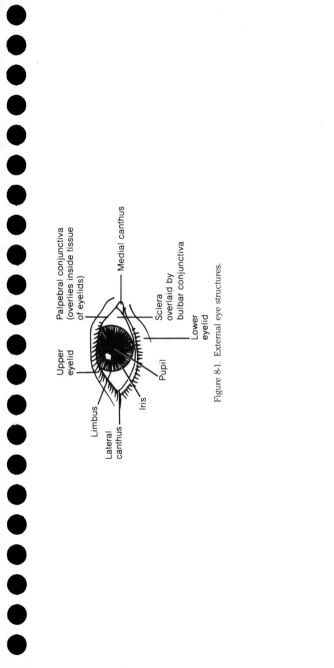

Figure 8-1. External eye structures.

Procedure	*Normal Findings*	*Deviations from Normal*
B. Inspect conjunctiva (bulbar and palpebral) and sclera for clarity and appearance by separating lids with thumb and index finger and asking the client to look up, down, and to either side.	Bulbar conjunctiva is clear with tiny vessels visible. Palpebral conjunctiva is pink with no discharge. Sclera is blue-white	Markedly reddened lids, lesions, nodules, discharge, crusting, foreign body present Sclera with petechiae; or marked jaundice
C. Inspect cornea (using oblique lighting) for appearance	Transparent, smooth, moist	Lesion, opacities, irregular light reflections, or foreign body present
D. Inspect iris and pupil for the following:		
1. Shape	Round	Irregular
2. Equality	Equal	Unequal
3. Color (iris)	Uniform color	Inconsistent color
E. Inspect lens for clarity	Clear	Cloudy
F. Inspect and palpate lacrimal apparatus (Fig. 8-2) for the following:		
1. Appearance	Puncta (small elevations on the nasal side of the upper and lower lids)—mucosa pink	Puncta markedly reddened and edematous
2. Response to pressure applied at nasal side of lower orbital rim	No tenderness or discharge noted when pressure is applied	Fluid or purulent discharge or pain on palpation

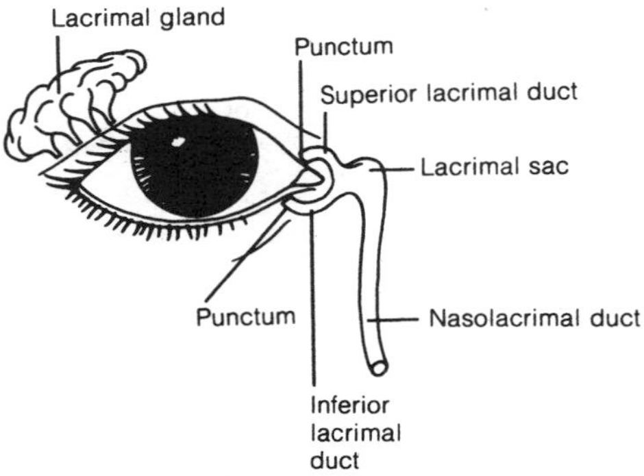

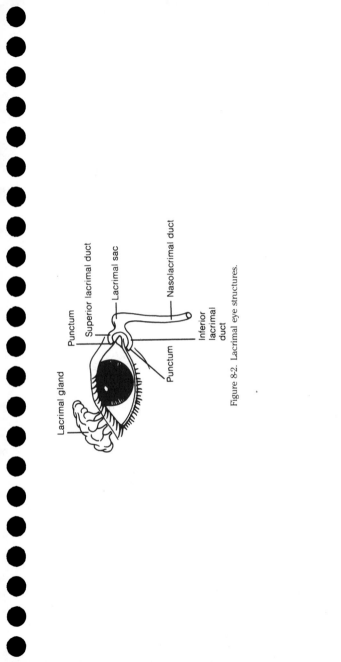

Figure 8-2. Lacrimal eye structures.

II. Objective Data: Assessment Techniques *(continued)*

Procedure	***Normal Findings***	***Deviations from Normal***
Testing Eye Function		
G. Inspect eye function as follows:		
1. Check visual acuity.		
a. Check for distance vision with Snellen chart 20 feet from client.	20/20 O.D. and O.S. with no hesitation, frowning, or squinting	Any letters missed on 20/20 line or above; reads chart by leaning forward, with head tilted, or squinting
b. Check near vision with newspaper approximately 14 inches from client's head. (See Appendix VII for Pocket Vision Screener.)	Reads print without difficulty at 14 inches	Reads print by holding it closer or farther away than 14 inches
2. Check peripheral vision: Face client at a distance of 2 to 3 feet. Client and examiner look directly ahead and cover eye directly opposite each other.	Client and examiner report seeing object at the same time as it approaches from the periphery.	Client does not report seeing object at the same time as the examiner.
3. Check accommodation (Fig. 8-3): Ask client to stare at an object 3 to 4 feet away, and move object in toward client's nose.	Pupils converge and constrict as object moves in toward the nose. Pupil responses are uniform.	Pupils do not converge or constrict. Pupil responses are unequal.

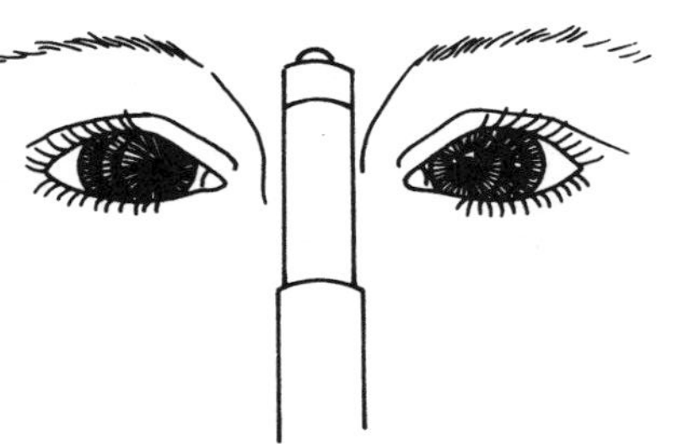

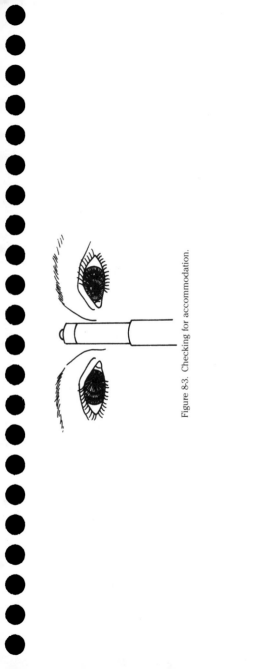

Figure 8-3. Checking for accommodation.

Procedure	*Normal Findings*	*Deviations from Normal*
4. Check extraocular movements (Fig. 8-4) by asking client to follow object as it is moved in six cardinal fields.	Both eyes move in a smooth, coordinated manner in all directions.	Jerky eye movements; failure to follow object with one or both eyes
5. Check response to light.		
a. Check corneal light reflex by asking client to look straight ahead and shining light toward facial midline (Fig. 8-5).	Reflections of light noted at same location on both eyes	Light reflections noted at different areas on both eyes
b. Check direct pupil response by asking client to look straight ahead and approaching each eye from the client's side with a penlight.	Illuminated pupils constrict.	Illuminated pupils fail to constrict.
c. Check consensual pupil response by asking the client to look straight ahead and approaching each eye from the client's side with a penlight.	Pupil opposite the one illuminated constricts simultaneously.	Pupil opposite the one illuminated fails to constrict.

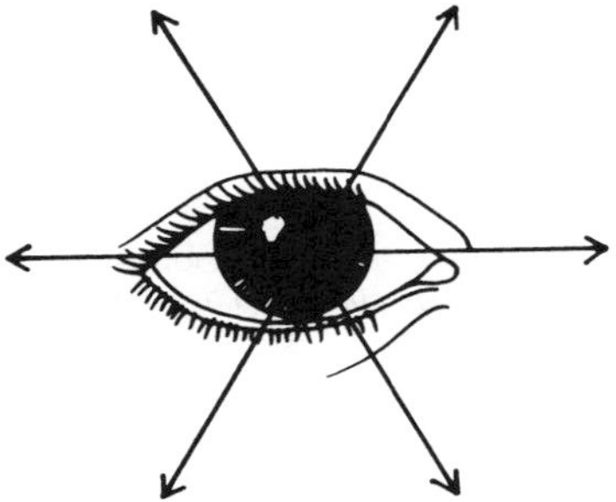

Figure 8-4. Six cardinal fields for checking extraocular movements.

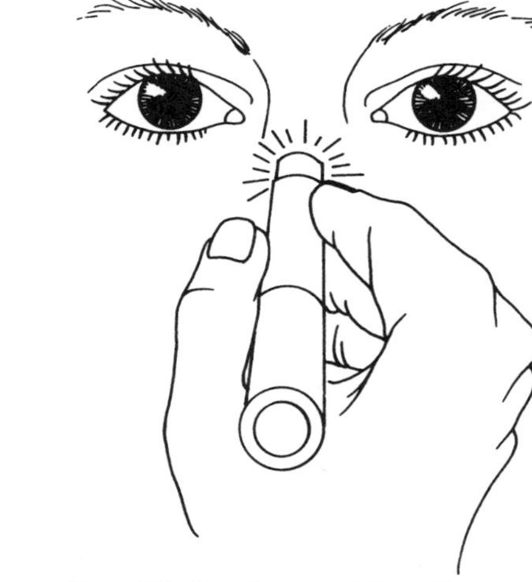

Figure 8-5. Checking corneal light reflex.

Procedure	***Normal Findings***	***Deviations from Normal***
6. Check for abnormal eye movement using cover-uncover test (Fig. 8-6): Ask client to look straight ahead, covering one eye with a cover card and observing uncovered eye for movement.	Uncovered eye does not move as opposite eye is covered. Covered eye does not move as cover is removed.	Uncovered eye moves to focus when opposite eye is covered. Covered eye moves to focus when cover is removed.
Ophthalmic Examination (use ophthalmoscope)		
H. Inspect the red reflex for shape and color	Round, red reflex is bright, with red-orange flow.	Red reflex has decreased color, dark spots, and abnormal shape.
I. Inspect the optic disc (Fig. 8-7) for the following:		
Shape	Round or slightly oval disc with sharply defined margins	Irregularly shaped disc, blurred margins
Color	Creamy pink (lighter than retina)	Pallor of entire disc or one section
Size	Approximately 1.5 mm size, symmetrical in both eyes	Size of disc not equal in both eyes

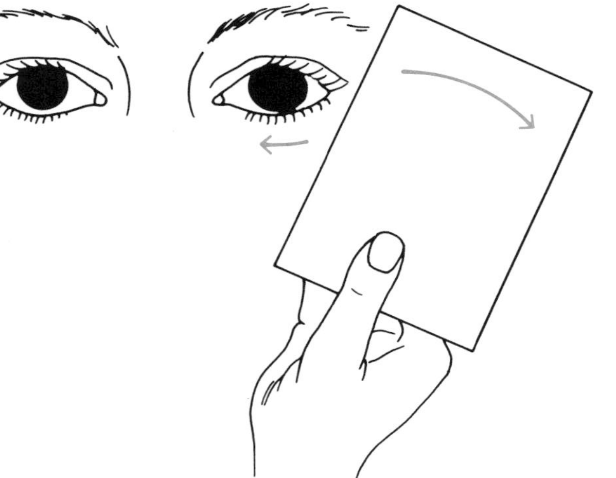

Figure 8-6. Uncover test for left eye demonstrating abnormal shift from lateral to central gaze.

Procedure	***Normal Findings***	***Deviations from Normal***
Physiological cup	Small area noted as paler than disc located just temporal of center of disc; occupies $\frac{4}{10}$ to $\frac{5}{10}$ of the diameter of the disc	Cup location and size not symmetrical in both eyes. Cup occupies more than $\frac{5}{10}$ diameter of the disc
J. Inspect the retinal vessels for the following:		
Appearance	Arteries, light red and smaller than veins; veins, darker in color and larger than arteries	Arteries less than $\frac{3}{5}$ size of veins; arteries pale
Distribution	Vessels regular in shape and decreasing in size as they branch and move toward the periphery; crossing of arteries and veins showing no changes in the diameter of the underlying vessel	Vessels irregular in shape and uneven in distribution; narrowing of underlying vessels at crossings of arteries and veins
K. Inspect retinal background for appearance.	Fine texture with pink, uniform color	Pallor of the fundus; soft or hard exudates; microaneurysms or hemorrhages present
L. Inspect macula for appearance	Darker than remainder of retina; fovea seen as a tiny bright light in the center of macula	Abnormalities in color or vessels; lesions present

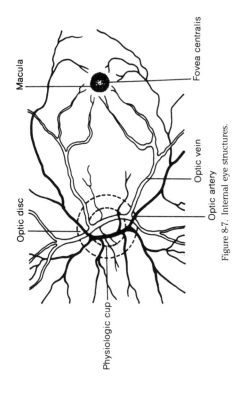

Figure 8-7. Internal eye structures.

Pediatric Variations

I. Preparation of Client

Explain procedure in order to decrease child's fear when room is darkened.

II. Objective Data: Assessment Techniques

Procedure	*Normal Findings*	*Deviations from Normal*
A. Inspect placement of light on cornea.	Light falls symmetrically within each pupil	Asymmetrical location of light reflection on pupil
B. Observe for placement/alignment of eyes (Fig. 8-8) by doing the following:		
1. Measuring inner canthal distance	Average distance 3 cm (1.2 inches)	
2. Assessing palpebral slant	Lie horizontally on imaginary line (except in Asian children)	Presence of upward slant in non-Asians
3. Observing placement of lids	With eye open, lids lie between upper iris and pupil.	Upper lid lies above iris (setting sun sign)
C. Inspect iris.	Color varies from brown to green to blue.	Black and white speckling of iris present (Brushfield spots)
D. Inspect lacrimal apparatus.	Lacrimal meatus not present until 3 months of age	

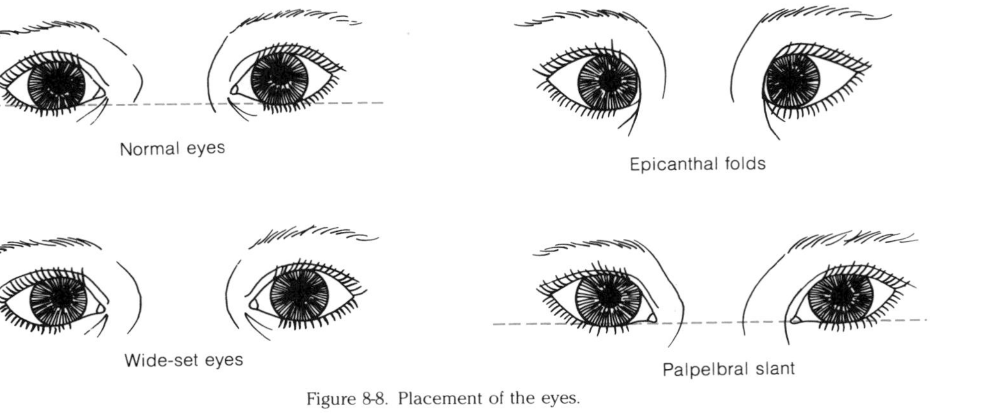

Figure 8-8. Placement of the eyes.

Geriatric Variations

External eye examination reveals:

- Conjunctiva thins and becomes yellowish
- White ring around iris (arcus senilis)
- Dry eyes due to decreased tear production
- Drooping eyelids (senile ptosis)
- Clouding of lens (cataracts)

Visual examination reveals:

- Presbyopia (decreased near vision due to decreased elasticity of lens)
- Slowed pupillary response and slowed accommodation

Visual field examination reveals:

- Decreased peripheral vision

Funduscopic examination reveals:

- Pale, narrowed arterioles

Cultural Variations

- Asians and some other groups may have common variation of epicanthic folds or narrowed palpebral fissures
- Dark-skinned clients may have sclera with yellow or pigmented freckles.

Possible Related Collaborative Problems

Potential complications:

Visual changes

Eye infections

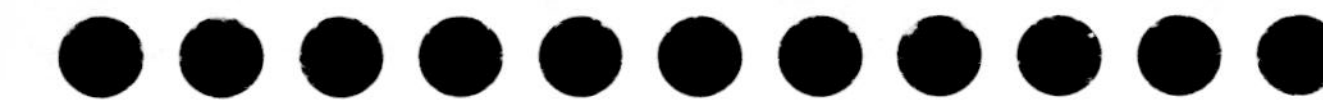

Cataracts
Glaucoma
Impaired functioning of lacrimal apparatus

Teaching Tips for Selected Nursing Diagnoses

Nursing Diagnoses	***Teaching Tips***
Adult Client NURSING DIAGNOSIS: Altered Health Maintenance related to lack of knowledge of necessity for eye examinations	Recommend the following guidelines for frequency of eye exams for individuals without symptoms: *Age* — *Frequency* 65 or older — Every 1–2 years 40–64 — Every 2–4 years 20–39 — Because of the high incidence and more aggressive course of glaucoma in blacks, even in the absence of visual or ocular symptoms, they should receive a comprehensive examination every 3–5 years. Other asymptomatic, otherwise normal, patients require a comprehensive evaluation less frequently. (Reprinted with permission from the American Academy of Ophthalmology 1992): Comprehensive Adult Eye Evaluation, Preferred Practice Pattern. American Academy of Ophthalmology, San Francisco, CA, 1992.

Teaching Tips for Selected Nursing Diagnoses *(continued)*

Nursing Diagnoses	***Teaching Tips***
NURSING DIAGNOSIS Altered Health Maintenance related to a knowledge deficit of care of eye infection	Instruct client on proper administration of eye drops and ointments. Discuss proper cleansing from inner to outer canthus and changing of cleansing cloth used to prevent cross-contamination (from eye to eye).
Pediatric Client	
NURSING DIAGNOSIS: Opportunity to enhance knowledge of eye care during the growing years.	*In the newborn nursery:* pediatricians or family physicians should examine all infants; ophthalmologists should examine all high-risk infants. *By age 6 months:* pediatricians or ophthalmologist should screen all infants. *At age $3\frac{1}{2}$ years:* pediatricians, family physicians, or ophthalmologists should examine all children. Focus should be on visual acuity. *At age 5 years and older:* pediatricians or family physicians should screen children for vision & motility annually if this is not provided by school personnel or volunteer organizations. Further screening should be done at routine school checks or after the appearance of symptoms. (Reprinted with permission of the American Academy of Ophthalmology, 1991).

Geriatric Client

NURSING DIAGNOSIS: Altered Protection related to decreased tear production secondary to the aging process	Instruct client on the use of artificial tears as necessary.
	Explore with client aids for independent living (e.g., magnifying glasses, cane). Encourage further evaluation if necessary. Instruct family to keep furniture in same place and to provide better lighting. Provide community resources (e.g., "talking" books and magazines available in libraries).
NURSING DIAGNOSIS: Altered Protection related to impaired vision secondary to the aging process	Adults 65 or over should have an ophthalmologic eye examination at least every two years. To promote this goal, the National Eye Care Project is a nationwide outreach program sponsored by the American Academy as a public service. It is designed to help the disadvantaged elderly obtain medical eye care. The toll free phone number is 1-800-222-EYES. To be eligible, a person must be a U.S. citizen or legal resident, age 65 or older, who does not have access to an ophthalmologist they may have seen in the past.

Nursing Diagnoses	*Teaching Tips*
	Adults with diabetes mellitus should have an ophthalmologic eye examination at the time of diagnosis and at medically appropriate intervals thereafter. Adults with risk factors such as a family history of glaucoma, cataract, retinal detachment, or degenerative eye disease should seek more frequent care, especially if they experience any of the following problems: • Blurry vision uncorrectable by lenses • Distorted or double vision • Dimming of vision that comes and goes, or sudden loss of vision • Red eye • Pain in or around the eyes • Excessive tearing or discharge from the eye • Swelling of the eyelids or protrusion of the eye • New floaters or flashes of light • Loss of side vision • Crossed, turned, or wandering eye • Halos (colored rays or circles around lights) (Reprinted with permission of the American Academy of Ophthalmology, 1991)

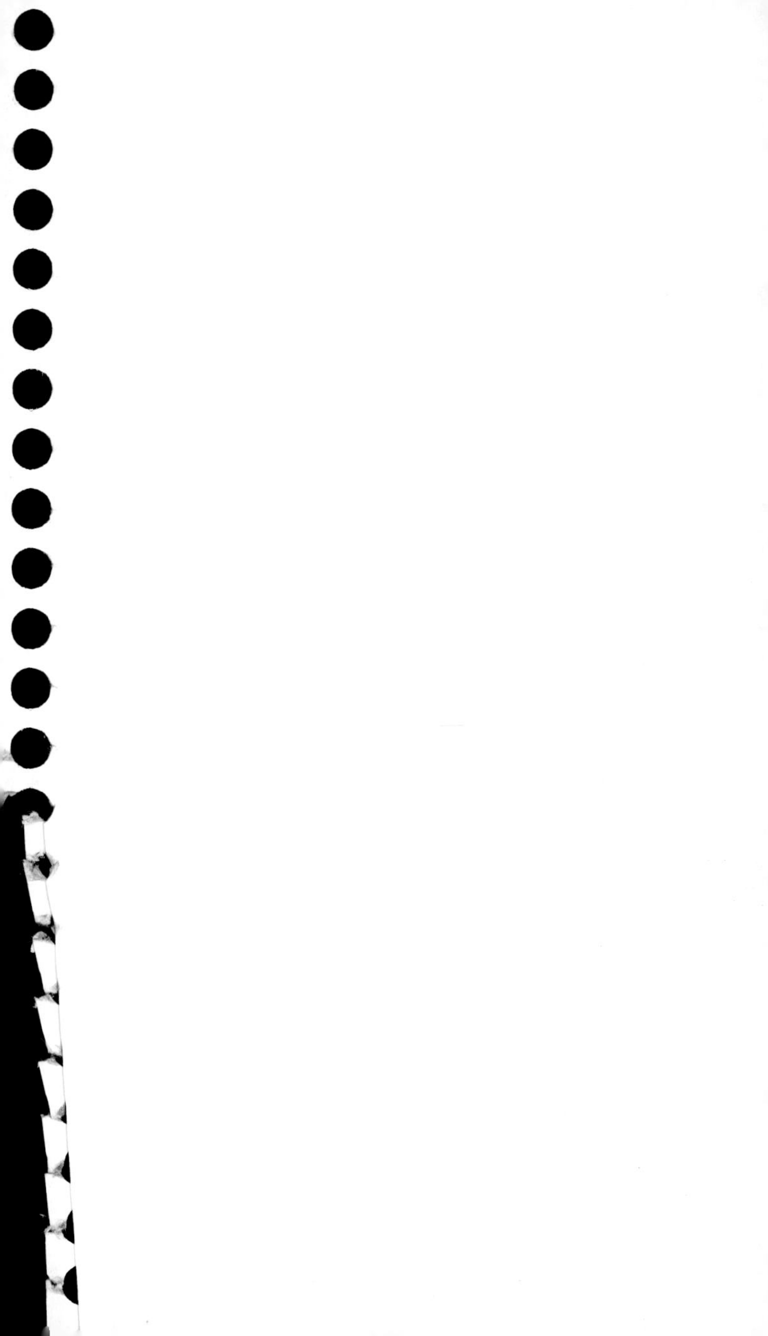

CHAPTER 9

Ear Asssessment

Equipment Needed

- Otoscope
- Tuning fork (512 or 1024hertz)

I. Subjective Data: Focus Questions

History of prior ear surgery? Trauma? Frequent infections? Ear pain? Drainage? Hearing loss? Tinnitus? Vertigo? Ototoxic medications? Last hearing examination?

II. Objective Data: Assessment Techniques

Client should be comfortably seated in such a way that you can easily visualize both ears. First, examine the external ear, then examine the ear canal and tympanic membrane with the otoscope, and finally assess hearing function, using the following guidelines:

Procedure	***Normal Findings***	***Deviations from Normal***
A. Inspect external ear (Fig. 9-1) for the following:		
Size and shape	Ears of equal size and similar appearance	Ears of unequal size or configuration
Position	Alignment of pinna with corner of eye and within 10-degree angle of vertical position	Pinna positioned below a line from corner of eye or unequal alignment
Lesions/discolorations	Skin smooth and without nodules; color pink	Erythema, edema, nodules, or areas of discoloration present
B. Palpate external ear	Nontender auricle	Painful auricle
C. Inspect auditory canal (using otoscope) (Fig. 9-2) for the following:		
Cerumen: Color, consistency, odor	Color: black, dark red, gray or brown Consistency: waxy, flaky, soft or hard Odor: none	Impacted cerumen (obstructs visualization of membrane), foul-smelling discharge

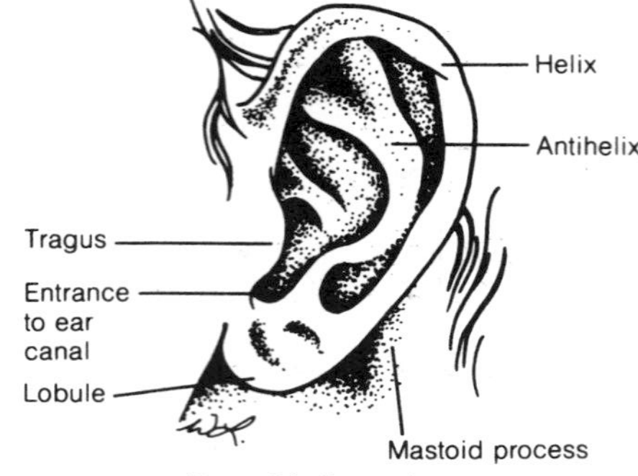

Figure 9-1. External ear.

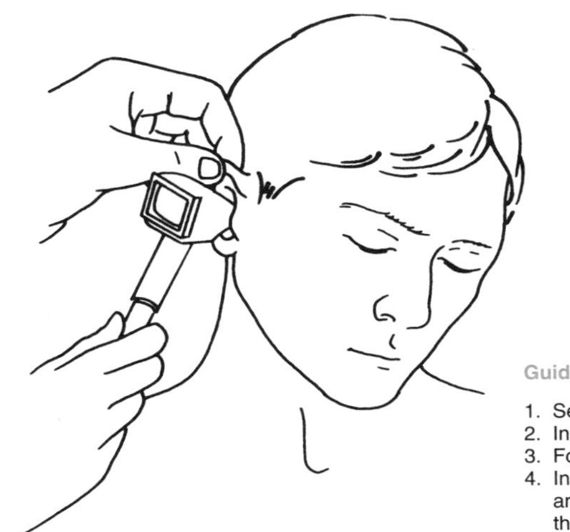

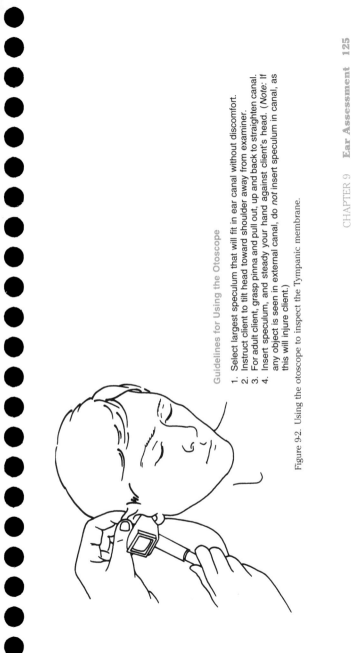

Guidelines for Using the Otoscope

1. Select largest speculum that will fit in ear canal without discomfort.
2. Instruct client to tilt head toward shoulder away from examiner.
3. For adult client, grasp pinna and pull out, up and back to straighten canal.
4. Insert speculum, and steady your hand against client's head. (*Note:* If any object is seen in external canal, do *not* insert speculum in canal, as this will injure client.)

Figure 9-2. Using the otoscope to inspect the Tympanic membrane.

Procedure	***Normal Findings***	***Deviations from Normal***
Appearance	Canal walls pink and uniform with tympanic membrane visible	Lesions, foreign body, erythema, or edema present in canal
Tenderness	Little or no discomfort on manipulation of pinna; inner two-thirds of canal very tender if touched with speculum	Moderate to severe pain when pinna is moved or otoscope speculum is inserted
D. Inspect tympanic membrane (TM), using otoscope (Fig. 9-2), for the following:		
Color	Pearly gray, shiny, and translucent	Dull appearance: blue (blood) or pink/red (inflammation)
Consistency	Intact; may show movement when swallowing	Perforations, scarring, or immobility
Landmarks (Fig. 9-3)	Cone of light, umbo, handle of malleus, and short process of malleus easily visualized	Retracted TM accentuates landmarks; bulging TM partially occludes landmarks.

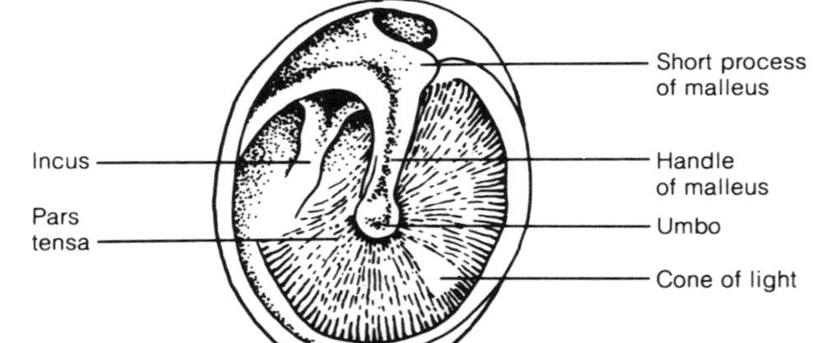

Figure 9-3. Normal Tympanic membrane.

II. Objective Data: Assessment Techniques *(continued)*

Procedure	*Normal Findings*	*Deviations from Normal*
E. Assess auditory function for the following:		
1. Gross hearing ability: Whisper words 1 to 2 feet behind client; hold watch 1 to 2 inches from client's ear.	Able to hear whispered words from 1 to 2 feet. Able to hear watch tick from 1 to 2 inches	Unable to hear whispered words or watch tick; unequal response
2. Lateralization of sound (Weber test): Place of activated tuning fork on center top of client's head (Fig. 9-4, A).	Vibration heard equally in both ears	Vibratory sound lateralized to poor ear in conductive loss and to good ear in sensorineural loss
3. Comparison of air conduction (AC) to bone conduction (BC)—Rinne's test: Place tuning fork on mastoid process until no longer heard, then move it to front of ear (Fig. 9-4, B, C).	AC > BC (air conduction is twice as long as bone conduction)	BC ≥ AC: 1. Bone conduction heard longer or equal to air conduction in conductive loss 2. Air conduction longer but not twice as long as bone conduction in sensorineural loss
F. Perform Romberg Test for Equilibrium by having client stand with feet together, first with eyes open, then with eyes closed. (Put your arms around client to prevent fall).	Client stands straight with minimal swaying	Client sways and moves feet apart to prevent fall

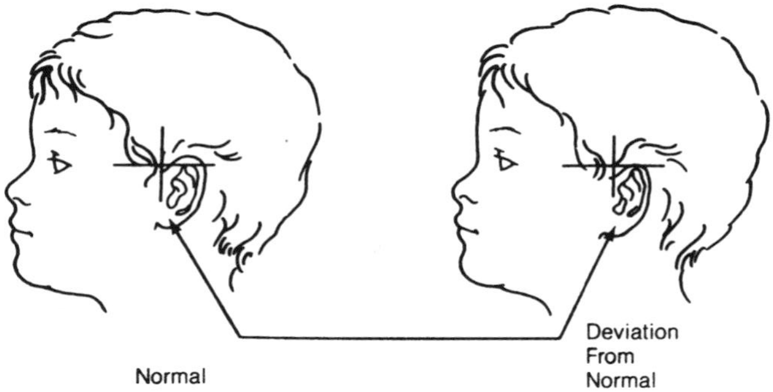

Figure 9-5. Placement and alignment of pinna in children.

Pediatric Variations *(continued)*

Procedure	Normal Findings	Deviations from Normal
C. To observe inner canal: Restrain child under 3 years; pull pinna downward and backward. For child over 3 years: pull pinna upward and backward. Inspect tympanic membrane using otoscope with pneumonic device.	TM moves with introduction of air.	TM does not move with introduction of air.

Geriatric Variations

- Elongated lobule
- Tuft of coarse hair may cover tragus
- Use 2028 Hz frequency test for screening high-frequency loss
- Perception of consonants (Z, T, F, G) and high-frequency sounds (S, Sh, Ph, K) decreases
- Dull retracted tympanic membrane
- Diminished hearing acuity (presbycusis)

Cultural Variations

- Ear wax varies. Dry, gray, flakey wax is usual in Asians and Native Americans. Light-honey to orange to dark-brown wax is most common in blacks and Caucasians.

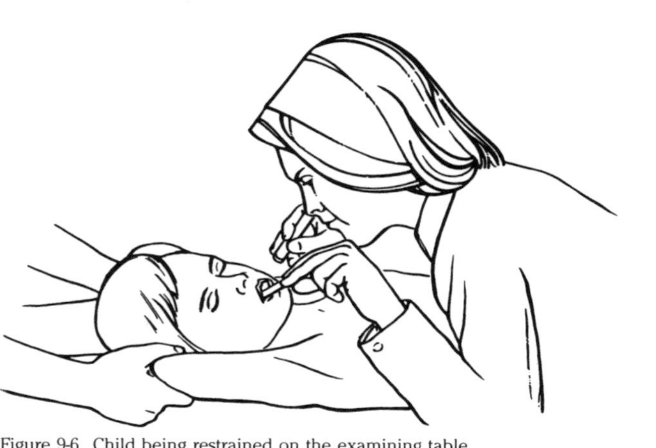

Figure 9-6. Child being restrained on the examining table.

Figure 9-7. Child being restrained in the upright position.

Possible Related Collaborative Problems

Potential complications:
Ear infection
Perforated eardrum
Hearing impairment

Teaching Tips for Selected Nursing Diagnoses

Nursing Diagnoses/ Collaborative Problems	***Teaching Tips***
Adult Client	
NURSING DIAGNOSIS: Risk for impaired sensory perception (hearing) related to working in loud, noisy environment	Teach client to wear protective hearing device when in environment with loud noises such as music, loud engines, aircraft, explosives, or firearms.
NURSING DIAGNOSIS: Sensory/Perceptual Alteration related to hearing impairment	Teach safety measures (e.g., burglar alarms, lights on telephone and alarms, phone designed for hearing impaired). Explore availability of resources for hearing aids, and refer client for reading or sign language learning if appropriate. Encourage client to ask others to repeat what is not heard.
NURSING DIAGNOSIS: Opportunity to enhance ear care	Teach client to cleanse ears with damp cloth and to avoid use of cotton-tipped applicators for cleaning internal auditory canal. Encourage use of sunscreen on external ear. Teach client to shake head to remove water in ear and dry ear after swimming to prevent swimmer's ear.

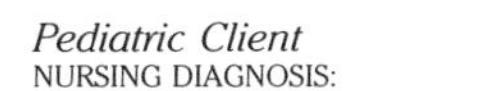

Pediatric Client

NURSING DIAGNOSIS:

Risk for Injury related to attempts to insert foreign objects in ear	Teach parents and child (as appropriate for age) dangers of insertion of foreign objects in ear. Teach parents to avoid toys with small removable parts Also, teach parents to avoid putting infant to bed with bottle filled with formula, juices, or sugar water, because this can settle in the oral pharynx and set up medium for bacteria to cause middle ear infections. Encourage yearly ear screening with physical examination during growing years.

Geriatric Client

NURSING DIAGNOSIS:

Sensory/Perceptual Alterations (auditory) related to aging process	Speak clearly, and allow client to see your lips. Speak within distance of 3–6 feet.

CHAPTER 10

Thoracic and Lung Assessment

Equipment Needed

- Stethoscope
- Tape measure

I. Subjective Data: Focus Questions

Coughing (productive, nonproductive)? Sputum (type and amount)? Allergies? Dyspnea or shortness of breath (at rest or on exertion)? Chest pain? History of asthma, bronchitis, emphyesema, tuberculosis? Cyanosis, pallor? Medications? Exposure to environmental inhalants (chemicals, fumes)? History of smoking (amount and length of time)?

II. Objective Data: Assessment Techniques

Expose anterior, posterior, and lateral chest with patient in sitting position. Locate landmarks (Fig. 10-1).

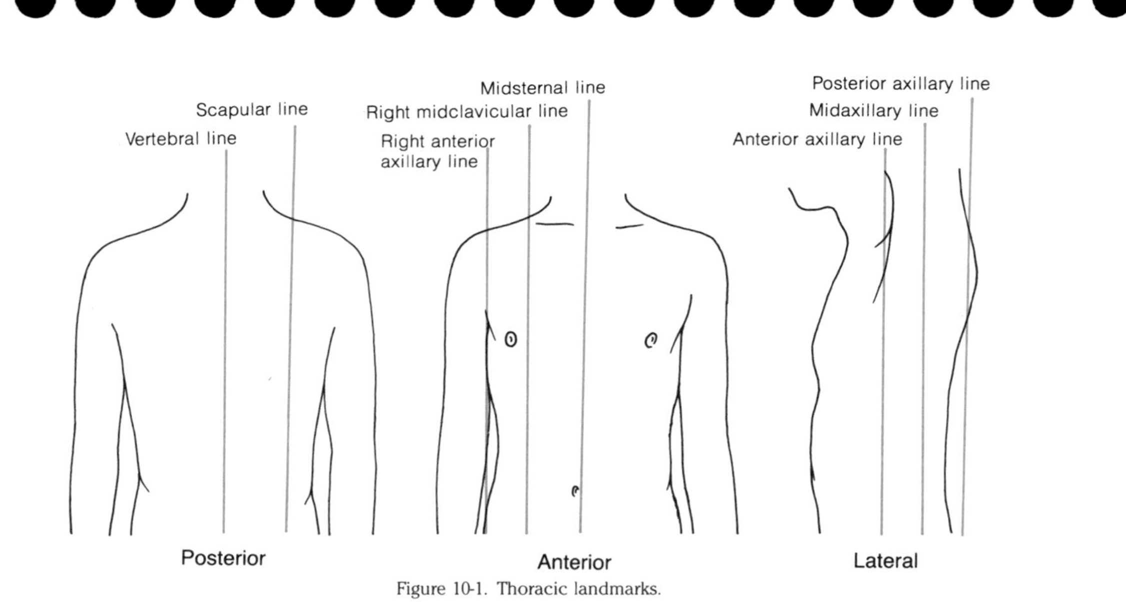

Figure 10-1. Thoracic landmarks.

Procedure	***Normal Findings***	***Deviations from Normal***
Inspection Inspect anterior, posterior, and lateral thorax for the following:		
Color	Pink	Pallor, cyanosis
Intercostal spaces	Even and relaxed	Bulging, retracting
Chest symmetry	Equal	Unequal
Rib slope	Less than 90 degrees downward	Horizontal or $\geq$90 degrees
Respirations (rate, rhythm, depth)	Even, 12–20/min, unlabored	Uneven; labored $<$12/min or $>$20/min; shallow; deep
Anterior-posterior to lateral diameter	1:2 ratio	Greater than 1:2 ratio (barrel chest) or less than 1:2 ratio
Shape and position of sternum	Level with ribs	Depressed or projecting
Position of trachea	Midline	Deviated to one side
Chest expansion	3 inches with deep inspiration	Less than 3 inches with deep inspiration

Palpation

Drape anterior chest and use finger pads or palms of hands to palpate posterior chest. Have client fold arms across anterior chest and lean forward to increase area of lungs. First palpate, percuss, and auscultate the posterior lungs and thorax while the client is sitting. Then palpate, percuss, and auscultate lateral lungs and thorax while the client is lying down in the supine position.

A. Palpate thorax at three levels for the following:		
1. Sensation	No pain or tenderness	Pain, tenderness
2. Vocal fremitus as client says "99"	Vibration decreased over periphery of lungs and increased over major airways	Vibration increased over lung with consolidation; vibration decreased over airway with obstruction
B. Palpate thorax for thoracic expansion by the following methods:	2- to 3-inch symmetrical thoracic expansion	Less than 2- to 3-inch thoracic expansion; asymmetrical expansion
1. Place hands on posterior thorax at level of 10th vertebra. Gently press skin between thumbs and have client take deep breath. Observe thumb movement (Fig. 10-2, *A*).	Symmetrical expansion (Thumbs move apart equal distance in both directions)	Asymmetrical expansion (Thumb movement apart unequal)
2. Anteriorly, press skin together at lower sternum and have patient take deep breath. Observe thumb movement (Fig. 10-2, *B*).	Symmetrical expansion (Thumbs move apart equal distance in both directions)	Asymmetrical expansion (Thumb movement apart unequal)

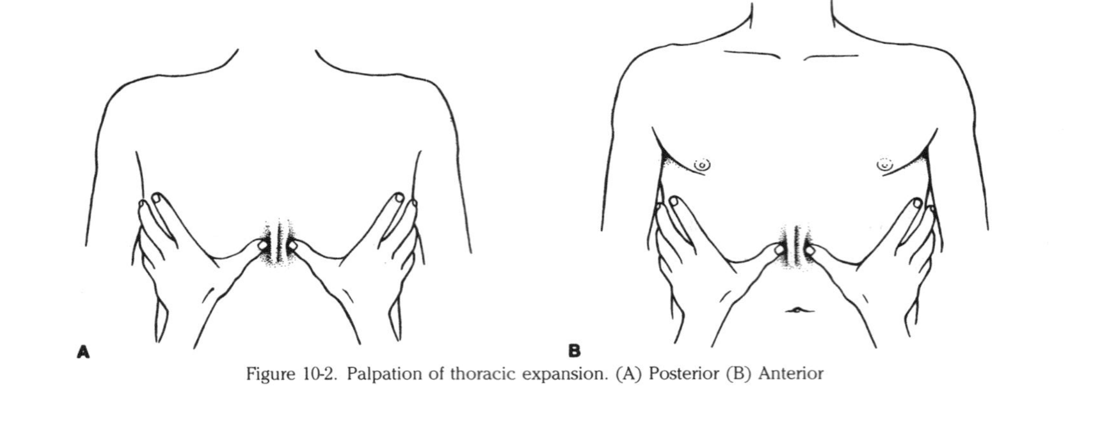

Figure 10-2. Palpation of thoracic expansion. (A) Posterior (B) Anterior

Procedure	Normal Findings	Deviations from Normal
Percussion		
Use mediate percussion over shoulder apices and intercostal spaces. Compare both for symmetry of percussion notes, while moving from apex to base of lungs as illustrated (see Fig. 10-3).		
A. Percuss over shoulder apices and at posterior, anterior, and lateral intercostal spaces as illustrated (Fig. 10-3). See Figure 10-4 to determine which underlying lung parts are being percussed.	Resonance	Hyperresonance heard over emphysematous lungs; dullness heard over solid masses or fluid.
B. Percuss for posterior diaphragmatic excursions bilaterally, as illustrated (Fig. 10-5).	Diaphragm descends 3 to 6 cm from T-10 (with full expiration held) to T-12 (with full inspiration held).	Diaphragm descends less than 3 cm or more than 5 cm.

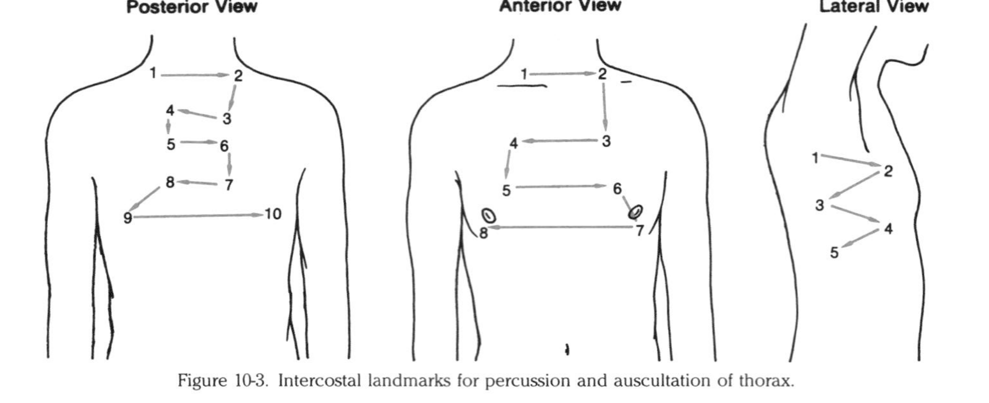

Figure 10-3. Intercostal landmarks for percussion and auscultation of thorax.

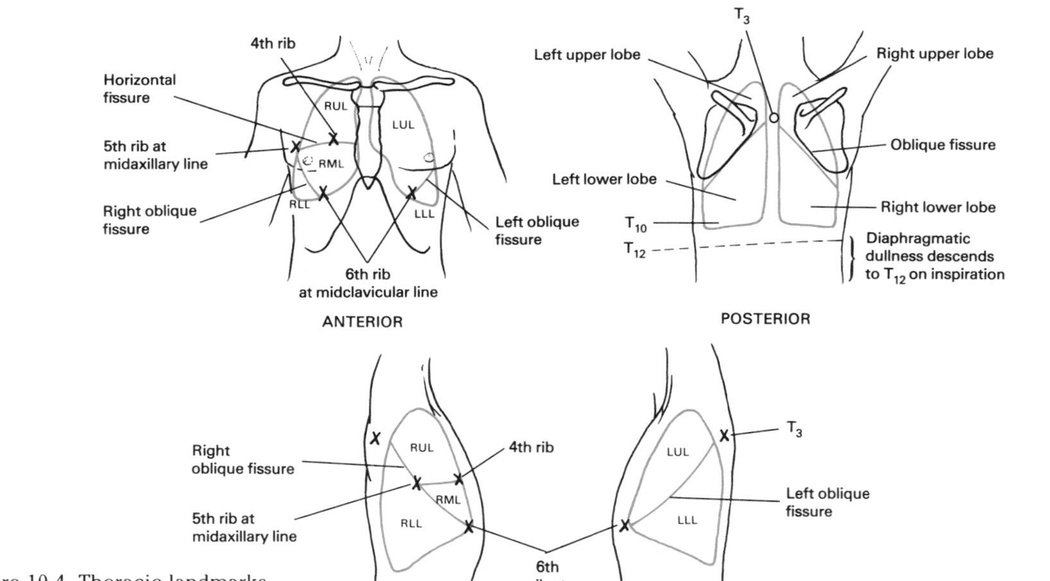

Figure 10-4. Thoracic landmarks of underlying lungs.

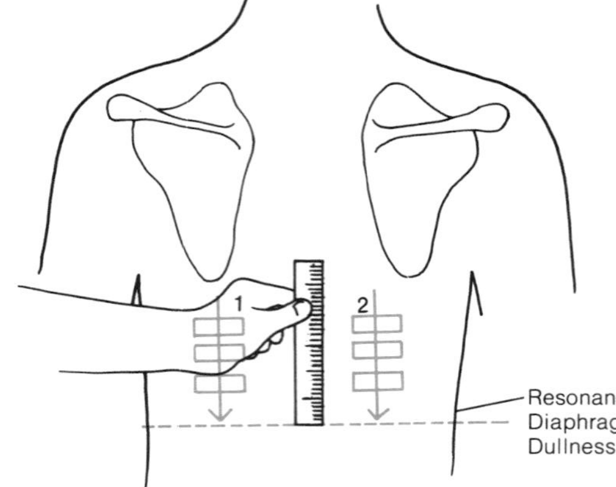

Figure 10-5. Percussing bilaterally for diaphragmatic excursions.

Procedure	Normal Findings	Deviations from Normal

Auscultation

Use diaphragm of stethoscope, exerting firm pressure over intercostal spaces. Instruct client to take slow, deep breaths through the mouth. Listen for two full breaths and compare symmetrical sides of thorax while moving stethoscope from apex to base of lungs, as illustrated in Figure 10-3.

Procedure	Normal Findings	Deviations from Normal
A. Auscultate breath sounds over the following:		
1. Trachea	Bronchial (tubular) breath sounds heard over trachea; expiration longer than inspiration.	Bronchial sounds heard over lung periphery

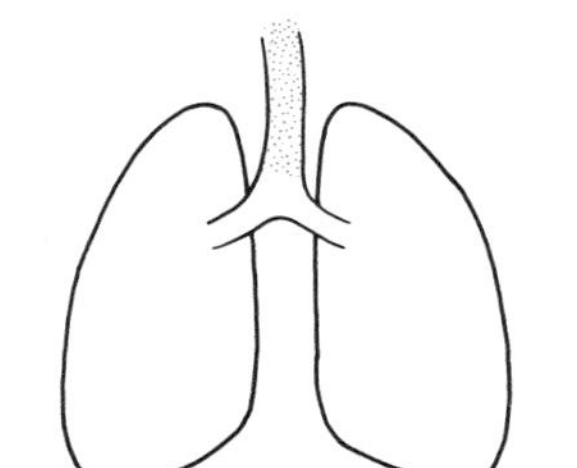

I E

Bronchial breath sounds

Procedure	***Normal Findings***	***Deviations from Normal***
2. Large-stem bronchi	Bronchovesicular breath sounds heard over main-stem bronchi: Below clavicles and between scapulae (inspiratory phase equals expiratory phase) I E Bronchovesicular breath sounds	Bronchovesicular breath sounds heard over lung periphery
3. Lung periphery	Vesicular (soft, breezy) breath sounds heard over lung periphery (inspiration longer than expiration) I E Vesicular breath sounds	Decreased breath sounds

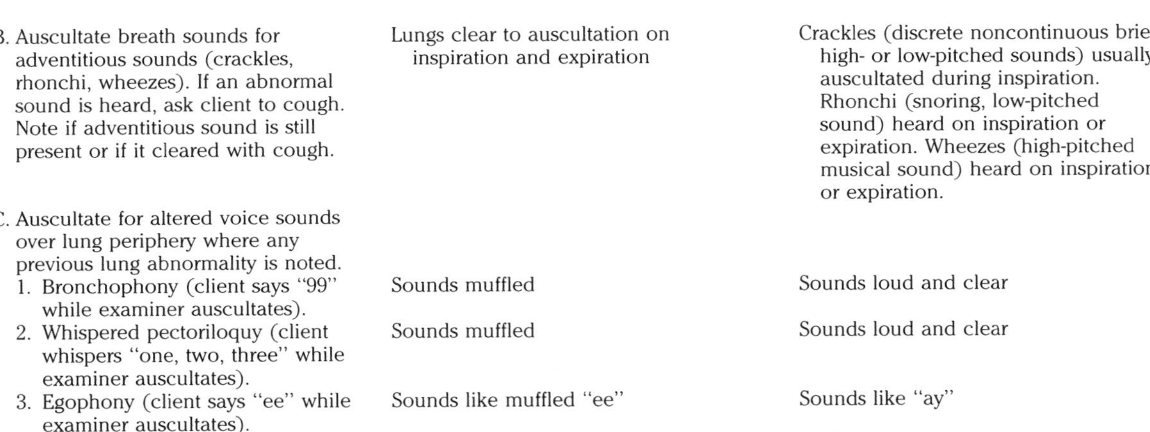

B. Auscultate breath sounds for adventitious sounds (crackles, rhonchi, wheezes). If an abnormal sound is heard, ask client to cough. Note if adventitious sound is still present or if it cleared with cough.	Lungs clear to auscultation on inspiration and expiration	Crackles (discrete noncontinuous brief high- or low-pitched sounds) usually auscultated during inspiration. Rhonchi (snoring, low-pitched sound) heard on inspiration or expiration. Wheezes (high-pitched musical sound) heard on inspiration or expiration.
C. Auscultate for altered voice sounds over lung periphery where any previous lung abnormality is noted.		
1. Bronchophony (client says "99" while examiner auscultates).	Sounds muffled	Sounds loud and clear
2. Whispered pectoriloquy (client whispers "one, two, three" while examiner auscultates).	Sounds muffled	Sounds loud and clear
3. Egophony (client says "ee" while examiner auscultates).	Sounds like muffled "ee"	Sounds like "ay"

(Adapted from Bates B: A Guide to Physical Examination and History Taking, 6th ed. Philadelphia, JB Lippincott, 1995.)

Pediatric Variations

I. Subjective Data: Focus Questions

History of wheezing, asthma, or other breathing problems?

II. Objective Data: Assessment Techniques

Inspection

Infancy: Anteroposterior diameter is equal to transverse diameter (1 : 1)—shape is nearly circular. Lateral diameter increases in proportion to anteroposterior diameter. Chest wall is thin with bony and cartilaginous rib cage soft and pliant. *Respirations:* Should be unlabored and quiet, with rate varying according to age (Table 10-1).

Percussion

Infancy and young children: Normally hyperresonant throughout. Any decrease in resonance is equal to dullness in the adult.

Table 10-1. Respiratory Rates in Children

Age	*Respiratory Rate*
Premature	40–90
Neonate	30–60
Infant	20–40
Young child	15–25
Adolescent	10–20

(Castiglia & Harbin: Child Health Care: Process and Practice, p 523. Philadelphia, JB Lippincott, 1992.)

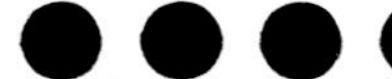

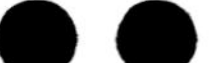

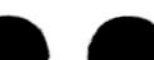

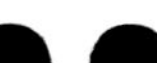

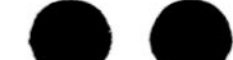
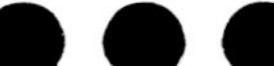

Auscultation
Bell or small diaphragm should be used to localize findings, especially in infants and young children. Breath sounds will be louder and harsher due to close proximity to origin of sounds. Wheezes and rhonchi occur more frequently in infants and young children.

Geriatric Variations

- Accentuated dorsal curve (kyphosis) of spine
- Hyperresonance of thorax due to age-related emphysemic changes
- Decreased breath sounds, and increased retention of mucus due to decreased pulmonary function
- Increased AP diameter
- Decreased ability to cough effectively

Cultural Variation

- Thoracic cavity size varies among cultural groups. The tendency is for Caucasians to have larger thoraxes than blacks, Asians, and Native Americans.

Possible Related Collaborative Problems

Potential complications:
Respiratory insufficiency/failure
Pneumonia
Pulmonary edema
Airway obstruction/atelectasis
Laryngeal edema
Pleural effusion
Oxygen toxicity
Carbondioxide toxicity
Pneumothorax
Respiratory acidosis
Respiratory alkalosis
Tracheal necrosis
Tracheobronchial constriction

Nursing Diagnoses	***Teaching Tips***
Adult Client	
NURSING DIAGNOSIS: Opportunity to enhance respiratory function	Encourage client to participate in a daily exercise program and to eat a well-balanced diet. Provide client with information on second-hand smoke-risks and how to decrease one's exposure. The Indoor Air Quality Information Clearinghouse provides free information (800)438-4318.
NURSING DIAGNOSIS: Ineffective Airway Clearance related to excessive mucus	Instruct client on effective deep breathing and coughing. Encourage liquid intake of 2–3 quarts/day. Caution client to use protective measures to prevent spread of infections.
NURSING DIAGNOSIS: Impaired Gas Exchange related to chronic lung tissue damage	Teach client diaphragmatic and pursed-lip breathing.
NURSING DIAGNOSIS: Ineffective Airway Clearance related to chronic allergy	Provide literature on environmental control. Assess whether client has kit to deal with emergencies (e.g., bee stings). If allergy is produced by unknown food, assist client with keeping a diary of allergy attacks to determine cause.

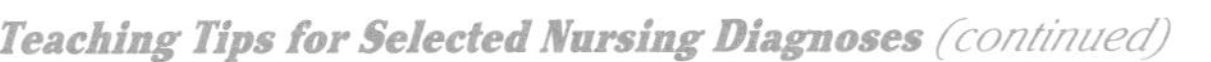

Teaching Tips for Selected Nursing Diagnoses *(continued)*

Nursing Diagnoses	Teaching Tips
NURSING DIAGNOSIS: Ineffective Breathing Pattern: hyperventilation related to hypoxia and lack of knowledge of controlled breathing techniques	Teach client how to become aware of breathing patterns and how to assess what aggravates hyperventilation (i.e., fatigue, stress). Teach controlled breathing techniques.
NURSING DIAGNOSIS: Impaired Gas Exchange related to smoking	Explain effects of smoking and that it is a primary risk factor for lung cancer. Assess client's desire to quit and refer to community agencies for self-help on smoking cessation programs. Discuss alternate methods of coping.
Pediatric Client	
NURSING DIAGNOSIS: Ineffective Airway Clearance related to bronchospasm and increased pulmonary secretions	Postural drainage and percussion may be used with children of various ages. Teach parents safety measures when using vaporizers. Teach alternate ways of humidifying air. For example, have parent run hot water in shower and close bathroom door. Sit with child in this room for approximately 10 minutes to liquefy secretions by steam. (Child must not be left alone in room.) Teach parents the importance of throat cultures for upper respiratory infections to identify streptococcus infections. *If child has asthma:* As asthma attacks decrease with increasing age of child, assist parents with letting child have more independence and avoiding overprotection. Teach family how to decrease allergens (i.e., dust) in home by using smooth surfaces that are easy to clean.

Nursing Diagnoses	***Teaching Tips***
Geriatric Client NURSING DIAGNOSIS: Impaired gas exchange related to poor muscle tone and decreased ability to remove secretions.	Teach client the importance of mobility and exercise to maintain adequate respiratory hygiene. Encourage client to discuss consideration of the "flu" shot with his/her physician.

CHAPTER 11

Cardiac Assessment

Equipment Needed

- Dual-head stethoscope

I. Subjective Data: Focus Questions

A. *Assessment of chief complaints*

1. Chest pain: Location? Radiation? Quality? Duration? What brings it on? What relieves it? Are there any other associated symptoms, such as nausea, vomiting, sweating?
2. Irregular heart beat: Does your heart pound or beat too fast? Does your heart skip or jump?

B. *Assessment of risk factors*

1. Do you have a history of hypertension, diabetes, rheumatic fever?
2. Is there a history in your family of heart attack, hypertension, stroke, diabetes?
3. Describe your nutritional intake. Have you ever been told you have a high cholesterol/ triglyceride level?
4. Do you smoke? how much? for how long?
5. How do you view yourself? What do you do to relax? How many hours a day do you work? How do you cope with stress?
6. Exercise: What do you do for exercise? How often?

II. Objective Data: Assessment Techniques

Procedure	Normal Findings	Deviations from Normal
Inspection Inspect the chest to identify landmarks that aid in assessment of the heart. Check for visibility of point of maximum impulse (PMI) and any *abnormal pulsations*.		
A. *Intercostal space (ICS):* Located by finding the sternal angle, which is felt as a ridge in the sternum approximately 2 inches below the sternal notch (Fig. 11-1). The adjacent rib is the second rib with the second ICS directly below it. Other ICSs can be identified by counting from the second ICS. The fifth ICS is at the junction of the sternum and the xiphoid process.	Small apical impulse (2.5 cm or less) at or medial to the left mid-clavicular line at the 4th or 5th intercostal space.	Impulses lateral to midclavicular line. Apical impulse on right side of chest. Bulging and/or prominent pulsations (>3 cm) at the point of maximal impulse (PMI).
B. *Midsternal line (MSL):* Imaginary line extending down the chest through the middle of the sternum. It divides the anterior chest in half (Fig. 11-1).		

Procedure	*Normal Findings*	*Deviations from Normal*
C. *Midclavicular line (MCL):* Imaginary line extending from middle of clavicle down the chest, dividing the left or right anterior chest into two parts (Fig. 11-1).		Prominent impulse at right sternal border in pulmonic or aortic area.
D. *Anterior axillary line (AAL):* Imaginary line extending along the lateral wall of the anterior chest and even with the anterior axillary fold (Fig. 11-1).		

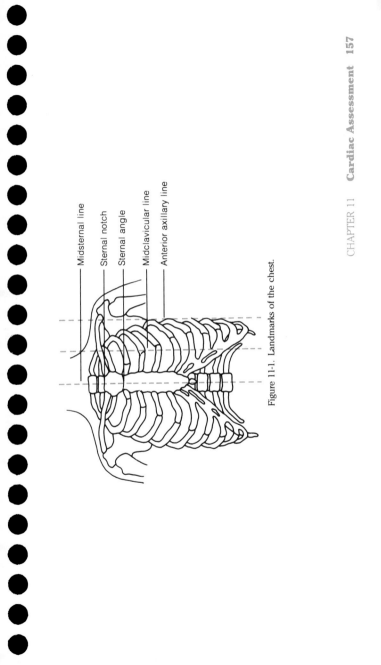

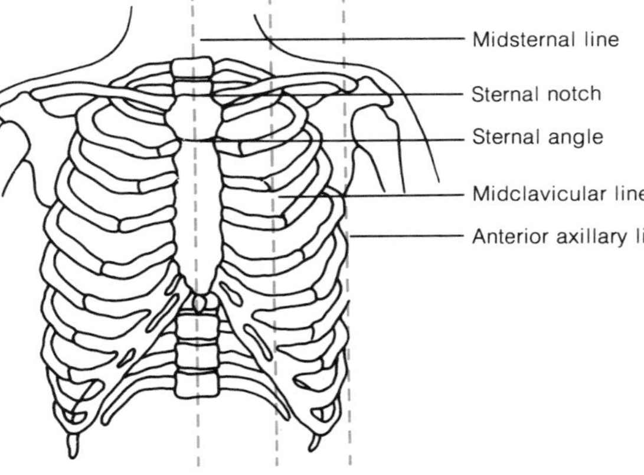

Figure 11-1. Landmarks of the chest.

Procedure	Normal Findings	Deviations from Normal
Palpation The client should be lying down. Palpate using the fingertips and palmar surfaces of the fingers in an organized fashion, beginning in the aortic area and moving down the chest toward the tricuspid area (Fig. 11-2).		
A. *Aortic area:* Palpate second ICS at right sternal border (Fig. 11-2).	No vibrations or pulsations palpated in aortic, pulmonic, or tricuspid area	Thrill, which feels similar to a purring cat, or pulsation in any of these areas except the mitral area
B. *Pulmonic area:* Palpate second ICS at left sternal border (Fig. 11-2).		
C. *Erb's point:* Palpate third ICS at left sternal border (Fig. 11-2).		
D. *Tricuspid area:* Palpate fifth ICS at lower left sternal border (Fig. 11-2).		
E. *Mitral area:* Palpate fifth ICS at the left MCL. This is also called the point of maximal impulse (PMI) (Fig. 11-2).	PMI is felt as a pulsation and is approximately the size of a nickel.	No pulsation. Area of pulsation is the size of a quarter or larger, or thrill is palpated.

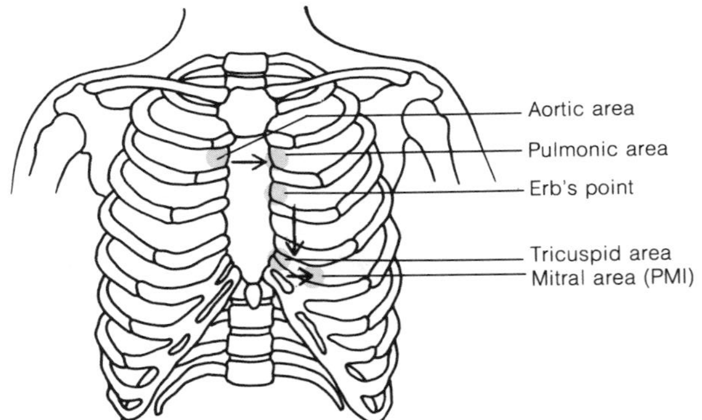

Figure 11-2. Areas to palpate on the chest.

Procedure	*Normal Findings*	*Deviations from Normal*
Percussion Percussion may be done to define cardiac borders by identifying areas of dullness, but it is generally unreliable. Size of the heart can be more accurately determined by chest x-ray.		
Auscultation Auscultate in an orderly, systematic fashion beginning with the aortic area. Move across and then down the chest. Focus on one sound at a time. Auscultate each area with the diaphragm of the stethoscope applied firmly to the chest. Repeat the sequence using the bell of the stethoscope applied lightly to the chest. Auscultate with the client in the supine position. Then listen specifically over the apex with the bell while the client is in the left lateral position. Assist the client to a sitting position, and auscultate the pericardium with the diaphragm. Then have the client lean forward and exhale while listening over the aortic area with the diaphragm.		
A. Auscultate to identify the first heart sound (S_1) or lub and the second heart sound (S_2) or dub (Fig. 11-3).	S_1 follows the long diastolic pause and precedes the short systolic pause and corresponds to each carotid pulsation. S_2 follows the short systolic phase and precedes the long diastolic phase.	
B. Auscultate for rate and rhythm.	Rate: 60–100 beats/min, regular rhythm	Bradycardia (heart rate below 60); tachycardia (heart rate above 100); rhythm irregular
C. Auscultate and focus on each sound and pause individually:	Crisp, distinct sound heard in each area but loudest at mitral and tricuspid areas	Split sound in middle-aged and older adults

1. Auscultate S_1: Heard best with diaphragm.	May become softer with inspiration. Split S_1 normal in children, young adults, and pregnant women.	
2. Auscultate S_2: Heard best with diaphragm.	Crisp, distinct sound heard loudest at the aortic and pulmonic areas. Split S_2 may be normal in adults if heard only during inspiration.	Split sound heard equally during inspiration and expiration
3. Auscultate systolic pause-space: Heard between S_1 and S_2 (Fig. 11-4)	Silent pause; should hear distinct end of S_1 and beginning of S_2 with nothing in between	*Murmur:* Swishing sound heard at beginning, middle, or end of systolic pause. (Note intensity, pitch, and quality—Table 11-1) *Click:* Sharp, high-pitched snapping sound heard immediately after S_1 or in the middle of the systolic pause
4. Auscultate diastolic pause-space heard between S_2 and the next S_1 (Fig. 11-4).	Silent pause; should hear distinct end of S_2 and distinct beginning of next S_1	*Murmur:* Swishing sound heard at beginning, middle, or end of diastolic pause. (Note intensity pitch, and quality—Table 11.1) *Snap:* High-pitched snapping sound heard after S_2 during the diastolic pause in the mitral or tricuspid areas

II. Objective Data: Assessment Techniques *(continued)*

Procedure	*Normal Findings*	*Deviations from Normal*
5. Auscultate S_3: Low, faint sound occurring at the beginning of the diastolic pause (Fig. 11-4).	S_3 auscultated in children and young adults but disappears upon standing or sitting up	S_3 auscultated in adults or that continues with standing or sitting in children and young adults
6. Auscultate S_4: Soft, low-pitched sound heard best with client in supine or left lateral position (Fig. 11-5)	Auscultated in infants, small children, and athletes	Auscultated in adults

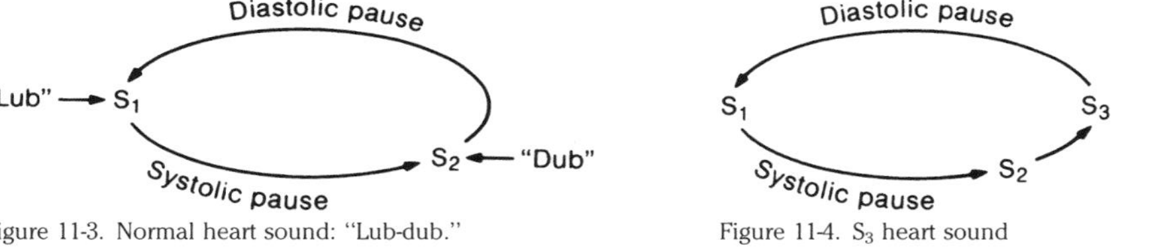

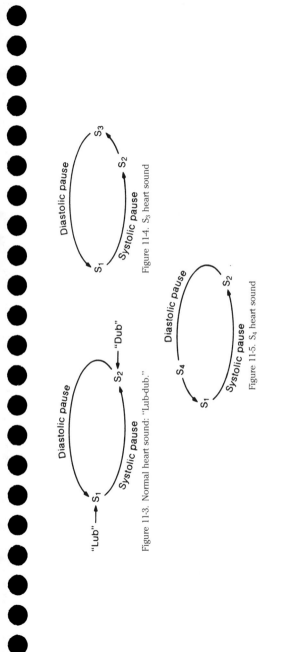

Figure 11-3. Normal heart sound: "Lub-dub."

Figure 11-4. S_3 heart sound

Figure 11-5. S_4 heart sound

Table 11-1. Classification for Intensity, Pitch, and Quality of Murmurs

Intensity

Grade 1—Very faint, heard only after the listener has "tuned in"; may not be heard in all positions
Grade 2—Quiet but heard immediately upon placing the stethoscope on the chest
Grade 3—Moderately loud
Grade 4—Loud
Grade 5—Very loud, may be heard with a stethoscope partly off the chest
Grade 6—May be heard with the stethoscope entirely off the chest

(Grades 5 and 6: Thrills are associated)

Pitch

High, medium, or low

Quality

Blowing, rumbling, harsh or musical

(Adapted from Bates B: A Guide to Physical Examination and History Taking, 6th ed. Philadelphia, JB Lippincott, 1995.)

Pediatric Variations

I. Subjective Data: Focus Questions

In addition to focus questions for adults, inquire about the following:

- Poor weight gain
- Signs of delayed development (e.g., slowed social development, language development, or motor skills)
- Difficulty in feeding (breast, bottle, acceptance of new foods)
- Inability to tolerate physical activity or play with peers
- Squatting behavior
- Excessive irritability or crying

II. Objective Data: Assessment Techniques

Procedure	*Normal Findings and Variations*
A. Inspect chest wall in semi-Fowler's position from an angle for PMI.	PMI easily visible because heart is larger in proportion to chest size (Fig. 11-6). Heart lies more horizontally up to age 5 to 6 years. Thus, the PMI may be lateral to the midclavicular line.
B. Palpate peripheral pulse points in relation to apical pulse and to each other: femoral, radial, brachial, and carotid.	Symmetrical and equal rate, strength, and rhythm

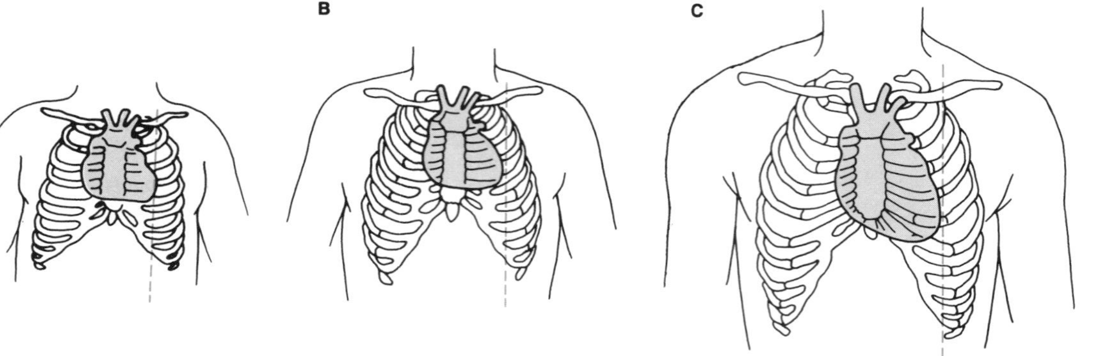

Age	*Location*
4 years	To left of midclavicular line
4–6 years	At midclavicular line
7–8 years	To right of midclavicular line

Figure 11-6. Location of apex of heart in (A) infant, (B) child, and (C) adult.

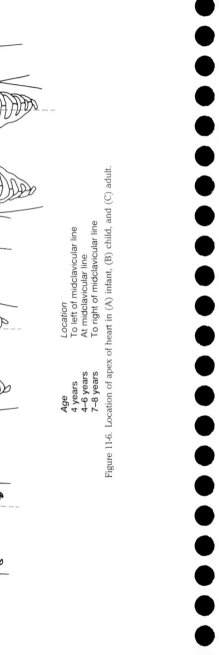

II. Objective Data: Assessment Techniques *(continued)*

Procedure	*Normal Findings and Variations*
C. Percuss heart size. (*Note:* This is rarely done due to the inaccuracy of the method.)	Percussion area is slightly larger because of horizontal position and overlying thymus gland.
D. Auscultate S_1 and S_2 at pulmonic area (Erb's point).	S_1 louder than S_2 or S_2 louder than S_1. Splitting of S_2 heard best at Erb's point (25%–33% of all children). Frequent site of innocent murmurs.
Tricuspid area	S_1 louder, preceding S_2
Mitral area	S_1 loudest
Sinus arrhythmia	Varies with respiration; very common and disappears with age
Rate	See Table 11-2 for normal pediatric pulse rates.

Table 11-2. Average Heart Rate of Infants and Children at Rest

Age	*Average Rate*	*Two Standard Deviations*
Birth	140	90–190
First 6 months	130	80–180
6–12 months	115	75–155
1–2 years	110	70–150
2–6 years	103	68–138
6–10 years	95	65–125
10–14 years	85	55–115

(Used with permission from Bates B: A Guide to Physical Examination and History Taking, 6th ed. Philadelphia, JB Lippincott, 1995.)

Geriatric Variations

- Thickening of heart walls
- Decreased elasticity of heart and arteries, reduced pumping ability of heart
- Decreased cardiac output and cardiac reserve
- Location of heart sounds and PMI may be varied due to kyphosis or scoliosis.
- Early and soft systolic murmurs are common.
- Atrial fibrillations often occur.
- Reduced maximum heart rate

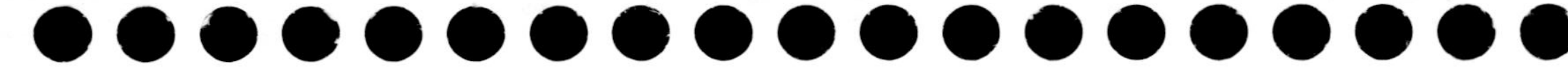

Possible Related Collaborative Problems

Potential complications:

Congestive heart failure	Cardiogenic shock	Endocarditis
Myocardial ischemia	Congenital heart disease	
Dysrhythmias	Angina	

Teaching Tips for Selected Nursing Diagnoses

Nursing Diagnoses/ Collaborative Problems	***Teaching Tips***
Adult Client NURSING DIAGNOSIS: Fear related to perceived increased risk of heart disease and family history of heart disease	Explain what you are doing when auscultating so that the client won't become alarmed by the length of time you are taking. Explain that vigorous exercise (20–30 minutes three times a week) may decrease serum triglycerides and cholesterol, and therefore prevent heart disease by increasing the working capabilities of the body and heart capillaries. Advise client to have a complete physical examination prior to starting a new fitness program.

Teaching Tips for Selected Nursing Diagnoses *(continued)*

Nursing Diagnoses/ Collaborative Problems	***Teaching Tips***
NURSING DIAGNOSIS: Ineffective Management of Therapeutic Regimen related to knowledge deficit: Taking pulse in order to assess heart rate prior to taking cardiac medications	Teach client correct method for taking pulse. Instruct on heart rate necessary for taking prescribed medication.
NURSING DIAGNOSIS: Altered Sexuality Patterns related to fear of injury post myocardial infarction	Instruct client to discuss limitations on sexual activities as recommended by physician. (Usually, a client can safely engage in sexual intercourse by the time he or she is permitted to walk up a flight of stairs.)
NURSING DIAGNOSIS: Ineffective Management of Therapeutic Regimen related to knowledge deficit: Optimal diet for coronary disease	Teach client the following dietary guidelines: • Total fat intake should be less than 30% of calories. • Saturated fat intake should be less than 10% of calories. • Polyunsaturated fat intake should not exceed 10% of calories. • Cholesterol intake should not exceed 300 mg/day. • Carbohydrate intake should constitute 50% or more of calories, with emphasis on complex carbohydrates. • Protein intake should provide the remainder of the calories. • Sodium intake should not exceed 3 g/day.

- Alcoholic consumption should not exceed 1–2 oz of ethanol per day. Two ounces of 100 proof whisky, 8 oz of wine, or 24 oz of beer each contain 1 oz of ethanol.
- Total calories should be sufficient to maintain the individual's recommended body weight.
- A wide variety of foods should be consumed.

(Reproduced with permission. "Dietary Guidelines for Healthy American Adults," 1988. Copyright © American Heart Association)

NURSING DIAGNOSIS:
Opportunity to enhance effective activity-exercise pattern

Teach client to seek physician's recommendation regarding an exercise plan and describe the following guidelines for healthy individuals.

1. Exercise only when feeling well. Wait until symptoms and signs of a cold or the flu (including fever) have been absent 2 days or more before resuming activity.
2. Do not exercise vigorously soon after eating. Wait at least 2 hours.
3. Adjust exercise to the weather. Exercise should be adjusted to environmental conditions. Special precautions are necessary when exercising in hot weather. If air temperature is over 70°F slow the pace, be alert for signs of heat injury, and drink adequate fluids to maintain hydration. If the air temperature is over 80°F exercise in the early morning or late afternoon to avoid the heat. Air-conditioned shopping malls are popular for walking.

Nursing Diagnoses/ Collaborative Problems	*Teaching Tips*
	4. Slow down for hills. When ascending hills decrease speed to avoid overexertion. 5. Wear proper clothing and shoes. Dress in loose-fitting comfortable clothes made of porous material appropriate for the weather. Use sweat suits only for warmth. 6. Understand personal limitations. Everyone should have periodic medical examinations. When under a physician's care, ask if there are limitations. 7. Select appropriate exercises. Cardiovascular (aerobic) exercises should be a major component of activities. However, flexibility and strengthening exercises should also be considered for a well-rounded program. 8. Be alert for symptoms. If the following symptoms occur, contact a physician before continuing exercise. Although any symptom should be clarified, these are particularly important: a. Discomfort in the upper body, including the chest, arm, neck, or jaw, during exercise. b. Faintness accompanying the exercise. c. Shortness of breath during exercise. d. Discomfort in bones and joints either during or after exercise. There may be slight muscle soreness when beginning exercise, but if back or joint develops discontinue exercise until after evaluation by a physician.

9. Watch for the following signs of overexercising:
   a. Inability to finish.
   b. Inability to converse during the activity.
   c. Faintness or nausea after exercise.
   d. Chronic fatigue.
   e. Sleeplessness.
   f. Aches and pains in the joints. Although there may be some muscle discomfort, joints should not hurt or feel stiff.
10. Start slowly and progress gradually. Allow time to adapt.

(Reproduced with permission. *Exercise Standards: A Statement for Healthcare Professionals* from the American Heart Association, 1995 Copyright © American Heart Association.)

CHAPTER 12

Peripheral Vascular Assessment

Equipment Needed

- Stethoscope
- Sphygmomanometer
- Tape measure
- Cotton (to detect light touch)
- Paper clip (tip used to detect sharp sensation—safer than pin tip)
- Tuning fork (to detect vibratory sensation)

I. Subjective Data: Focus Questions

Pain in calves, feet, buttocks, or legs? What aggravates the pain: Walking? Sitting long periods? Standing long periods? Sleep? What relieves the pain: Elevating legs? Rest? Lying down? Is there associated coldness, cyanosis, edema, varicosities, paresthesia, or tingling? Does client have well-fitting shoes? Does client wear constricting garments or hosiery? In what type of chair does client usually sit? Does he or she cross legs frequently? What is the amount and type of exercise the client does? Is client taking any drugs that may mimic arterial insufficiency?

II. Objective Data: Assessment Techniques

Procedure	Normal Findings	Deviations from Normal
Inspection, Palpation, and Auscultation of Circulation to Arms and Neck Inspection, palpation, and auscultation are performed together to assess the blood pressure and circulation to the upper extremities and neck while the client is in a sitting, then a standing position. A special maneuver (Allen's test) is used to detect arterial insufficiency of the hands.		
A. Palpate brachial artery; then auscultate arterial blood pressure in both arms with client sitting.	May be difference of 5–10 mm Hg between two arms *Systolic pressure:* 85–130 mm Hg with client sitting *Diastolic pressure:* <85 mm Hg* (see Table 4.2)	More than 10 mm Hg difference between two arms *Systolic pressure:* >140 or <95 mm Hg* *Diastolic pressure:* <60 or >90 mm Hg* (see Table 4-3)
B. Palpate brachial artery; then auscultate arterial blood pressure in both arms with client standing.	*Systolic pressure:* Difference between both arms of 15 mm Hg or less *Diastolic pressure:* Difference between both arms of 5 mm Hg or less	*Systolic pressure:* Difference between both arms of more than 15 mm Hg *Diastolic pressure:* Difference between both arms of more than 5 mm Hg
C. Palpate each carotid artery alternately for rate, rhythm, symmetry, strength, and elasticity.	60–90 beats/min; regular, equal, strong, and elastic	Less than 60 or more than 90 beats/min; irregular, unequal, weak and thready, bounding and firm, inelastic

* These values may vary with individuals.

Procedure	*Normal Findings*	*Deviations from Normal*
(*Caution:* Use *light* palpation over carotids since increased pressure may stimulate carotid sinus reflex and lower heart rate and blood pressure.)		
D. Auscultate carotid arteries with bell of stethoscope while patient holds breath.	No sound heard	Bruit (swishing sound)
E. Inspect and palpate upper extremities for the following:		
Color	Pink; pink or red tones visible under dark pigmentation	Pallor, cyanosis, rubor
Temperature	Warm	Cold
Sensation (scatter stimuli over trunk and upper extremities with client's eyes closed)	Client can identify light and deep touch; nontender	Paresthesia, tenderness, pain
Mobility	Mobile	Paralysis
Radial pulses (Fig. 12-1)	Bilateral pulses strong and equal	Bilateral/unilateral pulses weak, asymmetrical, or absent
Ulnar pulses (Fig. 12-2)	Bilateral pulses strong and equal	Bilateral/unilateral pulses weak, asymmetrical, or absent

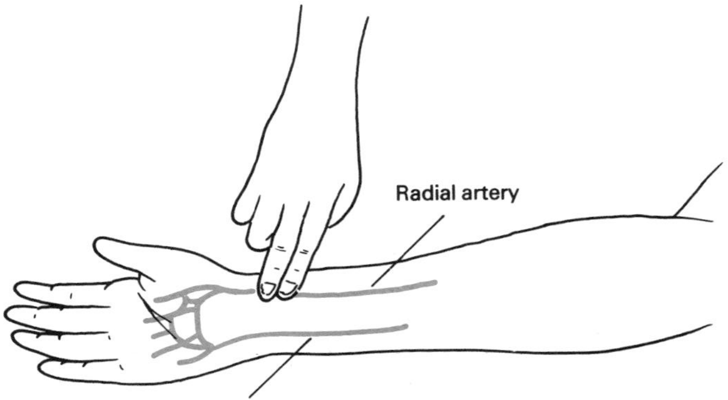

Radial artery

Ulnar artery

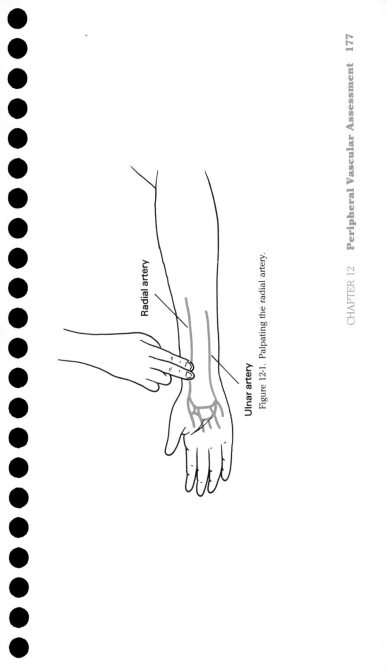

Figure 12-1. Palpating the radial artery.

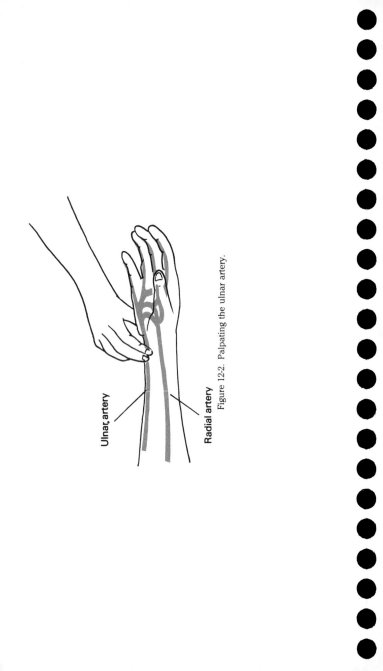

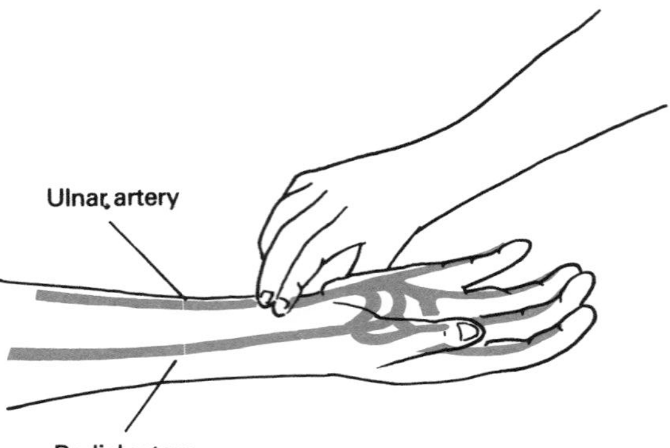

Figure 12-2. Palpating the ulnar artery.

II. Objective Data: Assessment Techniques *(continued)*

Procedure	Normal Findings	Deviations from Normal
F. Allen's test: If client has weak radial and ulnar pulses, perform Allen's test, a special maneuver (Fig. 12-3).	Full palm of hand becomes pink with release of ulnar or radial artery.	Only half of palm of hand becomes pink with release of ulnar or radial artery; other half of palm remains whitish.

Inspection and Palpation of Jugular Venous Pressure and Circulation of the Lower Extremities

Inspection and palpation are performed together to assess the jugular venous pressure and circulation of the lower extremities with the client in a supine position. Finally, two special maneuvers are performed to detect venous and arterial insufficiency of the legs.

Procedure	Normal Findings	Deviations from Normal
A. Inspect jugular veins with head elevated 45 degrees. Identify the highest point of venous wave (Fig. 12-4) in relation to the sternal angle. Measure in centimeters or inches.	Pulsation height $\leq$1 inch (3 cm)	Pulsation height $>$ 1 inch (3 cm)
B. Inspect and palpate legs for the following:		
Color	Pink; pink or red tones visible under dark pigmentation	Pallor, cyanosis, rubor
Temperature	Warm	Cold

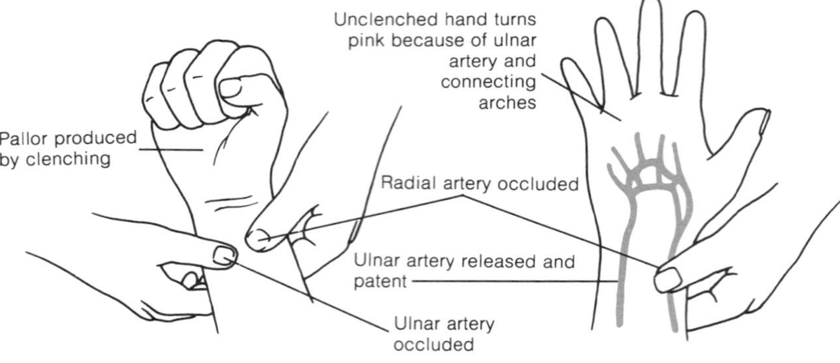

Guidelines to Perform Allen's Test

1. Ask client to make fist
2. Compress ulnar and radial arteries
3. Ask client to open hand
4. Release ulnar artery
5. Repeat with release on radial artery

Figure 12-3. Allen's test.

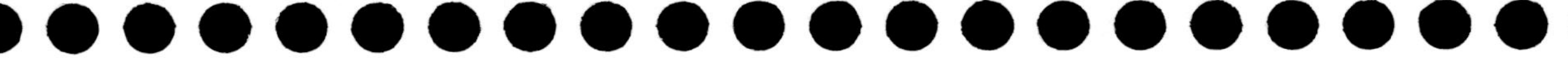

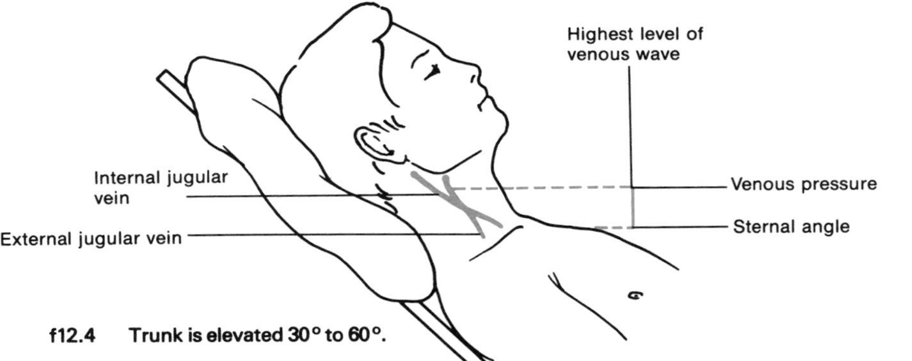

Figure 12-4. Inspection of jugular vein.

II. Objective Data: Assessment Techniques *(continued)*

Procedure	*Normal Findings*	*Deviations from Normal*
Sensation (scatter stimuli with client's eyes closed)	Client can identify light and deep touch; nontender	Paresthesia, tenderness, pain
Mobility	Mobile	Paralysis
Superficial veins	Slight venous distention with standing that collapses with elevation	Severe venous distention and bulging
Condition of skin	Intact	Lesions
Edema	Not present	Present
Femoral pulses (Fig. 12-5)	Bilateral pulses strong and equal	Bilateral/unilateral pulses weak, asymmetrical, or absent
Popliteal pulse (Have client bend knees or roll to stomach and flex leg 90 degrees. Press deeply to feel. See Fig. 12-6.)	Bilateral pulses strong and equal	Bilateral/unilateral pulses weak, asymmetrical, or absent
Dorsalis pedis pulse (Have client dorsiflex or extend foot. See Fig. 12-7.)	Bilateral pulses strong and equal (congenitally absent in 5%–10% of population)	Bilateral/unilateral pulses weak, asymmetrical, or absent
Posterior tibial pulse (located on medial malleolus of ankle; Fig. 12-8)	Bilateral pulses strong and equal	Bilateral/unilateral pulses weak or absent

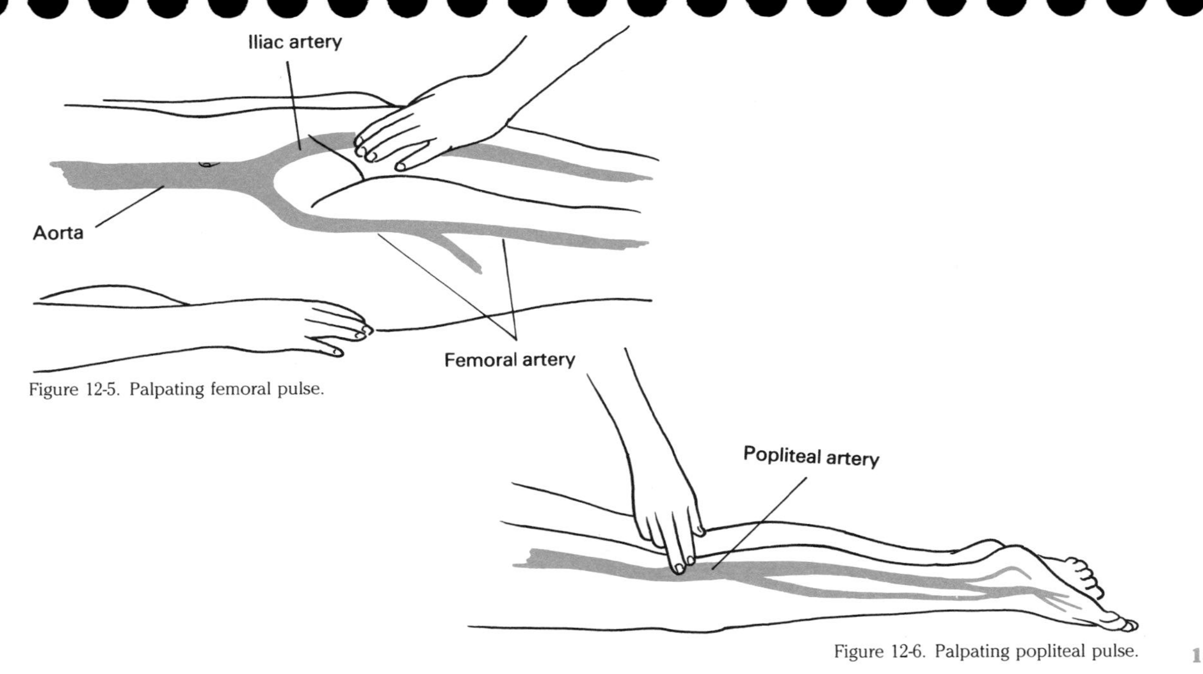

Figure 12-5. Palpating femoral pulse.

Figure 12-6. Palpating popliteal pulse.

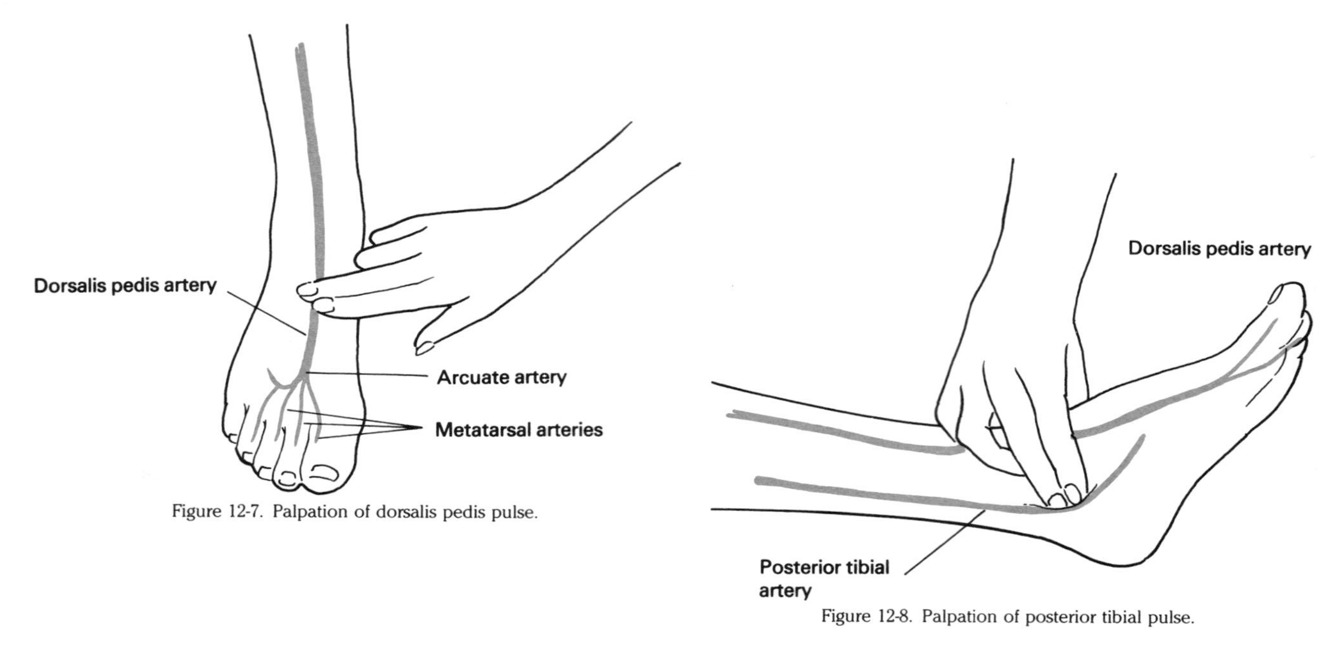

Figure 12-7. Palpation of dorsalis pedis pulse.

Figure 12-8. Palpation of posterior tibial pulse.

II. Objective Data: Assessment Techniques *(continued)*

Procedure	Normal Findings	Deviations from Normal
C. Special maneuvers:		
1. Check for deep phlebitis by quickly squeezing calf muscles against tibia.	Verbalizes no calf pain	Verbalizes painful calves
2. Check Homans' sign by extending leg and dorsiflexing foot.	Verbalizes no calf soreness or pain	Verbalizes soreness and pain in calves
3. Check for arterial insufficiency if leg pulses are decreased by instructing client to lie down on back while you support the client's legs 12 inches above heart level and:		
a. Have client move feet up and down at ankles for 60 seconds	Feet pink to slight pale color with this maneuver	Extensive pallor with this maneuver
b. Ask client to sit up and dangle legs in dependent position.	Pink color returns to tips of toes in 10 seconds. Veins on top of feet fill in 15 seconds.	Toes and feet are rubor (dusky red) color. Venous return to feet is delayed 45 seconds or more.
4. Check for competency of values (Trendelenburg test) if client has varicose veins: Feel dilated veins with one hand while using the other hand to compress veins firmly above level of the first hand.		
Palpate for impulse of blood flow.	No pulsation palpated	Pulsation felt

Procedure	*Normal Findings*	*Deviations from Normal*
D. Comparison of venous and arterial insufficiency of lower extremities (Fig. 12-9)		
	Arterial Insufficiency:	*Venous Insufficiency:*
Pulses	Decreased/absent	Present
Color	Pale on elevation; dusky rubor on dependency	Pink to cyanotic; brown pigment at ankles
Temperature	Cool, cold	Warm
Edema	None	Present
Skin	Shiny skin; thick nails; absence of hair; ulcers on toes; gangrene may develop	Ulcers on ankles; discolored, scaly
Sensation	Leg pain aggravated by exercise and relieved with rest. Pressure in buttocks or calves or cramps during walking, paresthesias.	Leg pain aggravated by long standing or sitting and relieved by elevation of legs, lying down, or walking. Also relieved with use of support hose.

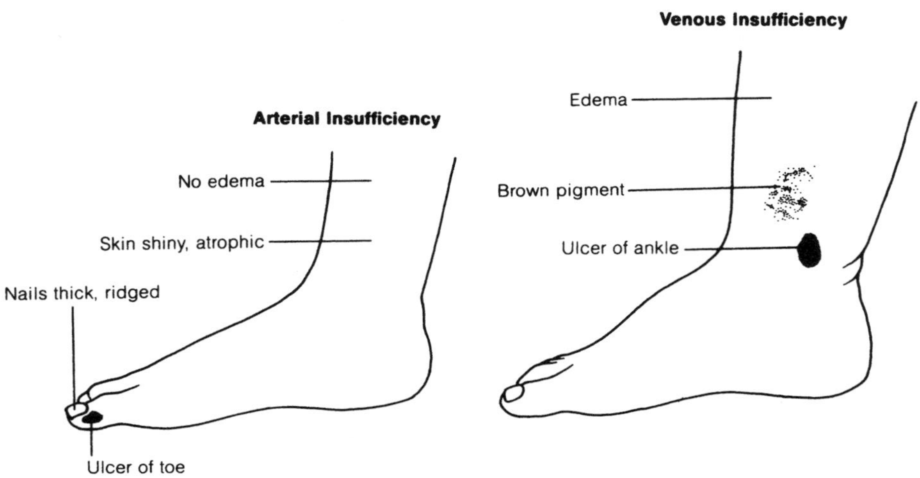

Figure 12-9. Comparison of arterial and venous insufficiency of lower extremities.

II. Objective Data: Assessment Techniques *(continued)*

Procedure	Normal Findings	Deviations from Normal
E. Auscultation of arteries. If arterial insufficiency is found in legs, auscultate over the following areas:		
Aorta	No sound	Bruits
Renal arteries	No sound	Bruits
Iliac artery	No sound	Bruits
Femoral artery (Fig. 12-10)	No sound	Bruits

Geriatric Variations

- Inspect for rigid, tortuous veins and arteries (decreased venous return and competency).
- Auscultate for increased systolic and diastolic blood pressure.

Possible Related Collaborative Problems

Potential complications

Hypertension
Thrombophlebitis
Arterial insufficiency
Peripheral neuropathy
Thrombosis/emboli
Venous insufficiency

Edema
Gangrene
Vasospasms
Claudication
Stasis ulcers

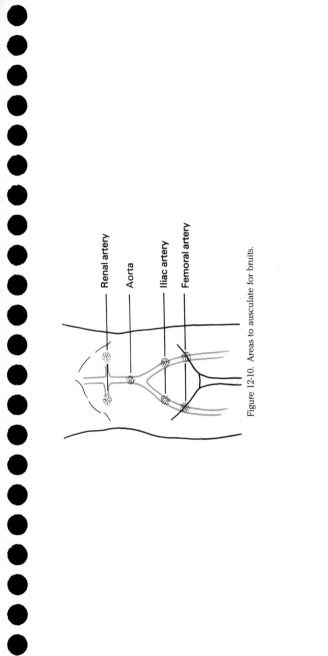

Figure 12-10. Areas to ausculate for bruits.

Nursing Diagnosis/Collaborative Problems	***Teaching Tips***
Adult Client	
NURSING DIAGNOSIS: Impaired Skin Integrity related to arterial insufficiency	Instruct client on importance of exercise and diet (eat foods high in protein, vitamins C and A, and zinc to promote healing) to aid healing of leg ulcers. Explain the importance of keeping area clean and dry.
NURSING DIAGNOSIS: Impaired Skin Integrity related to venous insufficiency	Instruct client on the importance of rest, avoidance of restrictive clothing, elevation of extremities to reduce edema, and proper diet to aid healing of leg ulcers.
NURSING DIAGNOSIS: Risk for Peripheral Neurovascular Dysfunction	Teach client how to assess condition of extremities (color, temperature, sensation, movement, swelling). Teach client how to modify activities of daily living in order to prevent injury and complications.
COLLABORATIVE PROBLEM: Potential complication: Hypertension	Explain the effects of diet (low fat and low cholesterol), reduction of stress, vigorous exercise, no smoking, and decreased use of alcohol on promotion of adequate circulation. Blood pressure checks should be done on a regular basis. Refer any client with a reading above 140/90.

CHAPTER 13

Breast Assessment

Equipment Needed

- Centimeter ruler
- Lubricant
- Small pillow

I. Subjective Data: Focus Questions

Tenderness? Pain? Swelling or change in size of breasts? Change in position of nipple or nipple discharge? Cysts? Lumps? Lesions? Breast self-examination (frequency and time performed)? Prior breast surgeries?

II. Objective Data: Assessment Techniques

Procedure	Normal Findings	Deviations from Normal

Inspection

The breast should be inspected with client in sitting position with arms at sides, with arms overhead, hands pressed on hips, and arms extended straight ahead as patient leans forward (Fig. 13-1). The areola and nipples should also be inspected.

A. Observe breasts for the following:

Procedure	Normal Findings	Deviations from Normal
Size and symmetry	Relatively equal with slight variation	Recent change to unequal size
Shape	Round and pendulous	
Color	Pink; striae with age and pregnancy	Redness; inflammation; blue hue; increased venous engorgement
Skin surface	Smooth	Retraction, dimpling, enlarged pores, "peau d'orange," edema, lumps, lesions, rashes, ulcers

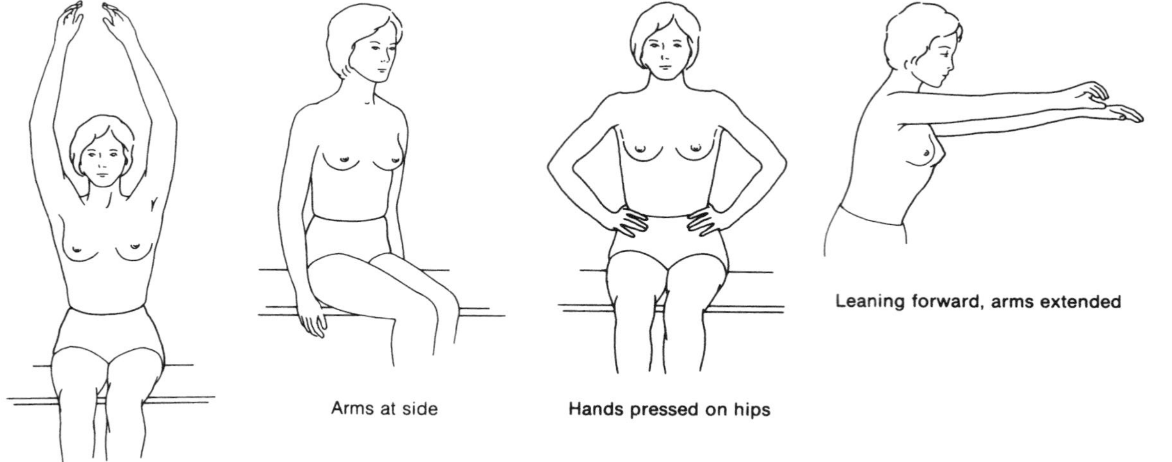

Figure 13-1. Positions for the client during breast inspection by the nurse.

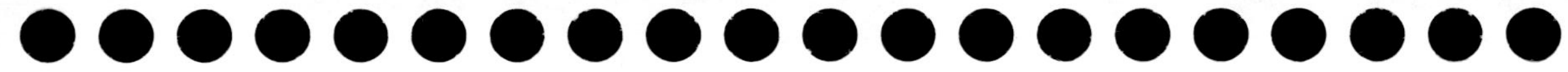

II. Objective Data: Assessment Techniques *(continued)*

Procedure	*Normal Findings*	*Deviations from Normal*
B. Observe areola and nipples for the following:		
Size	Relatively the same, slight variation	Large variation
Color	Pink to dark brown (varies with skin and hair color)	Inflamed
Shape	Round, oval, and everted	Inversion, if it occurs after maturation or changes with movement
Discharge	None; clear yellow 2 days after childbirth	Foul, purulent, sanguineous drainage
Texture	Small Montgomery tubercles present	Lesions, rashes, ulcers

Procedure	Normal Findings	Deviations from Normal

Palpation

Use the flat pads of three fingers to compress tissue against breast wall gently. Palpate with patient sitting. Then have patient lie down and place arm of side being examined over head with small pillow under upper back (Fig. 13-2). Palpate in circular motion starting at 12 o'clock and moving in concentric rings inward to areola and nipple (Fig. 13-3). Bimanual palpation may be used in large-breasted clients. A vertical or wedge pattern may be used if preferred (Fig. 13-3).

A. Palpate breasts for the following:

Procedure	Normal Findings	Deviations from Normal
Temperature	Warm	Erythema
Elasticity	Elastic	Lumpy
Tenderness	Nontender, slightly tender	Painful
Masses (note size, shape, mobility, consistency, and location—see landmarks below)	Bilateral firm inframammary transverse ridge at base of breasts	Masses or nodules present

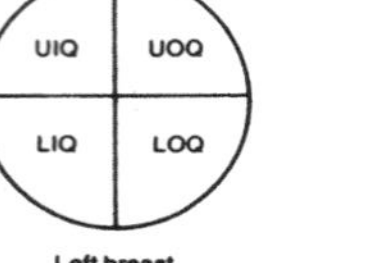

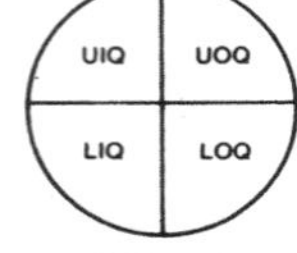

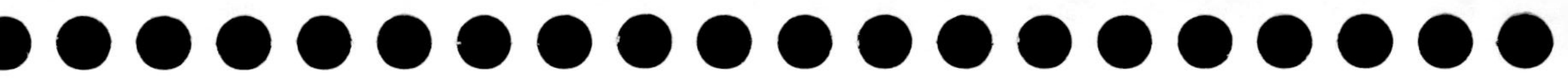

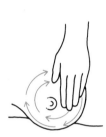

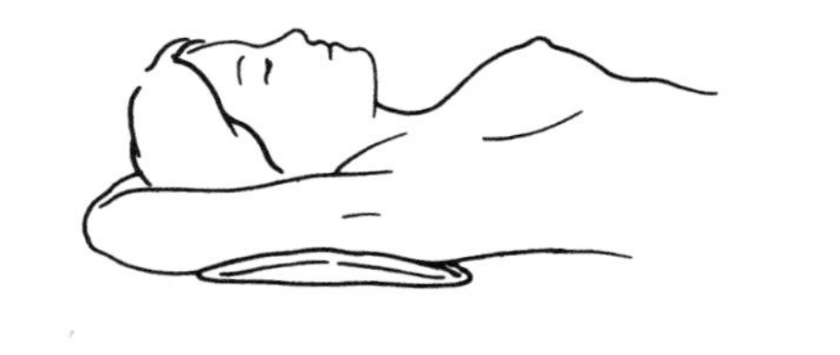

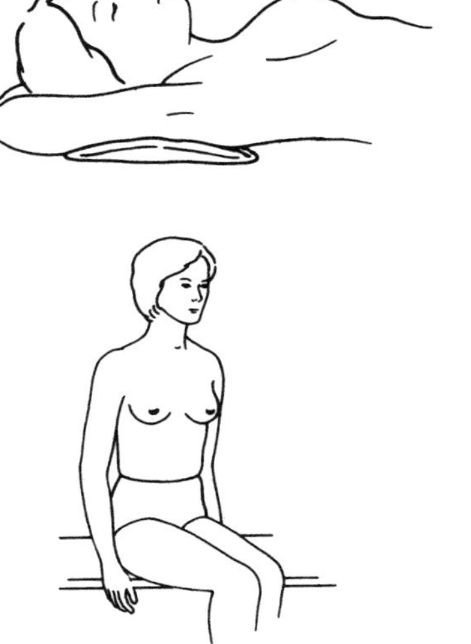

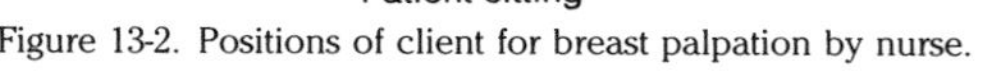
Figure 13-2. Positions of client for breast palpation by nurse.

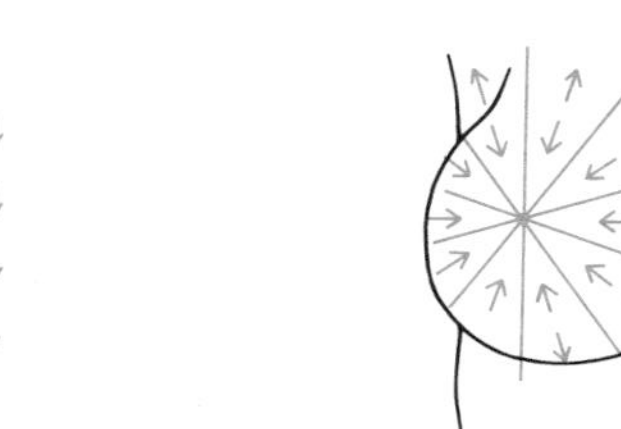

Figure 13-3. Patterns for breast palpation. Arrows indicate direction and areas for palpation.

II. Objective Data: Assessment Techniques *(continued)*

Procedure	*Normal Findings*	*Deviations from Normal*
B. Palpate nipple for discharge	None; clear yellow 2 days after childbirth	Discharge: unilateral serous, serosanguineous, clear, yellow, dark red
C. Palpate lymph nodes in the following areas: supraclavicular, subclavian, intermediate, brachial, scapular, mammary, internal mammary (Fig. 13-4).	None palpable	Palpable lymph nodes

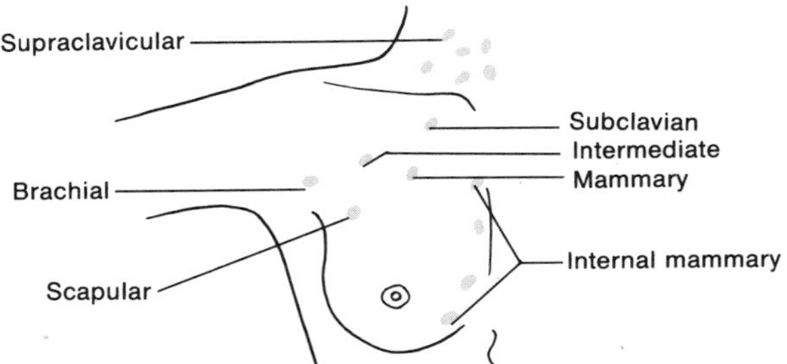

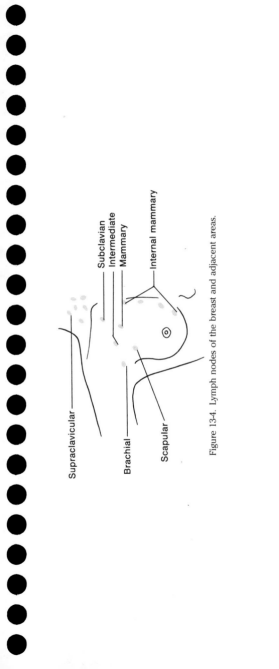

Figure 13-4. Lymph nodes of the breast and adjacent areas.

Variation for Men

Inspect and palpate breast with client seated, arms at sides. Palpate lymph nodes.

Pediatric Variations

Objective Data: Focus Questions

Asymmetrical growth? Girls prior to puberty: Pain or discomfort? Boys during adolescence: Abnormal increase in size? (See normal breast development in Chap. 15, Table 15-1; varies with age of child.)

Geriatric Variations

- Breasts less firm, pendulous, atrophied
- Coarser and more nodular tissue

Possible Related Collaborative Problems

Potential complications:
Infection (abscess)
Hematoma
Fibrocystic disease

Teaching Tips for Selected Nursing Diagnosis

Nursing Diagnosis	Teaching Tips
NURSING DIAGNOSIS: Ineffective Management of Therapeutic Regimen related to knowledge deficit of breast self-examination	Assess when and how client examines breasts. Instruct on correct technique and timing. (Breasts should be examined at the same time each month. If client has regular menstrual cycle, she should do examination right after menstruation when breasts are not swollen or tender.) Reinforce the following American Cancer Society recommendations: • Monthly breast self-examination for women age 20 years or older. • Breast clinical examination for women age 20–40 every 3 years and every year for women over 40 years. • Screening Mammography by age 40 and every 1–2 years age 40 to 49, and every year age 50 and over. Advise that cancer of the breast can be treated and often cured if detected early. (American Cancer Society, Cancer Facts and Figures, © 1996, p. 23)

CHAPTER 14

Abdominal Assessment

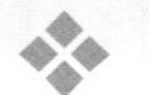

Equipment Needed

- Stethoscope (warm)
- Small ruler
- Marking pencil
- Small pillows
- Examiner should warm hands and have short fingernails

I. Subjective Data: Focus Questions

Nutritional history: Appetite, weight loss/gain? GI symptoms: dysphagia, nausea, vomiting, indigestion? Bowel habits: pattern, stool characteristics? Pain: Location, quality, pattern, relationship to ingestion of foods? Use of medications: aspirin, anti-inflammatory drugs, steroids? GI diagnostic tests? Surgeries?

II. Objective Data: Assessment Techniques

General Guidelines

The techniques used in assessment of the abdomen differ, in that inspection and auscultation precede percussion and palpation. This sequence allows accurate assessment of bowel sounds, and delays more uncomfortable maneuvers until last. The client is placed in the supine position, with small pillows under the head and knees. The abdomen is exposed from the breasts to the symphysis pubis.

Stand at the client's right side and carry out assessment systematically, beginning with the left upper quadrant (LUQ) and progressing clockwise through the four abdominal quadrants (Fig. 14-1). The bladder should be empty.

Procedure	***Normal Findings***	***Deviations from Normal***
Inspection		
A. Observe the skin for the following:		
Color	Normally paler, with white striae	Discolorations, red purple striae
Venous pattern	Fine veins observable	Engorged, prominent veins
Integrity	No rashes or lesions	Rashes, lesions
B. Special maneuver for prominent abdominal veins: Compress a section of vein with two fingers next to each other. Remove one finger and observe for filling. Repeat procedure, removing other finger.	Blood fills from above to lower abdomen.	Blood fills from lower to upper abdomen (obstructed inferior vena cava).

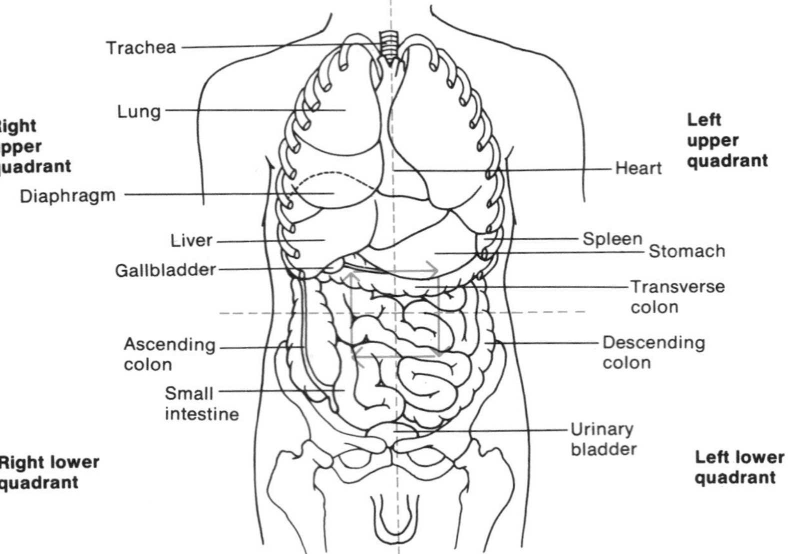

Figure 14-1. Anatomy of the abdomen: Anterior.

II. Objective Data: Assessment Techniques *(continued)*

Procedure	***Normal Findings***	***Deviations from Normal***
C. Observe the umbilicus for the following:		
Position	Sunken, centrally located	Abnormal placement, protrusion
Color	Pinkish	Inflamed, crusted; bluish color (Cullen's sign see in intraabdominal hemorrhage)
D. Observe the abdomen for the following:		
Contour	Rounded	Distended, scaphoid (sunken)
Symmetry	Symmetrical	Asymmetrical
Surface motion	No movement or slight peristalsis visualized over aorta	Bounding peristalsis, bounding pulsations
E. Observe color of stools	Brown to dark brown	Black, soft, tarry (melena); bright red
F. Observe color of emesis	Varies	Bloody (hematemesis)

II. Objective Data: Assessment Techniques *(continued)*

Procedure	***Normal Findings***	***Deviations from Normal***
Auscultation		
Using a warm stethoscope, auscultate for bowel sounds for up to 5 minutes in each quadrant, using the diaphragm and light pressure. Use the bell to auscultate vascular sounds.		
A. Auscultate for bowel sounds	High-pitched, irregular gurgles 5 to 35 times/min; present equally in all four quadrants	Absent, hyperactive (borborygmus); not present equally in each quadrant
B. Auscultate for vascular sounds	No bruits, no venous hums, no friction rubs	Bruits heard over aorta, renal arteries, or iliac arteries; venous hum auscultated over liver, spleen
Caution: If bruits are heard, do *not* palpate abdomen as part of the assessment. (Bruits may be indicative of a narrowed vessel or aneurysm.)		
Percussion		
Percussion notes will vary from dull to tympanic, with tympany dominating over the hollow organs. The hollow organs include the stomach, intestines, bladder, aorta, and gallbladder. Dull percussion notes will be heard over the liver, spleen, pancreas, kidneys, and uterus. Percuss from areas of tympany to dull to locate borders of these solid organs.		
A. Percuss all four quadrants for percussion tones (notes).	Generalized tympany over bowels	Increased dullness over enlarged organs
B. Percuss the liver for span (Fig. 14-2) as follows:	Liver span is 6–12 cm (2.5–5 inches) in the right MCL. *Note:* Span is greater in men.	Liver span is greater than 12 cm in the right MCL.

1. Percuss from below umbilicus at client's right midclavicular line (MCL), and percuss upward until you hear dullness. Mark this point.		
2. Percuss downward from lung resonance in the right MCL to dullness and mark.		
3. Repeat in midsternal line.	Liver span is 4–8 cm in midsternal line.	Liver span is greater than 8 cm in right midsternal line.
C. Percuss the spleen (Fig. 14-3) as follows:		
1. Percuss for dullness by percussing downward in left posterior axillary line, beginning with lung resonance until you hear splenic dullness.	Small area of dullness at sixth to tenth ribs	Dullness extends above sixth rib or covers larger area.
2. Splenic percussion sign: Ask client to inhale deeply and hold breath. Percuss lowest interspaces at left anterior axillary line.	Percussion note remains tympanic on inhalation.	Percussion note becomes dull on inhalation.

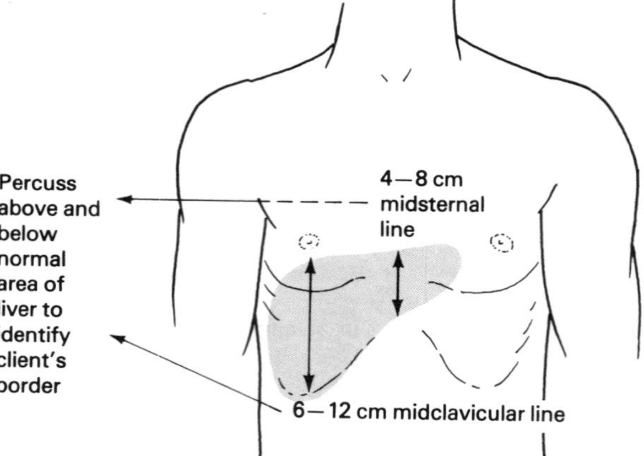

Figure 14-2. Normal liver span.

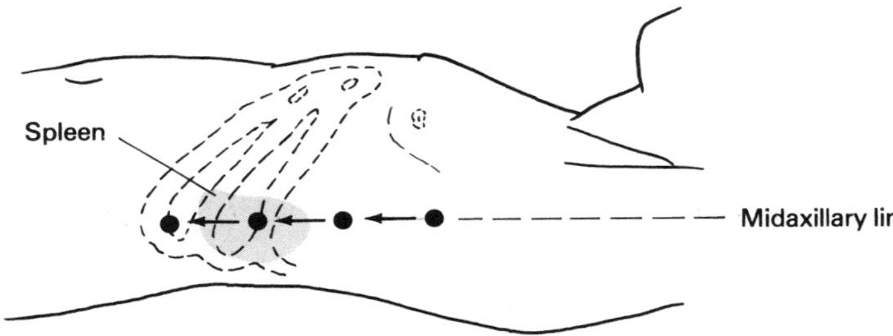

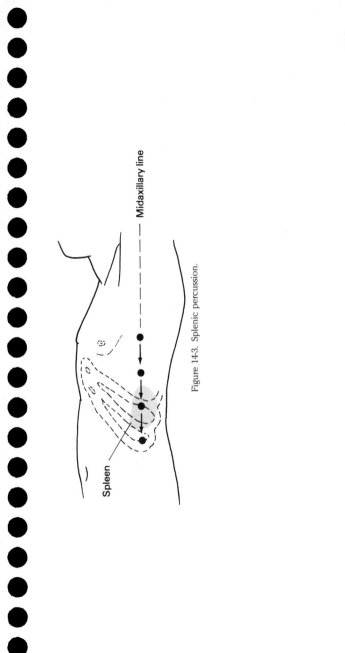

Figure 14-3. Splenic percussion.

Procedure	*Normal Findings*	*Deviations from Normal*
Palpation Light palpation precedes deep palpation to detect tenderness and superficial masses. Deep palpation is used to detect masses and size of organs. Watch the client's facial expressions and body posture carefully to help assess pain. Examine tender areas last. Never use deep palpation over tender organs in client with polycystic kidneys, after renal transplant, or after hearing an abnormal bruit. Use deep palpation with caution.		
A. Lightly palpate all four quadrants for the following:		
Tenderness	Nontender	Tender, painful
Guarding	Soft, nontender	Rigid, boardlike
Masses	No masses	Superficial masses (A superficial mass becomes more prominent against examiner's hand when client lifts head from examination table, whereas a deep abdominal mass does not.)
B. Palpate deeply in all four quadrants for the following:		
Tenderness	Mild tenderness over midline at xiphoid, cecum, sigmoid colon	Tenderness, severe pain

Guarding	Voluntary guarding	Involuntary guarding
Masses	No masses; aorta; feces in colon	Masses
C. Palpate deeply for liver border at right costal margin (Fig. 14-4) for the following:		
Tenderness	Nontender	Tenderness
Consistency	Smooth, firm sharp edge, no masses	Very enlarged lobe, irregular nodules, lobes
D. Palpate deeply for splenic border, using bimanual technique (Fig. 14-5). Check for the following:		
Size	Not normally palpable	Enlarged and palpable
Tenderness	Nontender	Tender
E. Palpate deeply for the kidneys by using bimanual technique (Fig. 14-6). Assess for the following:		
Size	Not normally palpable	Enlarged and palpable
Tenderness	Nontender	Tender
Masses	No masses	Masses

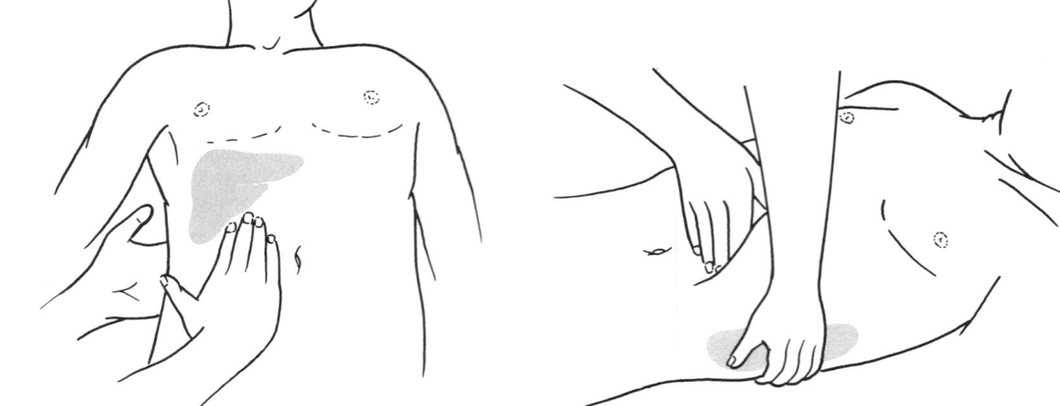

Guidelines for Liver Palpation

1. Stand at client's right side and place your left hand under clients back at the 11th and 12th ribs.
2. Place right hand parallel to right costal margin.
3. Ask client to breathe deeply, and press upward with your right fingers with each inhalation.

Figure 14-4. Guidelines for liver palpation.

Guidelines for Spleen Palpation

1. Stand at client's right side; reach across client to place your left hand under client's posterior lower ribs, and push up.
2. Place your right hand below rib margin.
3. Ask client to breathe deeply.
4. Press hands together to palpate spleen on inhalation.

Figure 14-5. Guidelines for spleen palpation.

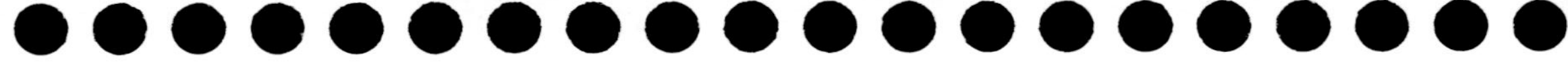

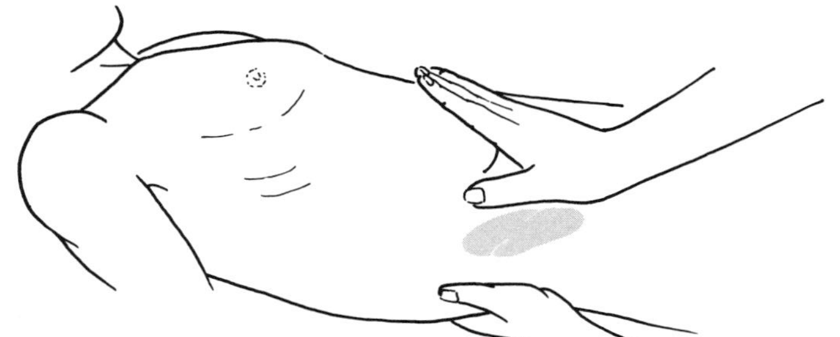

Guidelines for Kidney Palpation

1. Place one of your hands behind lower edge of rib cage and above iliac crest.
2. Place the other hand over corresponding anterior surface.
3. Instruct client to breathe deeply.
4. Lift up lower hand and push in with upper hand as client exhales.
5. Repeat on other side.

(*Note*: The kidneys are rarely palpable.)

Figure 14-6. Kidney palpation.

Procedure	***Normal Findings***	***Deviations from Normal***
F. Special maneuvers for ascites		
1. Measure abdominal girth at same point every day.	No increase in abdominal girth	Increase in abdominal girth
2. Fluid wave test: Place palmar surfaces of fingers and hand firmly on one side of abdomen. Tap with other hand on opposite abdominal wall side. Have assistant put lateral side of lower arm firmly on center of abdomen (Fig. 14-7).	No fluid wave transmitted	Fluid wave palpated
3. Shifting dullness: Place client in supine position and percuss from midline to flank, noting level of dullness. Then assist client to side position and percuss again for level of dullness.	Level of dullness does not change	Level of dullness is higher when client turns on side

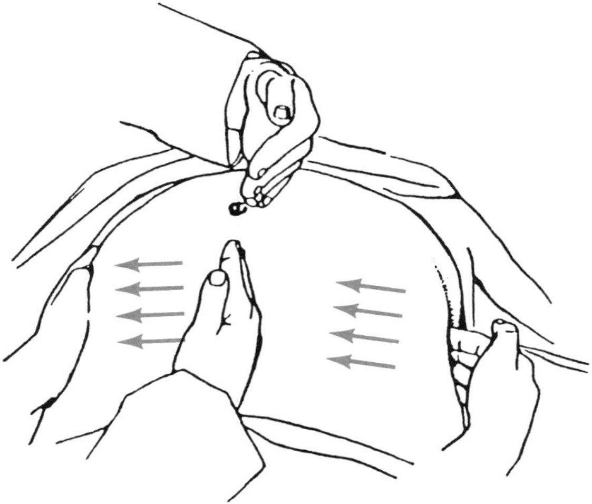

Figure 14-7. Test for ascites (fluid wave).

II. Objective Data: Assessment Techniques *(continued)*

Procedure	*Normal Findings*	*Deviations from Normal*
G. Special tests for appendicitis		
1. Rebound tenderness: Palpate deeply in one of client's four abdominal quadrants, and quickly withdraw palpating hand. Do this at end of abdominal exam.	No pain present	Pain present (Do not repeat if pain is present because of danger of rupture)
2. Psoas sign: Ask client to lie supine and raise right leg. Place pressure on client's thigh.	No abdominal pain present	Right lower abdominal pain present
3. Obturator sign: Ask client to flex right leg at hip and knee. Then rotate leg internally and externally.	No abdominal pain present	Lower abdominal pain present
H. Special tests for acute cholecystitis (Murphy's sign): Examiner places thumb below right costal margin and asks patient to inhale deeply.	Client has no increase in pain	Client has sharp increase in pain
I. Testing for asterixes (classic sign of hepatic coma): Dorsiflex client's wrist with fingers extended.	No tremor noted	Persistent involuntary flapping tremor

Pediatric Variations

I. Subjective Data: Focus Questions

Types of food, fluids, and formula? Ability to feed self? History of pica?

II. Objective Data: Assessment Techniques

Procedure	Normal Variations
Inspection	
A. Inspect contour and size of abdomen.	Prominent/cylindrical (potbelly) when erect, flat when supine. Superficial veins may be present in infants.
B. Inspect abdominal movement in children under 8 years.	Rises with inspiration in synchrony with chest; may have visible pulsations in epigastric region
Palpation	
A. Palpate liver border.	Normal, shortened liver span on percussion. May not extend below costal margin. *Infants and young children:* Liver may be felt 1–3 cm below costal margin; may descend with inspiration.
B. Palpate splenic border (may have child roll on right side).	*Infants and young children:* Spleen may be felt 1–3 cm below costal margin.
C. Palpate for abdominal tenderness.	Extremely difficult to assess in young children, who may confuse pressure of palpation with pain. Distraction is important.
D. Palpate kidney borders.	Difficult to locate except in newborns

Geriatric Variations

- Abdomen softer and organs more easily palpated due to a decrease in tone of abdominal musculature.
- Decreased production of saliva, decreased peristalsis, decreased enzymes, weaker gastric acid.
- Gastric mucosa and parietal cell degeneration results in a loss of intrinsic factor, which decreases absorption of vitamin B_{12}.
- Shortened liver span on percussion due to a decrease in liver size after age 50 years.
- Liver border more easily palpated.
- Decreased nerve sensation to lower bowel contributes to constipation.

Possible Related Collaborative Problems

Potential complications

Hemorrhage
Bowel strangulation
Ascites
Metabolic acidosis/alkalosis
GI bleeding
Gastric ulcers
Intestinal obstruction
Paralytic ileus
Diverticulitis
Hepatic failure
Evisceration

Teaching Tips for Selected Nursing Diagnoses

Nursing Diagnoses	*Teaching Tips*
Adult Client NURSING DIAGNOSIS: Altered Nutrition: More or less than body requirements	Discuss essential components of a well-balanced diet in relation to client's level of physical development and energy expenditure (basal metabolic rate). Teach client how to keep a daily food diary in order to assess intake. Discuss with client the following: • Decreasing calories • Increasing carbohydrates (whole grains and vegetables) • Decreasing saturated fats • Decreasing refined sugars • Decreasing cholesterol to 300 mg/day and salt to 5 g/day Provide information on support groups such as Weight Watchers, T.O.P.S. (Take Off Pounds Sensibly).
NURSING DIAGNOSIS: Constipation	Discuss bowel habits that are "normal for client." Caution against the overuse of laxatives. Discourage overuse of mineral oil as a laxative because it decreases absorption of vitamins A, D, E, and K. Explain the effects of nutrients, bulk, fluids, and exercise on elimination. The American Cancer Society (1996) recommends a high-fiber, low-fat diet that includes a variety of vegetables and fruits to reduce the risk of certain cancers. It is also recommended to limit consumption of salt-cured, smoked, and nitrite-cured foods, and to limit consumption of alcohol. Eat a varied diet and maintain a desirable weight.

Nursing Diagnoses	***Teaching Tips***
Pediatric Client NURSING DIAGNOSIS: Opportunity to enhance nutritional metabolic pattern of child	Teach parents nutritional needs of the child at various ages: *Infant:* Formula/breast feed first 6 months. Introduce one cereal at a time at 6 months. Introduce finger foods by 1 year. The American Academy of Pediatrics recommends that formula be fortified with iron. Breast-fed infants should get oral iron supplements. Fluoride supplements are also important. *Toddlers:* Food fads are common. Accept this as long as child gets balanced diet over period of days versus every day.
NURSING DIAGNOSIS: Fluid Volume Deficit related to vomiting or diarrhea	Teach parents to give child small amounts of clear liquids (approximately 1 ounce every hour for 8 hours) until symptoms subside. May recommend Pedialyte or Lytrem for fluid and electrolyte replacement.
NURSING DIAGNOSIS: Risk for Aspiration related to improper feeding and small size of stomach in newborns	Explain size of infant's stomach to parents (holds 60 cc), and demonstrate proper burping technique to use after every -ounce feeding.

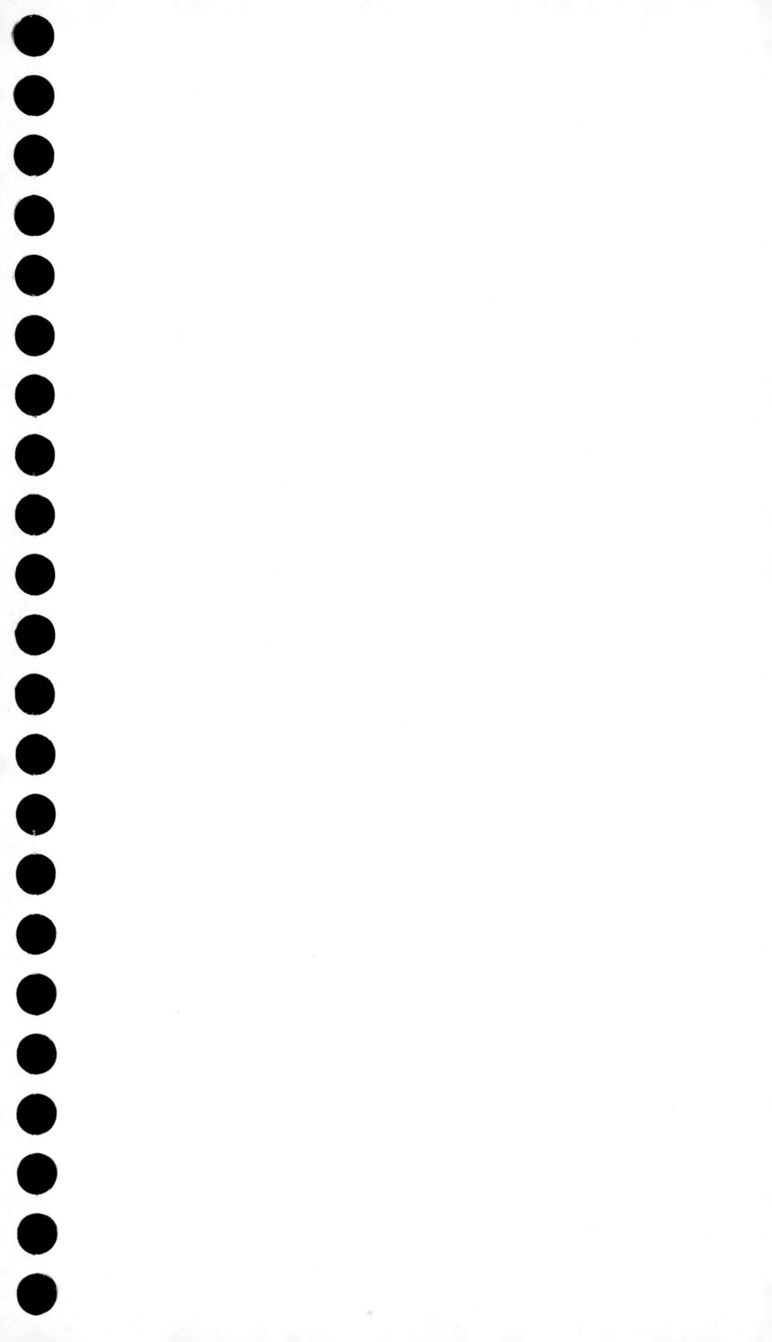

CHAPTER 15

Genitourinary–Reproductive Assessment

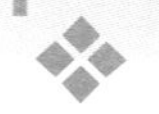

Assessment of Inguinal Area

Equipment Needed

- Gloves
- Private location

I. Subjective Data: Focus Questions

Any bulges or pain when straining or lifting heavy objects? Unusual drainage? Pain with urinating? Lower abdominal pain? Incontinence?

II. Objective Data: Assessment Techniques

Procedure	***Normal Findings***	***Deviations from Normal***
Inspection		
Have client stand so inguinal area is visible. Have client strain down.		
A. Inspect inguinal area	Smooth, symmetrical	Bulging on one or both sides that increases with straining
B. Inspect scrotum/labia	Symmetrical	Enlargement of scrotum/labia
Palpation		
Palpate inguinal area. Then have client strain down as you palpate inguinal area and scrotum/labia. Palpate for the following:		
Lymph nodes	Nonpalpable	Palpable, tender
Masses	Smooth, no masses	Bulge of soft tissue that increases with straining; may disappear when gently pushed in
Scrotum/labia	No change	Enlargement; mass felt increases with straining

Assessment of External Rectal Area

Nurses do not usually repeat the internal rectal examination that is done as a part of the medical examination unless there is a specific reason to do so, because it is uncomfortable and embarrassing for the client. For detailed information on technique, please see another source.

Equipment Needed

- Examination gloves
- Drape
- Pillow

I. Subjective Data: Focus Questions

Frequent loose stools? Constipation? Pain? Itching? Bleeding after stools?

II. Objective Data: Assessment Techniques

Procedure	***Normal Findings***	***Deviations from Normal***
Inspection Have client lie on left side with right leg flexed at hip and knee. Support leg on pillow if necessary. Provide a pillow for under the head. With one hand, gently separate buttocks so rectum is exposed.		
A. Inspect coccyx for the following:		
Hair	Normal distribution of body hair	Tufts or increase in body hair
Openings	None	Sinus tract

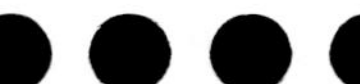

Color	Pink	Reddened
Drainage	None	Any drainage
B. Inspect rectum for the following:		
Color	Deep red	Shiny, blue
Mucosa	May have tags of skin; intact	Enlarged ovoid mass, hemorrhoids, prolapsed rectum rosette

Assessment of Female Genitalia

Equipment Needed

- Gown
- Drape
- Pillow
- Movable light source
- Gloves
- Lubricant

I. Subjective Data: Focus Questions

Pain or burning with intercourse or urination? Itching? Purulent or foul-smelling discharge? Amenorrhea or midcycle bleeding? Difficulty starting or stopping urinary stream? Stress incontinence?

II. Objective Data: Assessment Techniques

Procedure	*Normal Findings*	*Deviations from Normal*
Inspection Have client empty bladder and lie on her back with her head slightly elevated on a pillow. Knees should be bent and separated with feet resting on the bed. Light should be adjusted to provide good visualization of the genitalia (Fig. 15-1).		
A. Observe labia for the following:		
Size	Symmetrical	Swelling unequal
Skin texture	Smooth, lose skin	Vesicles, warts, open sores
Color	Pink	Blue, visible veins, shiny
Note: Using an examination glove, insert thumb and index finger between labia and separate.		
B. Observe urinary meatus for the following:		
Position	Anterior to vaginal orifice and in midline	Urinary meatus not visible; located within or near anterior surface of vaginal wall
Color	Pink	Red, inflamed

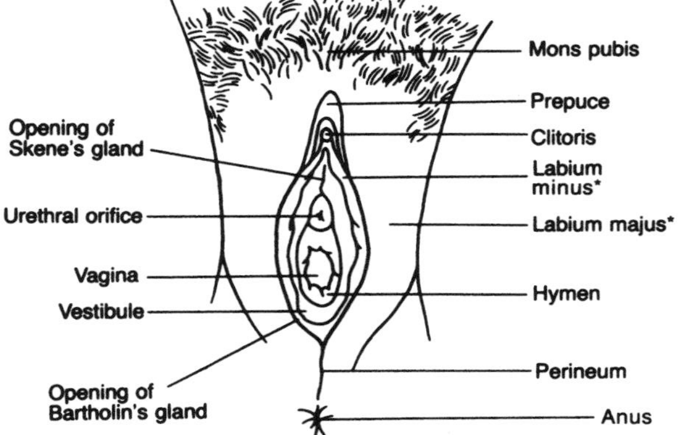

Figure 15-1. Female genitalia.

Procedure	*Normal Findings*	*Deviations from Normal*
C. Observe vaginal orifice for the following:		
Hymen	Absent; thin, elastic membrane that partially occludes orifice	Completely occludes orifice; thick
Discharge	Clear, milky, serosanguineous with menstrual cycle	Purulent, bloody, foul smelling
Note: Have client strain down.		
D. Observe vaginal wall for bulging	Slight movement	Bulging of anterior or posterior vaginal wall

Palpation

Don gloves. Using left thumb and index finger, gently separate labia and hold apart. Lubricate right index finger and insert into vaginal opening. Push up on anterior wall and "milk" toward opening. Push down on posterior wall and grasp tissue between thumb and index finger. Palpate tissue along entire lower half of vaginal orifice.

Procedure	*Normal Findings*	*Deviations from Normal*
A. Observe Skene's gland (see Fig. 15-1) for the following:		
Openings	Not visible	Visible openings
Discharge	None	Exudate from openings or urethra

B. Palpate posterior vaginal orifice for the following:

Swelling	None	Present
Lumps or nodules	Smooth, soft tissue	Hard, nonpliable tissue

Assessment of Male Genitalia

Equipment Needed

- Examination gloves

I. Subjective Data: Focus Questions

Pain? Tenderness? Discharge? Difficulty starting or stopping urinary stream? Rash? Lesions?

II. Objective Data: Assessment Techniques

Procedure	***Normal Findings***	***Deviations from Normal***
Inspection		
The male genitalia should be inspected with the client in a standing position. Privacy should be assured.		
A. Observe penis for the following:		
Urinary meatus	Located at tip of penis	Located on ventral or dorsal side of penis
Discharge	No discharge	Any drainage
Skin texture	Wrinkled	Nodules, growths, lesions
B. Observe scrotum for the following:		
Size	Left side lower than right	Unilateral or bilateral enlargement
Color	Pink or normal skin color	Red, shiny, bruised
Texture	Many skin folds	Lesions, ulcers, taut skin

Palpation

With client standing, gently palpate shaft of penis between gloved thumb and fingers. If foreskin is present, retract from tip of penis, then replace. Grasp each testicle between thumb and fingers. Gently roll testicle so all surfaces are palpated. Client may do self-examination with instructions and report findings (Fig. 15-2).

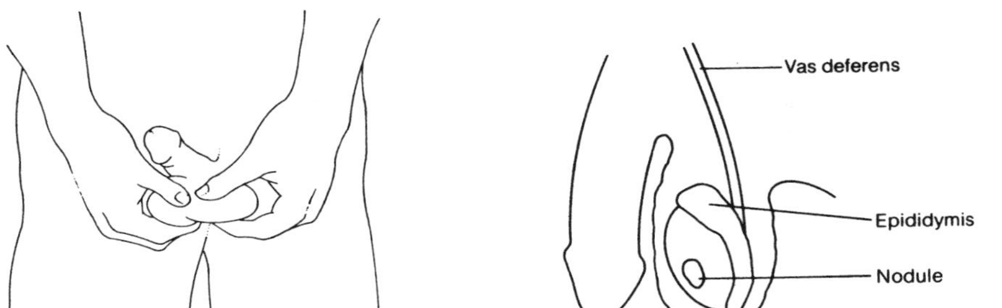

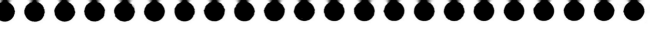

Figure 15-2. Testicular self-examination. Instruct client to gently roll each testicle between thumb and fingers of both hands, feeling for lumps or nodules.

II. Objective Data: Assessment Techniques *(continued)*

Procedure	*Normal Findings*	*Deviations from Normal*
A. Palpate penis for the following:		
Masses	None	Nodules, masses, or lesions anywhere on shaft or end
Tenderness	Slightly tender	Very tender or painful
Discharge	None	Clear or purulent from lesions or urinary meatus
Foreskin	May not be present; should retract and return easily with clean, smooth skin underneath	Unable to retract owing to phimosis or adherence to underlying tissue; any drainage or sores under skin
B. Palpate each testis for the following:		
Location	Both should be entirely in sac, left slightly lower than right.	One or both are absent or cannot be palpated above (partially descended).
Shape	Oval, symmetrical	Enlarged, different sizes
Texture	Smooth, firm	Grainy or coarse, lumps or nodules
Tenderness	Very tender	Pain; dull ache in lower abdomen or groin with feeling of heaviness

Pediatric Variations

I. Subjective Data: Focus Questions

During puberty: Development of secondary sexual characteristics? Previous education on sexual development and activities? Use of contraceptives? Type?

Females: Age of menarche? Frequency of menstrual periods? Amount of flow? Pain? Irregularities? Attitude toward menstrual cycle?

II. Objective Data: Assessment Techniques

Inspection and palpation of external male and female genitalia constitute the *total* genitourinary assessment until puberty. Assessment of the level of sexual development of girls and boys usually begins at approximately age 11 years. This determination involves assessment of secondary characteristics associated with sexual maturity. Tables 15-1 and 15-2 summarize the timing of sexual development for males and females.

Cultural Variations

Male and female genitalia are mutilated in pubertal rites in some cultures; for example, circumcision, removal of clitoris, or surgical incision along penile shaft and into its base for passage of urine and semen. Female pubic hair is shaved or plucked in some cultures.

Table 15-1. Classification of Sex Maturity Stages in Girls

Stage	*Pubic Hair*	*Breasts*
1	None	Elevation of papilla only
2	Sparse growth, long, slightly pigmented downy hair along the labia	Breast bud: elevation of breast and papilla as small mound; areolar diameter increased
3	Increased amount, darker and coarser; spread over junction of pubes	Enlargement of breast and areola; no contour separation
4	Resembles adult type, but less area covered	Separation of contour; areola and papilla form secondary mound
5	Adult quality and distribution	Mature breast contour. Projection of papilla only

(Adapted from Tanner JM: Growth at adolescence, 2nd ed. Oxford, Blackwell Scientific Publications, 1962; Daniel WA Jr: Growth of adolescence. Seminars in Adolescent Medicine, 1 (1), 15–24.)

Table 15-2. Classification of Genitalia Maturity Stages in Boys

Stage	*Pubic Hair*	*Penis*	*Testes*
1	None	Preadolescent	Preadolescent
2	Sparse growth, long, slightly pigmented	Slight enlargement	Scrotal reddening; coarse texture
3	Darker, more curled, small amount	Longer	Further increase
4	Resembles adult type, but less in quantity, no spread to medial thigh	Increase in width	Larger, scrotum dark
5	Adult quality and distribution	Adult size	Adult size

(Adapted from Tanner JM: Growth at Adolescence, 2nd ed. Oxford, Blackwell Scientific Publication, 1962; Daniel WA Jr: Growth of adolescence. Seminars in Adolescent Medicine, 1 (1), 15–24.)

Geriatric Variations

- Bladder capacity decreases to 250 mL due to periurethral atrophy
- 1–2 periods nocturice

Female

- Decrease in size and elasticity of labia, constriction of vaginal opening
- Diminished vaginal secretions and decreased elasticity of vaginal walls
- Shortened and narrowed vaginal vault

Male

- Decrease in size and firmness of testicles
- Loss of tone in musculature of scrotum
- Slowed erections and less forceful ejaculations
- Enlargement of median lobe of prostate

Cultural Variations

Both male and female genitalia are mutilated in some cultures pubertal rites. These include female circumcision, or removal of the clitoris, and creating a surgical slit at the base of the penis for the passage of urine and semen. Female pubic hair is shaved or plucked in some cultures.

Possible Related Collaborative Problems

Potential complications:

Bladder perforation
Urinary tract infection
Pelvic inflammatory disease
Genitalia ulcers or lesions
Obstruction of urethra
Hemorrhage
Hormonal imbalances
Renal failure
Renal calculi
Hypermenorrhea
Polymenorrhea

Teaching Tips for Selected Nursing Diagnoses/Collaborative Problems

Nursing Diagnoses	***Teaching Tips***
Adult Client NURSING DIAGNOSIS: Opportunity to enhance urinary elimination and reproductive pattern	Teach client to drink 8 glasses of fluid per day and to limit intake of alcohol, caffeine, and carbonated beverages. Teach client to avoid bubble bath and scented tissue that may irritate urethra. Teach female client to wear cotton underwear and to wipe perineum from front to back when cleansing.
NURSING DIAGNOSIS: Opportunity to enhance health-seeking behaviors: testicular self-examination	Instruct client on proper method of testicular self-examination to be performed once a month after a warm bath or shower. Instruct client to gently roll each testicle between thumb and fingers of both hands, feeling for lumps or nodules (Fig. 15-2). Have client demonstrate. Begin this at puberty, because it is one of the most common cancers in men aged 15–34 years.
NURSING DIAGNOSIS: Risk for infection (sexually transmitted disease)	Teach early warning signs and symptoms. Discuss methods of prevention (limit to 1 uninfected partner and use of condoms) and modes of transmission.

Nursing Diagnoses	*Teaching Tips*
NURSING DIAGNOSIS: Risk for altered health maintenance management related to a lack of knowledge of birth control methods.	Teach alternate forms of birth control, proper use of methods, and advantages and disadvantages of each. Discuss the importance of increasing vitamin B_6 and folic acid in the diet because of malabsorption of these vitamins while taking birth control pills. Instruct on use of alternate birth control for 3 months after discontinuing the pill to reestablish menstrual cycle before attempting to conceive.
NURSING DIAGNOSIS: Opportunity to enhance health maintenance during menopause	Inform client that pregnancy may still occur during early menopausal years. Instruct to consume 1500 mg calcium/day along with a well-balanced diet. Explain that water-soluble lubricant may be used for vaginal dryness if intercourse is painful. Explain ways to help client cope with hot flashes (i.e., use of cool clothing, fans, showers, cool drinks; avoidance of red wine, aged cheeses, and chocolate—these contain tyramine, which can trigger hot flashes). Teach male clients about the male climacteric period (during the fifties or sixties) during which time sexual hormones are reduced. Symptoms of hot flashes, sweating, headaches, dizziness, and heart palpitations may be experienced.

NURSING DIAGNOSIS: Altered health maintenance related to knowledge deficit of need for colorectal and pelvic examinations and Pap smears	Explain procedure. Teach relaxation. Approach sexuality as a normal part of activities of daily living. Prepare adolescent girl for first pelvic examination. The American Cancer Society (1996) recommends that women who are or have been sexually active or are 18 years old should have an annual Pap test and pelvic examination. After a woman has had three or more consecutive satisfactory and normal annual examinations, the Pap test may be performed less frequently at the physician's discretion. Women at high risk for endometrial cancer (history of infertility, obesity, failure to ovulate, abnormal uterine bleeding, or unopposed estrogen or tamoxifen therapy) should have an endometrial tissue sample at menopause and thereafter at the physician's discretion (American Cancer Society, 1995, p. 24). *For both men and women without symptoms:* A digital rectal exam is recommended every year after age 40, and a stool blood test every year after age 50, in addition to a sigmoidoscopy examination preferably flexible, every 3 to 5 years after age 50. (American Cancer Society, 1996).
NURSING DIAGNOSIS: Sexual dysfunction: impotence related to unknown etiology	Explore possible etiologies and alternate forms of sexual satisfaction. Refer to urologist for information on penile implants, surgery, and other alternatives.
NURSING DIAGNOSIS: Sexual dysfunction related to ineffective individual coping pattern	Teach effects and benefits of exercise. Explore communication with partner. Refer to counselor (psychiatric, sexual, marriage) as needed. Provide adequate literature on sex and health teaching for client.

Teaching Tips for Selected Nursing Diagnoses/Collaborative Problems *(continued)*

Nursing Diagnoses	Teaching Tips
NURSING DIAGNOSIS: Sexual dysfunction related to loss of body part or physiological limitations (e.g., dyspareunia with aging)	Explore prior sexual patterns. Explore alternatives. Provide resource material on self-help groups (e.g., Ostomy Association, Reach for Recovery). Suggest use of foreplay and lubricants to increase secretions as necessary. Provide literature and referrals.
Pediatric Client NURSING DIAGNOSIS: Risk for altered elimination pattern related to parental knowledge deficit of toilet training techniques.	Teach parents the importance of physiological and psychological readiness in toilet training. Explain use of "potty chairs" and that bowel control precedes bladder control. Inform parents of the benefits of positive reinforcement and that noctural enuresis may persist up to age 4 to 5 years.
NURSING DIAGNOSIS: Opportunity to enhance sexual function.	Sexual education is recommended in the early school years. Assess what child already knows and what he or she is ready to know. *Fourth to fifth grade:* Interested in conception and birth. *Fifth to sixth grade:* Interested in their bodies and opposite sex changes. Education on birth control may be appropriate because of early experimentation. Discuss normal development of secondary sexual characteristics and the normal psychological changes associated with puberty.

Geriatric Client

NURSING DIAGNOSIS:	
Alteration in urinary elimination: Incontinence	Explain to family how to decrease environmental barriers (offer bedpan frequently, proper lighting, availability and proximity of commode) for functional incontinence. Teach client cutaneous triggering mechanisms for reflex incontinence. Teach client Kegel exercises to strengthen pelvic floor muscles (i.e., tightening of buttocks and practicing starting and stopping stream) for stress incontinence.
COLLABORATIVE PROBLEM:	
Potential complication: Prostate hypertrophy	Teach client about effects of normal enlargement of prostate on urination (frequency, dribbling and nocturia). Encourage yearly rectal exams and prostate-specific antigen on men 50 years and older.

CHAPTER 16

Musculoskeletal Assessment

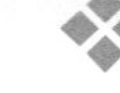

Equipment Needed

- Tape measure
- Goniometer

I. Subjective Data: Focus Questions

Pain: At rest? With exercise? Changes in shape or size of an extremity? Changes in ability to carry out activities of daily living, sports, work? Stiffness: Time of day, relation to weight-bearing/exercise? Decreased/altered/absent sensations? Redness or swelling of joints? History of fractures, orthopedic surgery? Occupational and recreational history?

II. Objective Data: Assessment Techniques

Inspection and palpation are performed while the client is standing, sitting, and supine. Range of motion (ROM) can be measured by degrees, using approximation or a goniometer. (Normal shoulder ROM is given as an example—Fig. 16-1). In assessing muscle weakness or swelling, size is compared bilaterally by measuring circumference with a tape measure. Joints should not be forced into painful positions. Muscle strength can be estimated using a muscle strength scale (Table 16-1).

Inspection: Observe for ROM, swelling, deformity, atrophy, condition of surrounding tissues, and pain.

Palpation: Palpate for heat, strength, tone, edema, crepitus, and nodules. (*Note:* Dominant side is normally stronger in muscle strength and tone.)

Procedure	Normal Findings	Deviations from Normal
Inspection of Gait and Stance		
Observe gait and stance as the client enters and walks around the room.		
A. Inspect the stance for the following:		
Base of support	Weight evenly distributed	Uneven base, with unequal weight bearing
Weight-bearing stability	Able to stand on right/left heels, toes	Weakness or inability to use either extremity
Posture	Erect	Stooped
B. Inspect the gait of the following:		
Position of feet	Toes point straight ahead	Toes point in or out
Posture	Erect	Stooped
Stride	Equal on both sides	Wide-based,propulsive, shuffling or limping

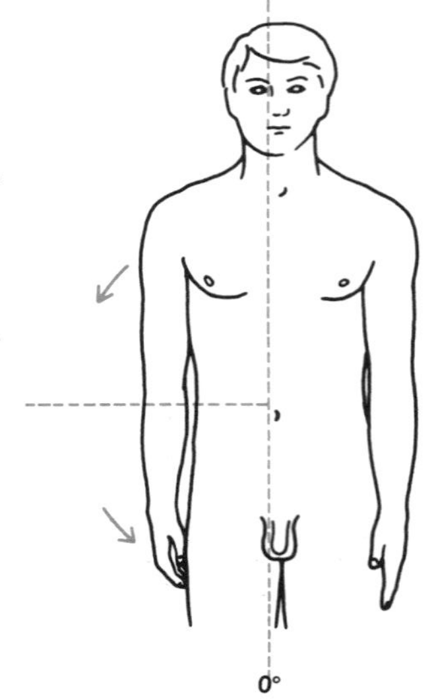

Figure 16-1. Normal shoulder range of motion, illustrating degrees.

Table 16-1. Scale for Muscle Strength

Scale	
0	No muscular contraction
1	Bare flicker of contraction
2	Active movement with gravity removed
3	Active movement against gravity
4	Active movement against gravity and some resistance
5	Active movement against full resistance with no fatigue; normal muscle strength

Normal strength ranges from 3 to 5.
(Adapted from Bates B: A Guide to Physical Examination and History Taking, 6th ed., p. 513. Philadelphia: JB Lippincott, 1995.)

II. Objective Data: Assessment Techniques *(continued)*

Procedure	Normal Findings	Deviations from Normal
Inspection and Palpation of the Spine, Shoulder, and Posterior Iliac Crest		
Inspection		
With client standing, observe in the erect position and as the client bends forward to touch toes. Stabilize client at the waist, and evaluate ROM of the upper trunk.		
Inspect the spine for the following:		
Curves	Cervical concave; thoracic convex; lumbar concave (Fig. 16-2)	Kyphosis, scoliosis, lordosis (Fig. 16-2)
Posture	Erect	Stooped
ROM: Flexion, lateral bending, rotation, extension (Fig. 16-3)	Full ROM	Limited ROM with pain or crepitation
Palpation		
With client in standing or sitting position, palpate the paravertebral muscles, using both moderate pressure and gentle sweeping motions. Ask client to shrug shoulders against resistance.		
A. Palpate the paravertebrals for the following:		
Muscle strength and tone	Equally strong	Weak, spasm
Temperature	Warm	Hot and swollen
Sensation	Nontender	Tender, painful

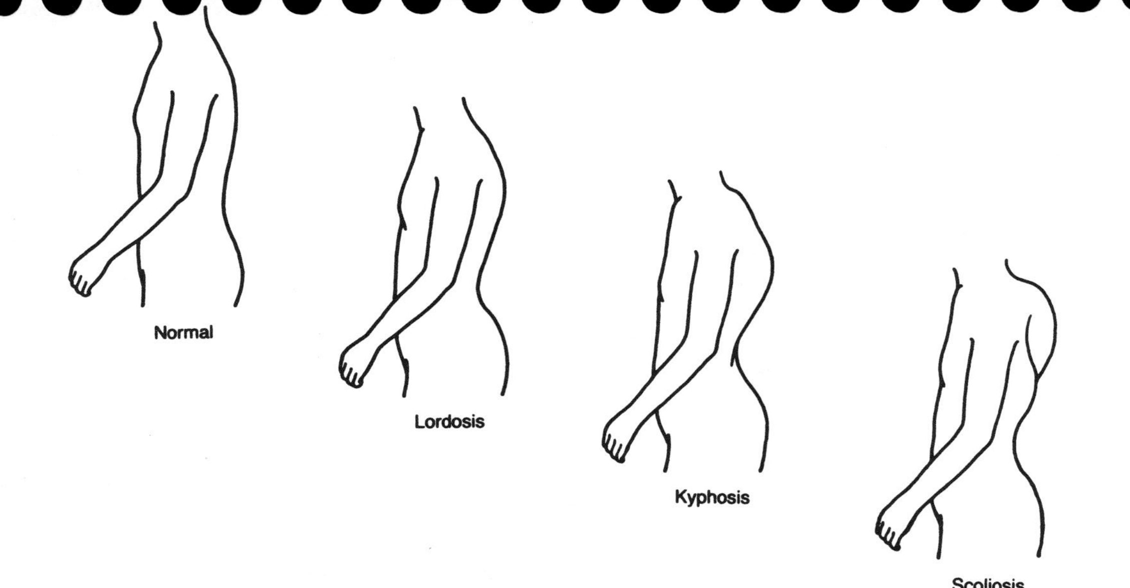

Figure 16-2. Normal and abnormal spinal curves.

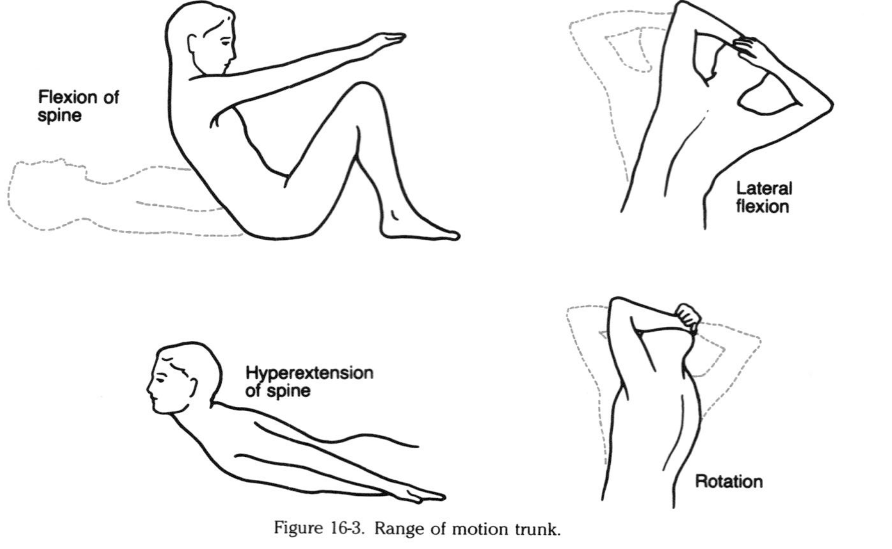

Figure 16-3. Range of motion trunk.

II. Objective Data: Assessment Techniques *(continued)*

Procedure	*Normal Findings*	*Deviations from Normal*
B. Palpate the shoulder (trapezius muscle) for the following:		
Muscle strength and tone	Able to shrug shoulders against resistance (3 to 5)	Weakness with shrugging of shoulders; pain (0 to 2)
Sensation	Nontender	Tender, painful
C. Palpate the shoulder, scapula, and posterior hip for the following:		
Bony prominences	Smooth and nontender, no swelling	Bony enlargement and tenderness, swelling, pain
Muscle size, strength, and tone	Equal in size bilaterally; equally strong (3 to 5)	Muscle atrophy, weakness, flabbiness, or swelling (0 to 2)
Temperature	Warm to cool	Hot

II. Objective Data: Assessment Techniques *(continued)*

Procedure	Normal Findings	Deviations from Normal
Inspection and Palpation of the Head, Neck, and Thorax		
Inspection With client in sitting position facing you, inspect body parts. Ask client to open and close mouth to assess temporomandibular joint (TMJ) function.		
A. Observe the head for the following:		
Facial structure and muscle development	Symmetrical structure and development of muscles	Asymmetrical structure and development of muscles
TMJ function	Can open mouth 2 inches	Limited ROM; audible crepitation, click; trismus (muscle spasms)
B. Observe the thorax for posture	Erect, slight kyphosis	Stooped; abnormal spinal curves
C. Observe the neck for ROM: Flexion, extension, rotation, lateral bending (Fig. 16-4)	Full ROM	Limited ROM with crepitation or pain; nuchal rigidity
Palpation While inspecting the TMJ, palpate it bilaterally anterior to the tragus of the ear as client opens mouth and clenches teeth. Ask client to turn head laterally against resistance.		

A. Palpate the TMJ for the following:		
Joint function	Smooth movement bilaterally on opening, with no clicks or pain	Palpable click, pain
Joint contour	Symmetrical	Asymmetrical
Temperature	Warm	Hot and swollen
B. Palpate the neck (sternocleidomastoid) for muscle strength and tone	Can turn head laterally against resistance without pain (3 to 5)	Weakness or pain when turning head against resistance (0 to 2)

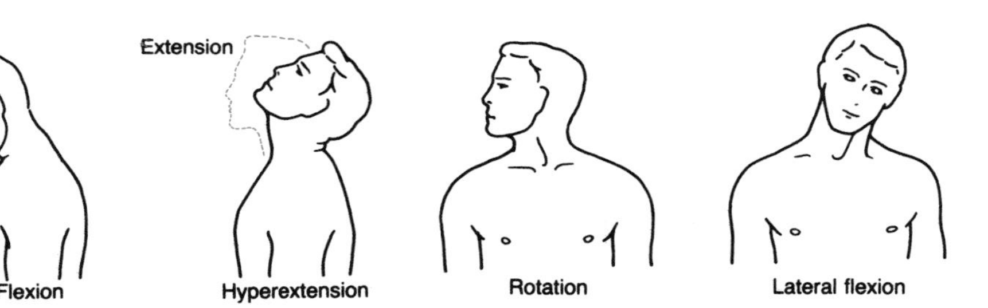

Figure 16-4. Range of motion of neck.

Procedure	Normal Findings	Deviations from Normal

Inspection and Palpation of the Upper Exremities

Inspection

Position client in the sitting position facing you, with the upper extremities exposed. Inspect each joint and determine ROM. Both active and passive ROM may be assessed. It is easier for the client to carry out ROM if you demonstrate movements first.

Procedure	Normal Findings	Deviations from Normal
A. Observe the shoulder, elbow, wrist, hand, and fingers for bone structure, bony prominences, muscle mass, joint structure, and symmetry.	Bilaterally symmetrical	Bony deformity, muscle atrophy, swelling, deviation, contractures, nodes, tophi
B. Observe the shoulder, elbow, wrist, and fingers for ROM.	Full ROM	Limited ROM with crepitation or pain

Normal ROM for each joint:

Shoulder	*Elbow*	*Wrist*	*Fingers*
Flexion	Flexion	Flexion	Flexion
Extension	Extension	Extension	Extension
Abduction	Supination	Deviation	Opposition
Adduction	Pronation	Radial	
Rotation		Ulnar	

See Figure 16-5.

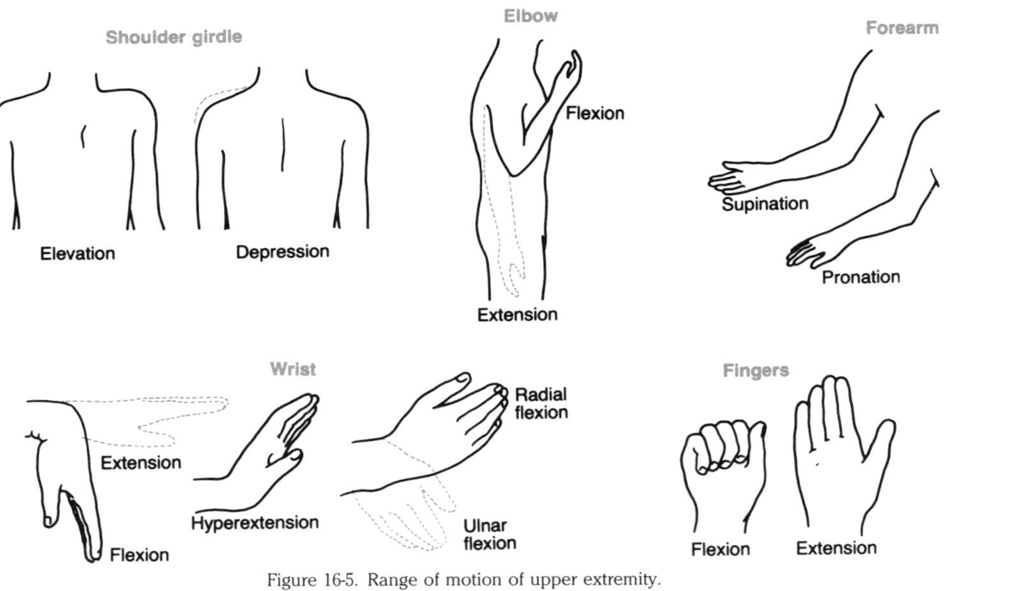

Figure 16-5. Range of motion of upper extremity.

Procedure	Normal Findings	Deviations from Normal
Palpation As the musculoskeletal structure of the upper extremity is going through active or passive ROM, palpate bones, muscles, tendons, and joints. Assess muscle strength and tone.		
A. Palpate the arm (biceps, triceps) for muscle strength and tone.	Can flex and extend arm against resistance (3 to 5)	Weakness, paralysis (1 to 2)
B. Palpate the hand for the following:		
Muscle strength, tone	Grip is firm and equal	Weakness, paralysis
Sensation	Nontender (3 to 5)	Tenderness, pain (1 to 2)
C. Palpate the elbow, wrist, hand, and fingers for the following:		
Bony landmarks	Nontender, smooth	Bony enlargement
Muscle size	Regular and equal bilaterally	Muscle atrophy
Joint structure	Symmetrical and equal	Loss of joint structure; joint bogginess; nodules, swelling
Strength	Equally strong (3 to 5)	Unilateral or bilateral weakness (0 to 2)
Temperature	Warm	Hot
Sensation	Nontender	Tender, painful

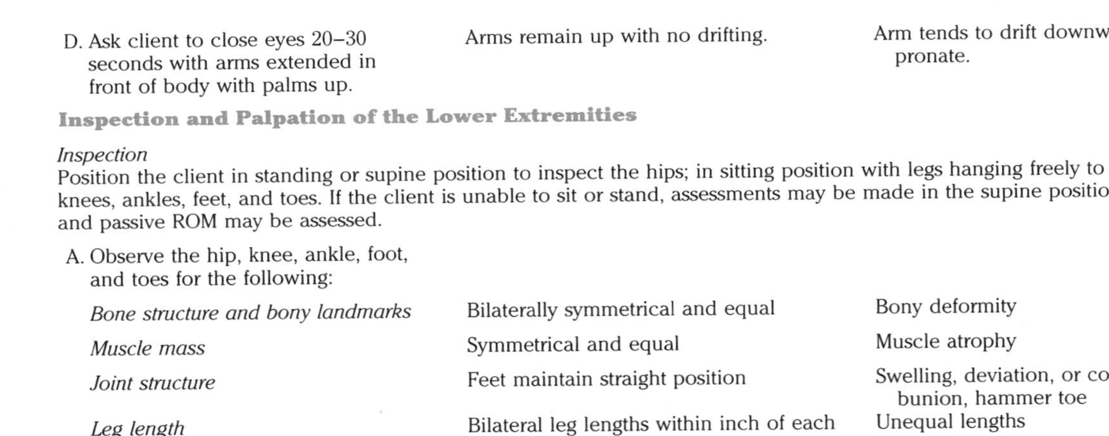

D. Ask client to close eyes 20–30 seconds with arms extended in front of body with palms up.	Arms remain up with no drifting.	Arm tends to drift downward and pronate.

Inspection and Palpation of the Lower Extremities

Inspection

Position the client in standing or supine position to inspect the hips; in sitting position with legs hanging freely to inspect the knees, ankles, feet, and toes. If the client is unable to sit or stand, assessments may be made in the supine position. Both active and passive ROM may be assessed.

A. Observe the hip, knee, ankle, foot, and toes for the following:		
Bone structure and bony landmarks	Bilaterally symmetrical and equal	Bony deformity
Muscle mass	Symmetrical and equal	Muscle atrophy
Joint structure	Feet maintain straight position	Swelling, deviation, or contractures; bunion, hammer toe
Leg length	Bilateral leg lengths within inch of each other	Unequal lengths

B. Observe the hip, knee, ankle, and toes for ROM (Fig. 16-6).

Full ROM

Limited ROM with crepitation or pain

Normal ROM for each joint:

Hip	*Knee*	*Ankle*	*Toes*
Rotation	Flexion	Dorsiflexion	Flexion
Flexion	Extension	Plantar flexion	Extension
Extension		Inversion	
		Eversion	

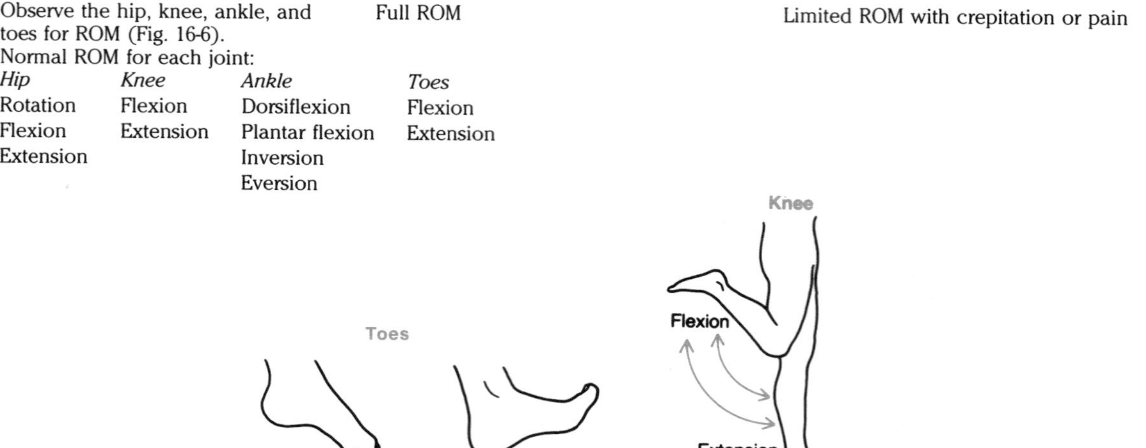

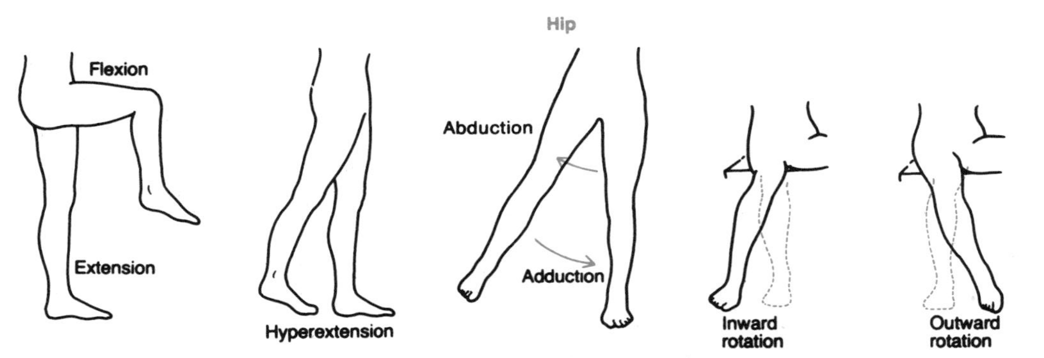

Figure 16-6. Range of motion of lower extremity.

Palpation
As the musculoskeletal structure of the lower extremity is going through active or passive ROM, palpate bones, bony landmarks, muscles, joints. Assess muscle strength and tone.

Procedure	*Normal Findings*	*Deviations from Normal*
Palpate the hip (quadriceps, gastrocnemius) for the following:		
Bony landmarks	Bilaterally symmetrical and equal	Bony enlargement
Muscle size and strength	Smooth, regular, strong (3 to 5)	Muscle atrophy and weakness (0 to 2)
Joint structure	Bilaterally symmetrical; strong	Loss of joint structure; joint bogginess
Temperature	Warm	Hot and swollen
Sensation	Nontender	Tenderness, pain

Pediatric Variations

Procedure	*Normal Variations*
Infancy	
A. Inspect lower extremities.	A distinct bowlegged growth pattern persists and begins to disappear at 18 months. At 2 years, a knock-kneed pattern is common (Fig. 16-7), persisting until age 6 to 10, when legs straighten. A greater ROM in joints is present in infants. Legs are wide set until the child begins walking; weight is borne on the inside of the feet.

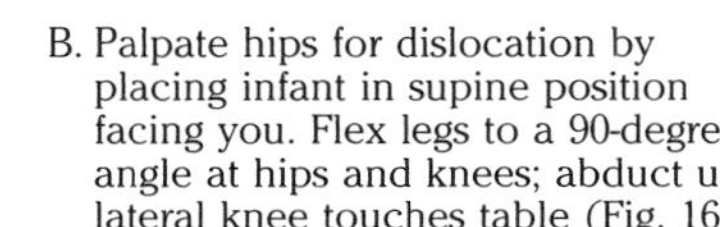

B. Palpate hips for dislocation by placing infant in supine position facing you. Flex legs to a 90-degree angle at hips and knees; abduct until lateral knee touches table (Fig. 16-8).	Hips should not click or snap when abducted.
Over age 2	
A. Inspect gait.	Wide-based gait common until age 2
B. Measure distance between knees with ankles together.	Less than 2 inches
Over age 7	
Measure distance between ankles with knees together. Longitudinal arch of foot is often obscured by adipose until age 3, and infant appears flatfooted.	Less than 3 inches
4–13 years of age	
(See also Appendix II for developmental milestones.)	
Inspect curvature of spine:	
A. Stand behind erect child and note asymmetry of shoulders and hips.	Shoulders symmetrical, parallel with hips
B. Have child bend forward at waist until back is parallel to floor. Observe from side, looking for asymmetry or prominence of rib cage.	Shoulders, scapula, iliac crests symmetrical

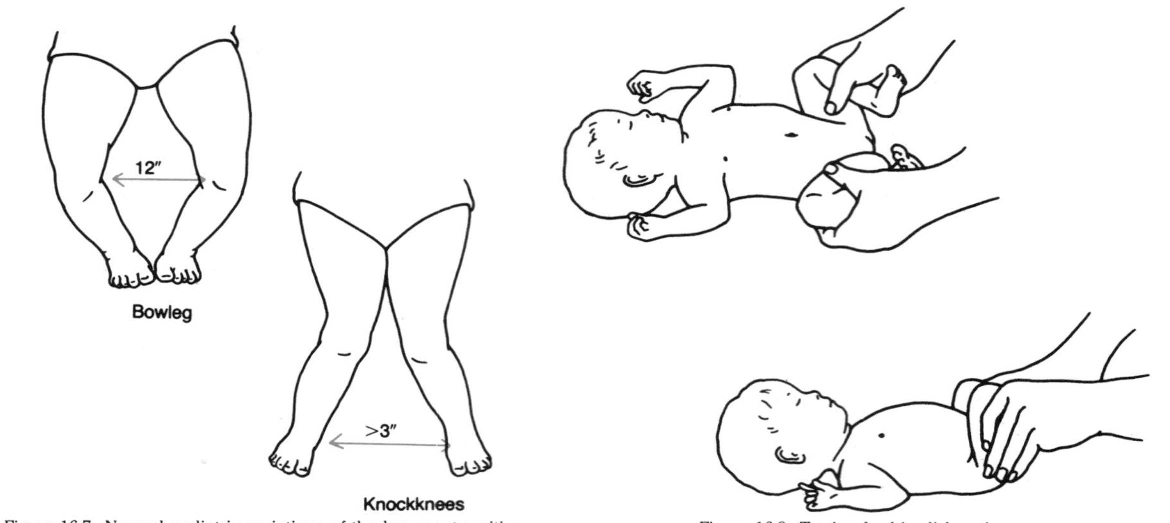

Figure 16-7. Normal pediatric variations of the lower extremities.

Figure 16-8. Testing for hip dislocation.

Geriatric Variations

- Decrease in total bone mass due to decreased activity level, change in hormones, and bone resorption. This results in weaker, softer bones.
- Accentuated dorsal spinal curve (kyphosis)
- Loss of muscle bulk and tone
- Decreased ROM of spine, neck, extremities
- Decrease in height (1.2 cm of height is lost every 20 years)
- Shoulder width decreases
- Chest and pelvis width increase

Cultural Variations

- Some variation in muscle size and mass in different racial/ethnic groups may have absence of peroneus tertius in foot or palmaris longus muscles in wrist.
- Blacks tend to be advanced in and Asians tend to fall behind in the growth and development norms established for U.S. Caucasians.

Possible Related Collaborative Problems

Potential complications:
Bone fractures
Sprains
Contractures of joints
Osteoporosis

Dislocation of Joints
Compartmental Syndrome

Teaching Tips for Selected Nursing Diagnoses

Nursing Diagnoses	*Teaching Tips*
Adult Client NURSING DIAGNOSIS: Opportunity to Enhance Mobility	Teach client the importance of maintaining an ideal weight. Explain the importance of doing weight-bearing and muscle-toning exercises at least 3 times per week. Encourage client to wear seatbelts in vehicles, to wear low well-fitted shoes, and to use walking aids (cane) as needed to prevent injury.
NURSING DIAGNOSIS: Chronic Pain in the muscles and joints	Discuss independent pain measures the client may find useful (e.g., massage, relaxation, distraction). Weight loss may also reduce discomfort if obesity is straining the bones, muscles, and joints. Explain use and side effects of pain medications.
NURSING DIAGNOSIS: Risk for Injury related to excessive exercise/improper body mechanics	Caution the client against the dangerous effects of excessive exercise. Teach proper body mechanics and correct posture.
Pediatric Client NURSING DIAGNOSIS: Risk for Injury related to premature physical developmental level	Caution parents on home safety precautions (e.g., gates at stairways, removal of objects that may cause unnecessary falls, and avoiding leaving child near water alone), based on child's level of musculoskeletal development. Develop home safety checklist with parents. Teach normal milestones of musculoskeletal development, and advise parent to encourage these skills as appropriate.

Geriatric Client

NURSING DIAGNOSIS: Risk for Injury related to decalcification of bones secondary to sedentary lifestyle and postmenopausal state	Discuss importance of calcium supplements in diet for postmenopausal women. Explain effects of exercise on decreasing bone decalcification.
NURSING DIAGNOSIS: Risk for Injury related to unstable gait secondary to aging process	Explain correct use of aids (e.g., crutches, canes, walkers) and other prostheses. Use referrals as necessary. Instruct client on measures to prevent falls (e.g., adequate lighting, avoidance of loose board ends and scatter rugs on floor). Discourage use of sleeping pills and suggest alternate methods of promoting sleep (e.g., watching TV, reading, warm bath, music, warm milk).
NURSING DIAGNOSIS: Impaired Physical Mobility related to decreased activity secondary to aging process	Instruct client on the hazards of immobility and methods to prevent complications (e.g,. turning, coughing, deep breathing, repositioning, ROM, adequate diet, plentiful fluid intake, and diversional activities). Encourage mild exercise to loosen joint stiffness.
NURSING DIAGNOSIS: Self-Care deficit related to impaired mobility and/or weakness	Assess safe level of activity with client, and teach methods to increase activity gradually to that level. Explore alternate self-help methods of maintaining self-care (e.g., feeding aids, wheelchairs, crutches, hygienic aids). Assist client with identifying and utilizing services and groups to assist with activities of daily living (e.g., Meals on Wheels). Support and teach family caregivers.

CHAPTER 17

Neurological Assessment

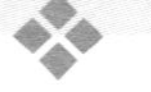

The neurological assessment is performed last because several of its components may have been integrated into previous parts of the examination. For example, the eighth cranial nerve may have been tested during the ear examination and therefore will not need to be tested again.

The neurological assessment consists of six parts: (1) mental status, (2) cranial nerves, (3) sensory function, (4) motor function, (5) cerebellar function, and (6) reflexes.

Equipment Needed

- Penlight
- Tuning fork
- Reflex hammer
- Cotton wisp
- Paper clip (for detection of sharp–dull sensations)
- Salt
- Sugar
- Cotton-tipped applicators
- Glass of water
- Tongue blade
- Ophthalmoscope

Subjective Data: Focus Questions

Loss of consciousness? Dizziness?Fainting? Headaches: Precipitating factors, location, duration, frequency, relieving factors? Convulsions: Type, precipitating factors, duration?

Numbness? Tingling? Paralysis? Neuralgia? Loss of memory, confusion? Visual loss, blurring, pain? Facial pain, weakness, twitching? Speech problems (aphasia: expressive/receptive)? Swallowing problems? Drooling? Neck weakness, spasms?

Mental Status Assessment

Assessment of mental status is performed by observing the client and asking him or her questions. Much of this information may have already been assessed during the interview and physical assessment.

Objective Data: Assessment Techniques

Procedure	***Normal Findings***	***Deviations from Normal***
A. Observe appearance and movement:		
Posture	Relaxed, with shoulders back and both feet stable	Tense, rigid, slumped, asymmetrical posture
Gait	Coordinated and smooth	Uncoordinated: staggering, shuffling, stumbling

Objective Data: Assessment Techniques *(continued)*

Procedure	***Normal Findings***	***Deviations from Normal***
Motor movements	Smooth, coordinated movements; client alters position occasionally	Jerky, uncoordinated; tremors, tics, fast or slow movements
Dress	Clothes fit and are appropriate for occasion and weather	Clothes extra large or small and inappropriate for occasion
Hygiene	Skin clean, nails clean and trimmed	Dirty, unshaven; dirty nails; foul odors
Facial expression	Good eye contract, smiles/frowns appropriately	Poor eye contact; no expression or exaggerated expression
Speech	Clear with moderate pace	High pitched; monotonal; hoarse; very soft or weak
B. Observe mood:		
Feelings	Responds appropriately to topic discussed; expresses feelings appropriate to situation	Expresses feelings inappropriate to situation (extreme anger or euphoria)
Expressions	Expresses good feelings about self, others, and life; verbalizes positive coping mechanisms (talking, support systems, counseling, exercise, etc.)	Expresses dissatisfaction with self, others, and life in general; verbalizes negative coping mechanisms (use of alcohol, drugs, etc.)

C. Observe thought process and perceptions:		
Clarity and content	Expresses full and free-flowing thoughts during interview	Thoughts expressed are jumbled, confusing, and not reality oriented
Perceptions	Follows directions accurately	Is unable to follow through with directives
	Perceptions realistic and consistent with yours	Perceptions unrealistic and inconsistent with yours and others
D. Observe cognition:		
Level of consciousness (examiner can deduce this information from interview conversation) *Note:* If client is not responding verbally, do the following:	Aware of self, others, place and time; follows instructions	Unable to express where he or she is, time, and who others are; does not follow instructions
• Ask client to squeeze your hand	Squeezes hand	No response
• Ask client to nod head when you touch him or her	Nods head	No response
• Squeeze client's finger firmly	Pulls finger away	No response

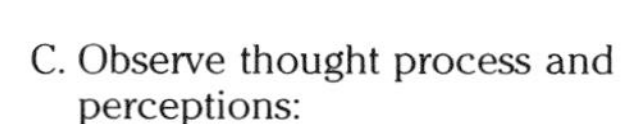

Objective Data: Assessment Techniques

Procedure	Normal Findings	Deviations from Normal
Length of concentration	Listens to you and responds with full thoughts	Fidgets; does not listen attentively to you; expresses incomplete thoughts
Memory	Correctly answers questions about current day's activities; recalls significant past events	Unable to recall any current or past events
Abstract reasoning: Ask client to explain a proverb, e.g., "A stitch in time saves nine."	Explains proverb accurately	Unable to give abstract meaning of proverb
Ability to make sound judgments: Ask client questions such as, "Why did you come to the hospital?" or "What do you do when you have pain?"	Answers to questions based on sound rationale	Answers to questions are not based on sound rationale
Ability to identify similarities: Ask client questions such as, "How are birds and bees alike?"	Identifies similarity	Unable to identify similarity
Sensory perception and coordination: Ask client to write name and draw circle.	Client writes name and draws circle accurately.	Client does not write name or draw circle accurately.

Pediatric Variations

Subjective Data: Focus Questions

Excessive difficulty in relationships with siblings, peers, parents, and teachers? Sudden changes in activities such as play or school activities? Excessive fears? Change in attention span?

Normal Variations

Abstract reasoning is not possible before ages 10 to 12. Judgment ability varies with level of development.

Birth to 11 years: Knowledge of normal development is most important in evaluating cognition. Cues for evaluating cognition in infants and young children are primarily *not* valid. Awareness, attention to mother, and a parent's report on the infant's attentiveness are also important. Play activities or games can be used to elicit many desired responses. For example, a young child can be asked to recall three to four numbers in sequence as a test of memory.

Birth to 6 years: Objective findings can be determined using the Denver Developmental Screening Test.

Geriatric Variations

- Slowed thought processes
- Slowed responses to questions
- Decreased ability to recall directions
- Slowed reaction time
- Decreased sleep intervals

Possible Related Collaborative Problems

Potential complications:

Depression	Suicide attempts
Alcohol abuse	Drug abuse

Teaching Tips for Selected Nursing Diagnoses

Nursing Diagnoses	***Teaching Tips***
Adult Client	
NURSING DIAGNOSIS: Altered Thought Processes related to altered physiological processes (aging, head injury, stroke, etc.)	Inform client of the purpose and benefits of community agencies that offer support. Refer client as necessary. Assist family in coping, and explain how to communicate accurately using short sentences.
NURSING DIAGNOSIS: Ineffective Individual Coping related to excessive stressors	Teach client the use of appropriate stress-reducing measures (e.g., relaxation techniques, biofeedback, exercise, hobbies). Inform client of beneficial effects of decreasing coffee, sugar, and salt in diet and maintaining adequate B and C vitamins in diet for adequate functioning of the endocrine and nervous systems. Refer client to community agencies and support groups as necessary.
Impaired Memory	Teach client memory enhancing techniques.
Opportunity to enhance critical thinking	Teach client critical thinking skills. Assist client to obtain resources to enhance critical thought processes.

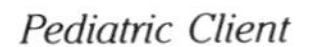

Pediatric Client

NURSING DIAGNOSIS:
Ineffective Family Coping related to difficulty with child's behaviors

Discuss social development of the child.

Infant: "Stranger anxiety" is normal. Teach parents ways to assist infant to warm up to strangers. Encourage verbalization, reassurance, and cuddling. Help parent assess child's readiness to begin school and to verbalize any school problems with child.

Cranial Nerve Assessment

Various techniques are used to assess cranial nerve (CN) functioning.

Objective Data: Assessment Techniques

Procedure	***Normal Findings***	***Deviations from Normal***
Assess CN I through XII.		
1. *CN I—Olfactory:* Hold scent (e.g., coffee, orange) under each nostril with other occluded while client closes eyes.	Identifies scent correctly with each nostril	Unable to identify correct odor

Objective Data: Assessment Techniques *(continued)*

Procedure	*Normal Findings*	*Deviations from Normal*
2. *CN II—Optic:* a. Assession vision. b. Assess visual fields. c. Do fundoscopic examination for direct visualization of optic nerve.	See Chapter 8, Eye Assessment.	See Chapter 8, Eye Assessment.
3. *CN III—Oculomotor* *CN IV—Trochlear* *CN VI—Abducens:* a. Assess extraocular movements. b. Assess PERRLA (pupils equally round and reactive to light and accommodation).	See Chapter 8, Eye Assessment.	See Chapter 8, Eye Assessment.
4. *CN V—Trigeminal:* a. Assess sensory function by		
• Touching cornea lightly with wisp of cotton. (Fig. 17-1)	Eyelids blink bilaterally	Absent or unilateral blinking of eyelids
• Testing client's ability to feel light touch, dull, and sharp facial sensations. (Fig. 17-2)	Identifies light touch, dull and sharp sensations to forehead, cheeks, and chin	Unable to identify or feel facial sensations

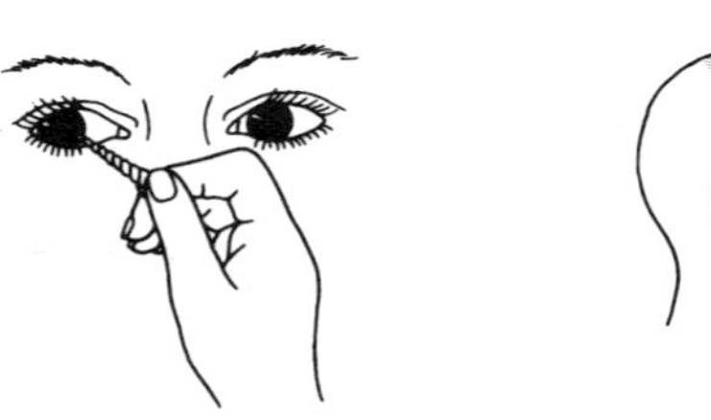

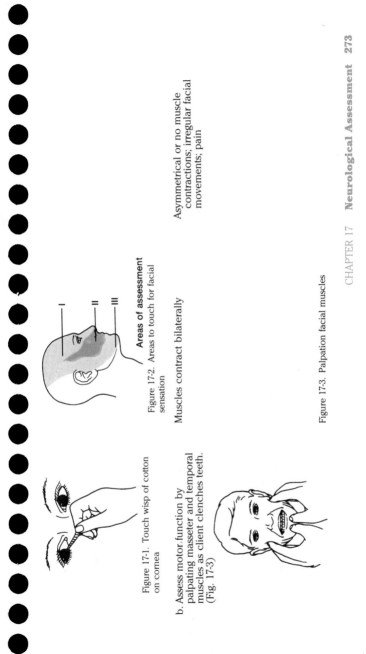

Figure 17-1. Touch wisp of cotton on cornea

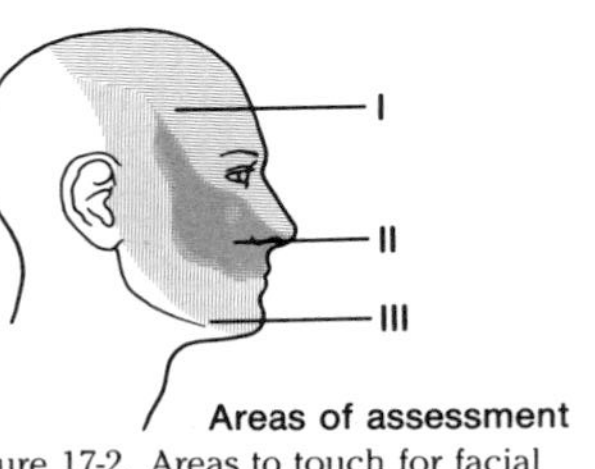

Figure 17-2. Areas to touch for facial sensation

b. Assess motor function by palpating masseter and temporal muscles as client clenches teeth. (Fig. 17-3)	Muscles contract bilaterally	Asymmetrical or no muscle contractions; irregular facial movements; pain

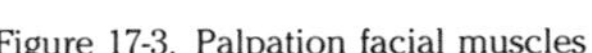

Figure 17-3. Palpation facial muscles

Procedure	***Normal Findings***	***Deviations from Normal***
c. Assess jaw jerk.	Mouth opens slightly	No response, or mouth opens widely
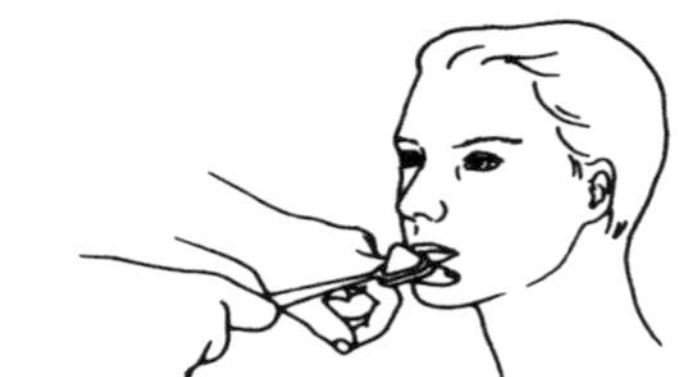 Figure 17-4. Jaw jerk		
5. *CN VII—Facial:*		
a. Assess sensory function by asking client to identify sugar, lemon, salt on anterior two-thirds of tongue, with eyes closed and tongue protruded.	Identifies taste correctly	Unable to taste or to identify taste correctly
b. Assess motor function by asking client to do the following: • Smile • Frown • Show teeth	 Smiles Frowns Shows teeth	 Unable to perform facial movements as instructed, or movements asymmetrical

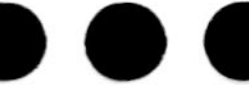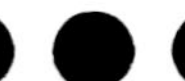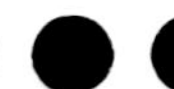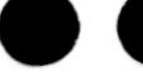

• Blow out cheeks • Raise eyebrows and tightly close eyes	Blows out cheeks Raises eyebrows and closes eyes tightly as instructed Facial movements symmetrical	
6. *CN VIII—Acoustic:* Assess hearing.	See Chapter 9, Ear Assessment.	See Chapter 9, Ear Assessment.
7. *CN IX—Glossopharyngeal and CN X—Vagus:* Ask client to a. Open mouth and say "ah."	Bilateral, symmetrical rise of soft palate and uvula	Unequal or absent rise of soft palate and uvula

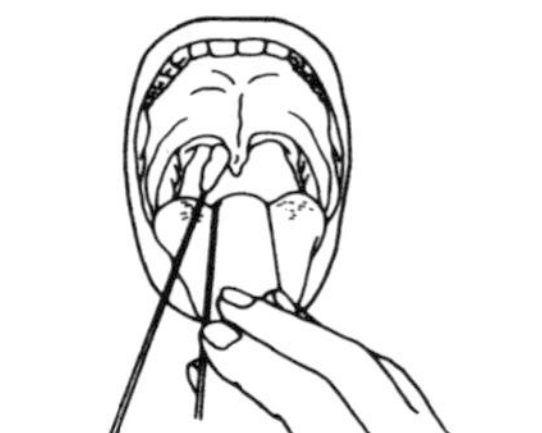

Figure 17-5. Stimulating gag reflex

b. Touch back of tongue or soft palate with tongue blade.	Gag reflex present	Gag reflex absent

c. Identify sugar, lemon juice, and salt taste on posterior one-third of protruded tongue, with eyes closed.	Identifies correct taste	Unable to identify correct taste
8. *CN XI—Spinal Accessory:*		
a. Palpate strength of trapezius muscles by asking client to shrug shoulders against your hands.	Symmetrical, strong contraction of trapezius muscles	Asymmetrical, weak, or absent contraction of trapezius muscles

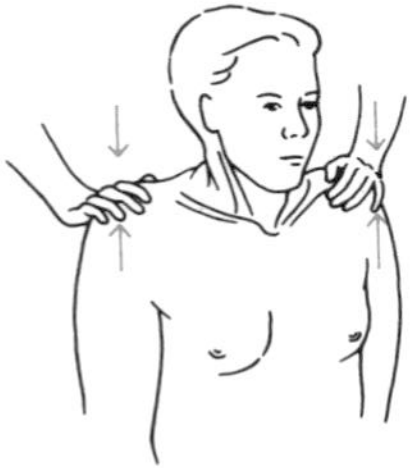

Figure 17-6. Palpating trapezius muscles

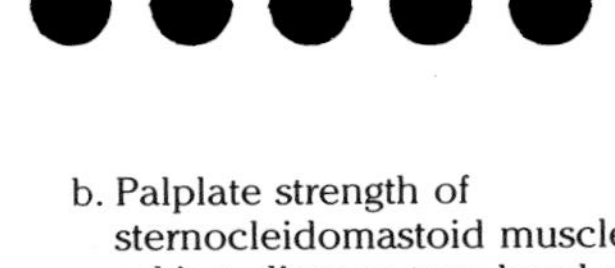

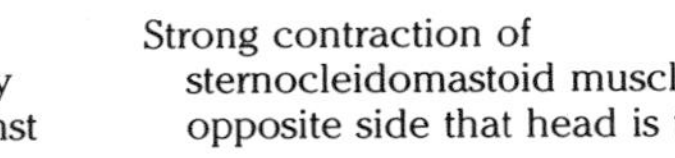

b. Palplate strength of sternocleidomastoid muscles by asking client to turn head against your hand.

Strong contraction of sternocleidomastoid muscle on opposite side that head is turned

Weak or absent contraction of sternocleidomastoid muscle on opposite side that head is turned

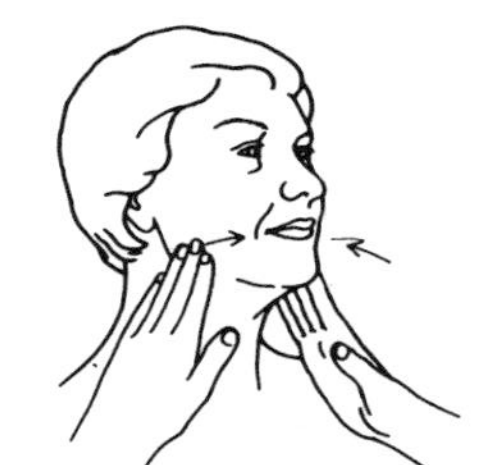

Figure 17-7. Palpating sternocleidomastoid muscles

9. *CN XII—Hypoglossal Nerve:*
Ask client to protrude tongue and move it to each side against tongue blade.

Symmetrical tongue with smooth outward movement and bilateral strength

Asymmetrical tongue; deviation to one side, unequal, or no strength

Geriatric Variations

- Decreased ability to see, hear, taste, and smell

Possible Related Collaborative Problems

Potential complications:
Cranial nerve impairment
Corneal ulceration
Increased intra-ocular pressure

Teaching Tips for Selected Nursing Diagnoses

Nursing Diagnosis	***Teaching Tip***
Sensory-perceptual alterations related to injury or aging	Explain to family the use and benefits of sensory therapy. Refer for hearing/visual aids as necessary. Teach client slowly and concisely. Speak clearly and demonstrate instructions from client's best side for hearing and seeing. Teach client how to prevent thermal injuries.

Sensory Nerve Assessment

In order to test the client's ability to perceive various sensations over the extremities and abdomen, stimuli must be scattered to cover all the dermatomes. The client is asked to close his or her eyes and identify the type of sensation perceived and the body area where it was felt. If a perceptual deficit is identified, the area is mapped out to determine the extent of impaired sensation.

Objective Data: Assessment Techniques

Procedure	Normal Findings	Deviations from Normal
A. Test for primary sensations with client's eyes closed by touching client with the following:		
1. Piece of cotton	Identifies area of light touch	Unable to identify location or light touch sensation
2. Alternately with sharp tip and dull tip of paper clip	Identifies area touched and differentiates between sharp and dull sensations	Unable to identify location or differentiate touch sensation
3. Vibrating tuning fork on major distal bony prominences of wrist, sternum	Identifies vibratory sensation	Unable to identify vibratory sensation
B. Test for cortical and discriminatory sensation with client's eyes closed by asking client to identify the following:		

Procedure	*Normal Findings*	*Deviations from Normal*
1. The number of points touching him or her while you touch him or her with two points simultaneously (two-point discrimination)	Identifies two points on: • Forearm at 40 mm apart • Back at 40–70 mm apart • Dorsal hands at 20–30 mm apart • Fingertips at 2–5 mm apart	Unable to identify two points at normal ranges
Figure 17-8. Two point discrimination		
2. The object (e.g., a coin) you place in his or her hand (stereogenesis)	Identifies correct object	Unable to identify object
3. A number you write on his or her palm with a tongue blade (graphesthesia)	Identifies correct number	Unable to identify number

4. The direction you move a part of his or her body (e.g., move great toe up or down; kinesthesia)	Identifies correct direction body part is moved	Unable to identify direction in which body part is moved

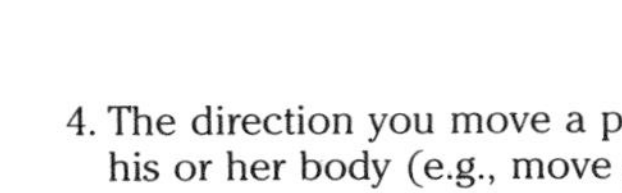

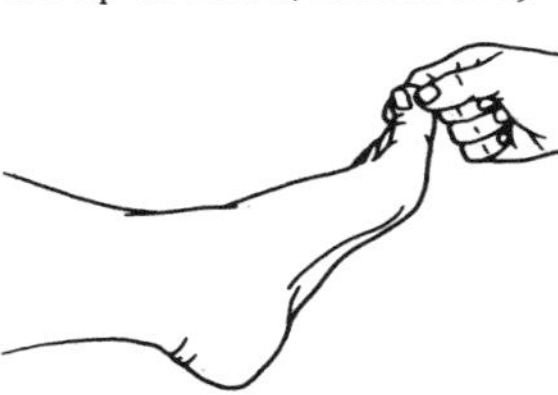

Figure 17-9. Kinesthesia

Geriatric Variations

- Generalized decreased sensations due to atrophy of peripheral nerve endings
- Decreased pain perception

Possible Related Collaborative Problems

Peripheral nerve impairment
Neuropathies
Teaching Tips for Selected Nursing Diagnoses

Nursing Diagnosis	***Teaching Tips***
Risk for Injury related to decreased tactile sensations	Instruct on proper inspection and protective care of extremities. Caution client on dangers of exposure to extreme hot and cold temperatures, contact with sharp objects, and wearing tight-fitting shoes or garments.

Motor Assessment

Assess muscle size, tone, movement, voluntary movements, and strength. See Chapter 16, Musculoskeletal Assessment.

Cerebellar Assessment

Ask the client to perform the following actions, after you demonstrate them, in order to assess coordination.

Objective Data: Assessment Techniques

Procedure	*Normal Findings*	*Deviations from Normal*
Ask client to do the following:		
1. Close eyes, and hold arms over head and straight out in front.	Holds arms over head and straight out steadily for 20 seconds	Downward drift; a flexion of one or both arms
2. With arms extended to the sides, touch each forefinger alternately to nose, first with eyes open and then with eyes closed.	Smooth accurate movements while touching finger to nose	Uncoordinated jerky movements; inability to touch nose

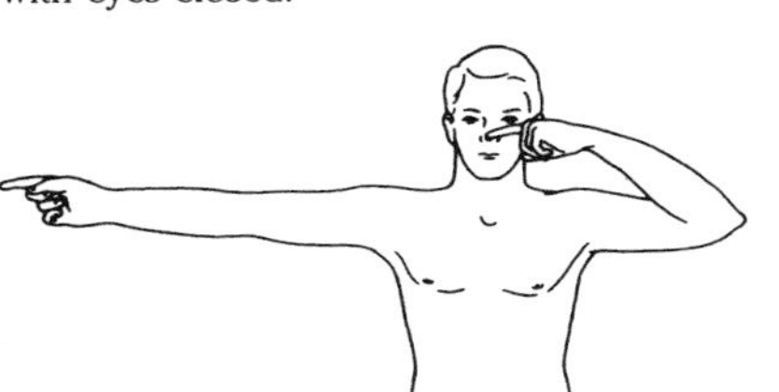

Figure 17-10. Finger-to-nose procedure

Procedure	*Normal Findings*	*Deviations from Normal*
3. Tap forefinger to thumb rapidly.	Rapidly taps forefinger to thumb	Jerky, uncoordinated movements of forefinger and thumb
4. Touch each finger to thumb.	Rapidly touches each finger to thumb	Spastic, awkward movements

Figure 17-11. Finger-to-thumb procedure

Procedure	*Normal Findings*	*Deviations from Normal*
5. Button and unbutton coat/shirt.	Buttons and unbuttons clothes smoothly	Clumpsy attempts to button/unbutton clothes
6. Run heel down each shin.	Runs each heel smoothly down each shin	Unable to place heel on shin and move it down shin with coordination

Figure 17-12. Heel-to-shin procedure

7. Stand erect with feet together and arms at sides, first with eyes open and then with eyes closed. (Put your arms around client to prevent falls—Romberg test.)	Stands straight with minimal swaying	Sways, moves feet out to prevent fall
8. Walk naturally.	Steady gait with opposite arm swing	Unsteady gait, uncoordinated arm swing; uses wide foot stance; shuffles or drags feet; lifts feet high off ground; crosses feet when walking
9. Walk in a heel-to-toe fashion (tandem walk).	Maintains balance with tandem walk	Unsteady tandem walk; unable to walk tandem style

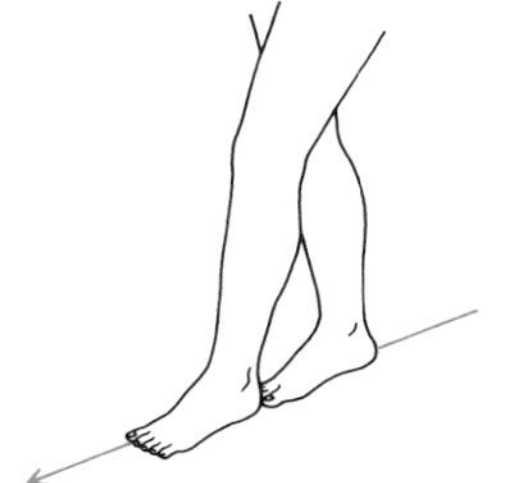

Figure 17-13. Tandem walk

Objective Data: Assessment Techniques *(continued)*

Procedure	Normal Findings	Deviations from Normal
10. Stand on each foot (one at a time).	Stands on one foot at a time	Unable to stand on one foot at a time
11. Hop on each foot (one at a time).	Hops on each foot without losing balance	Inadequate strength or balance to hop on each foot
12. Walk on heels, then toes.	Walks on heels, then toes	Unable to walk on heels or toes.

Geriatric Variation

- Slowed coordination and voluntary movements
- Decreased fine motor coordination

Reflex Assessment

Objective Data: Assessment Techniques

To elicit deep tendon reflexes: Attempt to distract the client away from the area being examined (to decrease tension and facilitate the reflex arc) by the following maneuvers:

- When testing upper extremities, have client clench teeth.
- While testing lower extremities, have client interlock hands and pull (see Figure 17-14) while you briskly tap specific tendons with a reflex hammer to elicit deep tendon reflexes.

Deep tendon reflexes are rated as follows:

4+ hyperactive (disease)
3+ brisk
2+ normal
1+ sluggish
0 no response

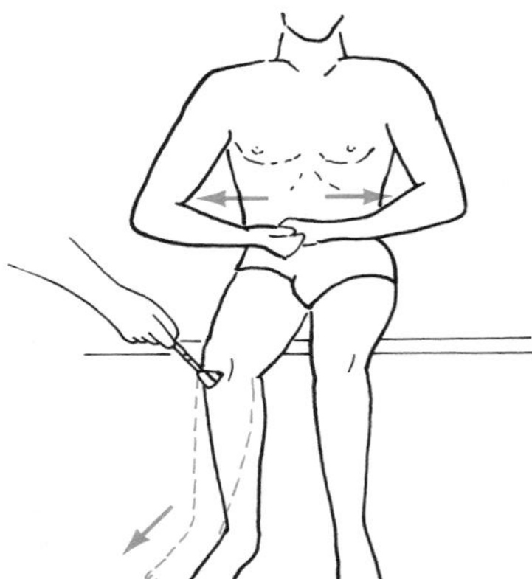

Figure 17-14. Eliciting deep tendon reflexes

To elicit superficial reflexes: Lightly stroke the skin with a moderately sharp instrument (e.g., key, tongue blade). Finally, certain maneuvers are performed to elicit any pathological reflexes.

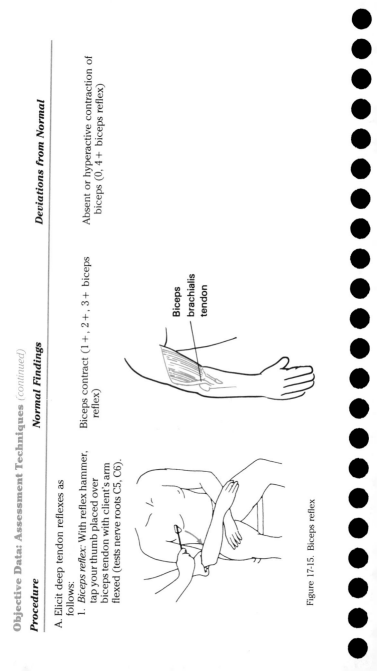

Procedure	Normal Findings	Deviations from Normal
A. Elicit deep tendon reflexes as follows:		
1. *Biceps reflex:* With reflex hammer, tap your thumb placed over biceps tendon with client's arm flexed (tests nerve roots C5, C6).	Biceps contract (1+, 2+, 3+ biceps reflex)	Absent or hyperactive contraction of biceps (0, 4+ biceps reflex)

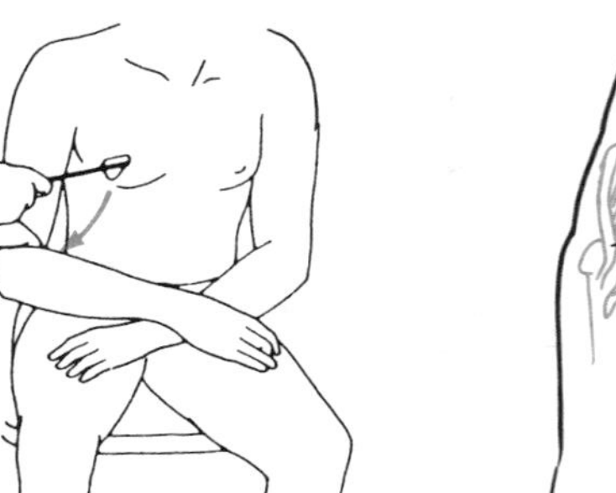

Figure 17-15. Biceps reflex

2. *Brachioradialis reflex:* Tap brachioradialis tendon just above wrist on radial side with client's arm resting midway between supination and pronation (tests nerve roots C5, C6).	Elbow flexes with pronation of forearm (1+, 2+, 3+ brachioradialis reflex)	Absent or hyperactive flexion of elbow and forearm pronation (0+, 4+ brachioradialis reflex)

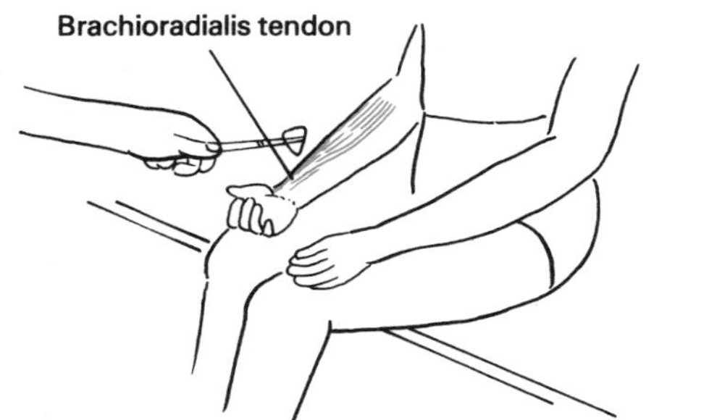

Figure 17-16. Brachioradialus reflex

Procedure	*Normal Findings*	*Deviations from Normal*
3. *Triceps reflex:* Tap triceps tendon (just above elbow) with client's arm abducted and forearm hanging freely (tests nerve roots C6, C7, C8).	Elbow extends (1+, 2+, 3+ triceps reflex)	Absent or hyperactive elbow extension (0, 4+ triceps reflex)

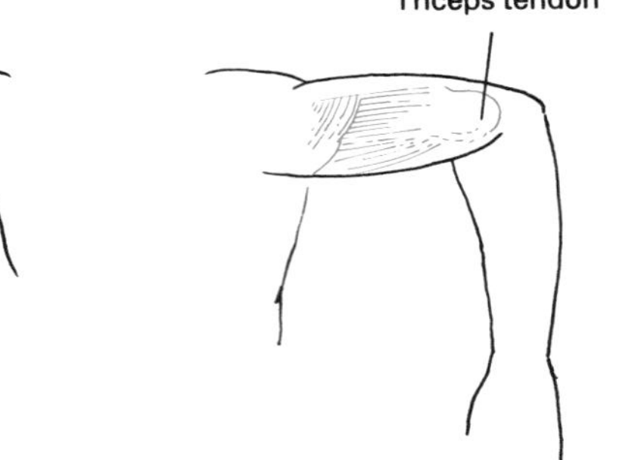

Figure 17-17. Triceps reflex

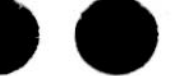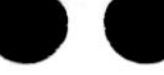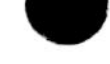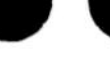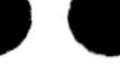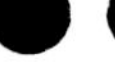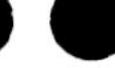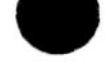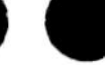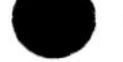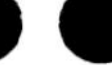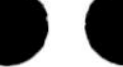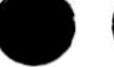

4. *Patellar reflex:* Tap patellar tendon with client's knee flexed and thigh stabilized (tests nerve roots L2 and L3).	Extension of knee (1+, 2+, 3+ patellar reflex)	Absent or hyperactive extension of knee (0, 4+ patellar reflex)

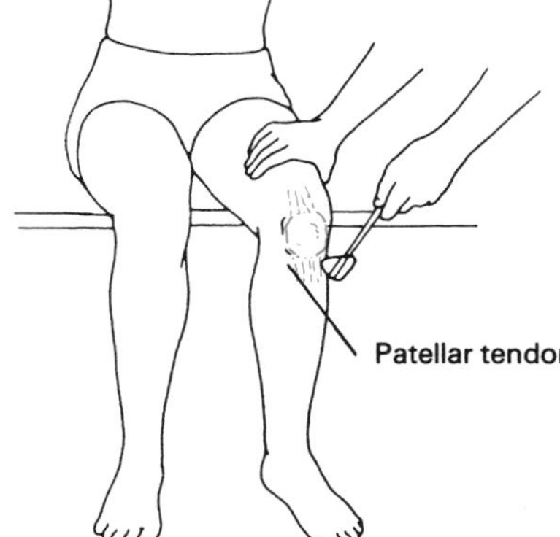

Figure 17-18. Patellar reflex

Procedure	Normal Findings	Deviations from Normal
5. *Achilles reflex:* Tap Achilles tendon with client's foot slightly dorsiflexed and stabilized (tests nerve roots S1, S2).	Plantar flexion of foot (1+, 2+, 3+ Achilles reflex)	Absent of hyperactive plantar flexion of foot (0, 4+ plantar flexion)

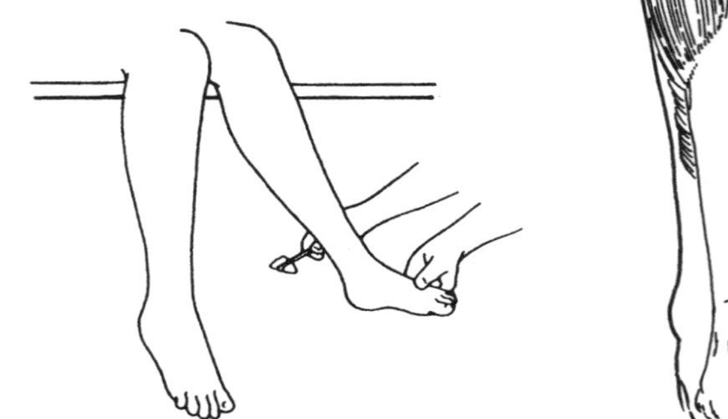

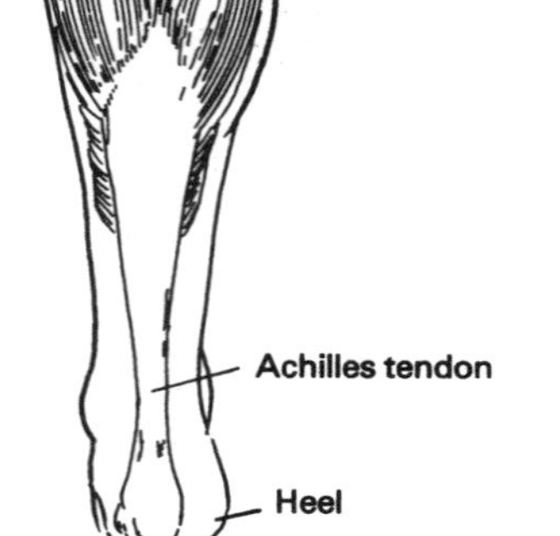

Figure 17-19. Achilles reflex

B. Elicit superficial reflexes as follows:		
1. Lightly stroke each side of abdomen above and below umbilicus (umbilicus reflexes).	Bilateral upward and downward movements of umbilicus toward stroke; abdomen contracts	Absent or unilateral movement of umbilicus; no abdominal contraction

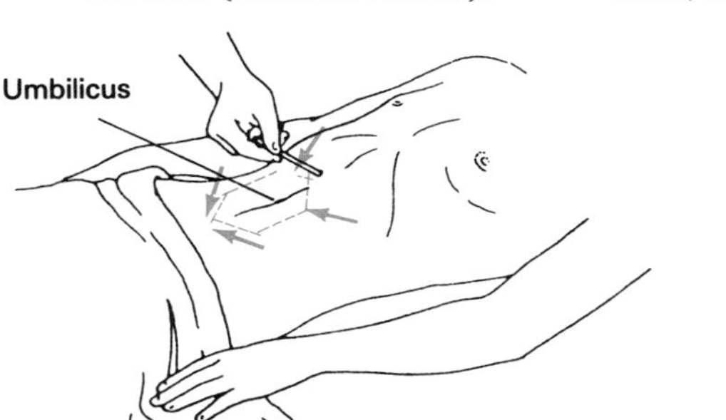

Figure 17-20. Umbilical reflex

2. Stroke gluteal area.	Anal sphincter contracts	Absent contraction of gluteal reflex
3. Stroke inner upper thigh of males.	Scrotum elevates on side stimulated	No elevation of scrotum

Procedure	***Normal Findings***	***Deviations from Normal***
C. Assess for pathological reflexes as follows:		
1. *Babinski reflex:* Use tongue blade to stroke lateral aspect of sole from heel to ball of foot.	Flexion of all toes (plantar response—negative Babinski reflex in adults)	Great toe extends and other toes fan out (positive Babinski reflex in adults) *Note:* This positive Babinski reflex is normal in the first 12 months of life (see Pediatric Variations)

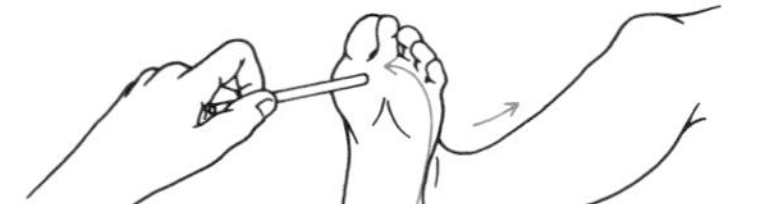

Figure 17-21. Babinski reflex

Procedure	***Normal Findings***	***Deviations from Normal***
2. *Ankle clonus:* Sharply dorsiflex foot with knee supported and partially flexed, and hold this way.	Foot stays dorsiflexed with no movement	Foot oscillates between dorsiflexion and plantar flexion

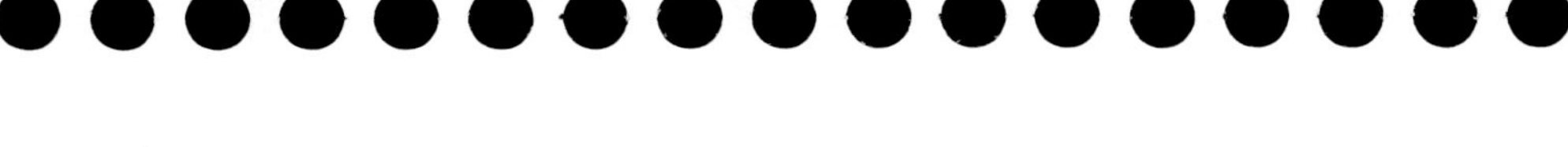

Figure 17-22. Ankle clonus

3. *Brudzinsky's sign:* Have client lie flat and flex neck forward.	No pain, resistance, or hip-knee flexion accompanies maneuver.	Pain, resistance and hip-knee flexion occur in response to maneuver.

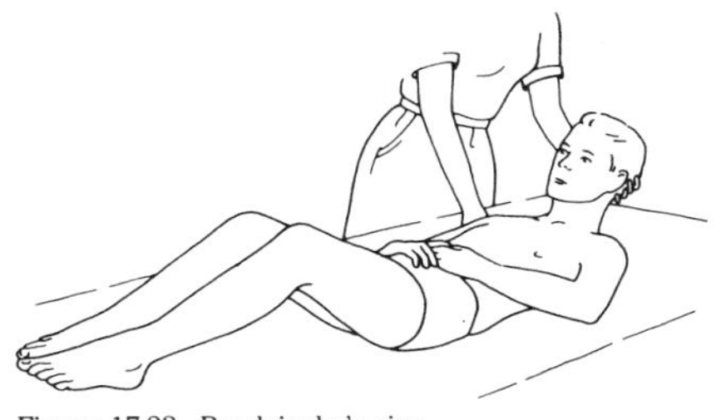

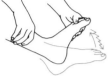

Figure 17-23. Brudzinsky's sign

Procedure	*Normal Findings*	*Deviations from Normal*
4. *Kernig's sign:* Have client lie flat and flex one knee and hip on same side.	No pain or resistance to maneuver	Pain and resistance to maneuver

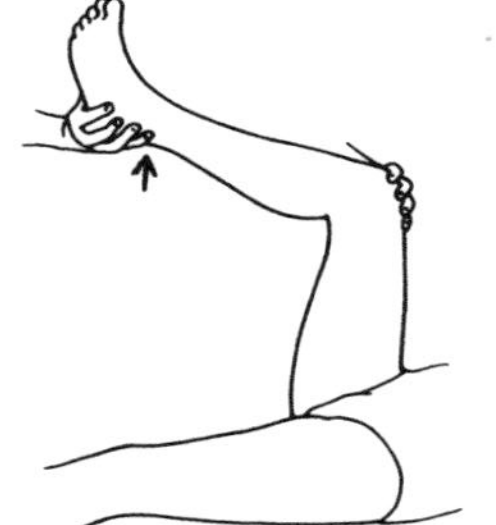

Figure 17-24. Kernig's sign

5. *Decortication:* Observe posture.	Normal posture	Abnormal flexion in response to pain or spontaneously

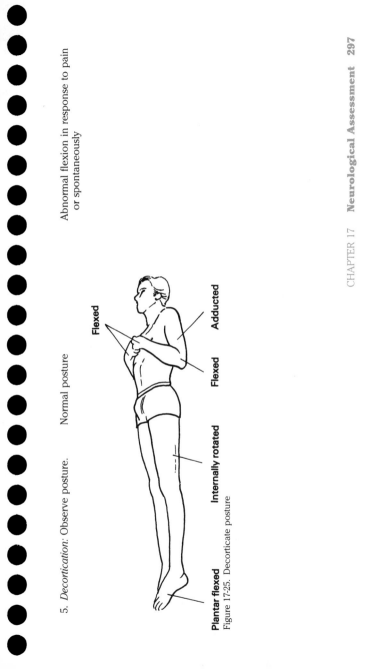

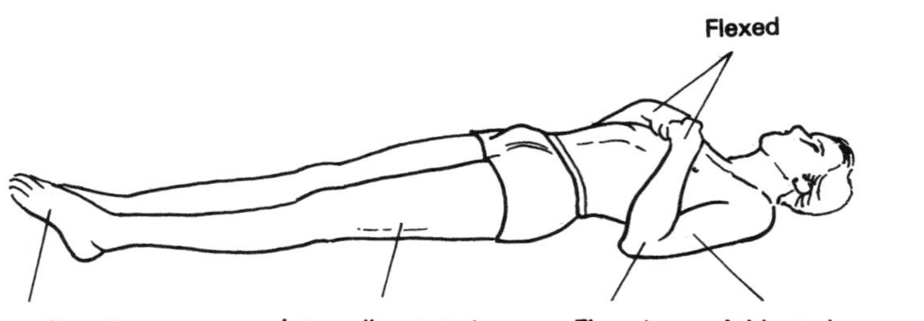

Figure 17-25. Decorticate posture

Objective Data: Assessment Techniques *(continued)*

Procedure	Normal Findings	Deviations from Normal
6. *Decerebration:* Observe posture.	Normal posture	Abnormal extension response to pain or spontaneously

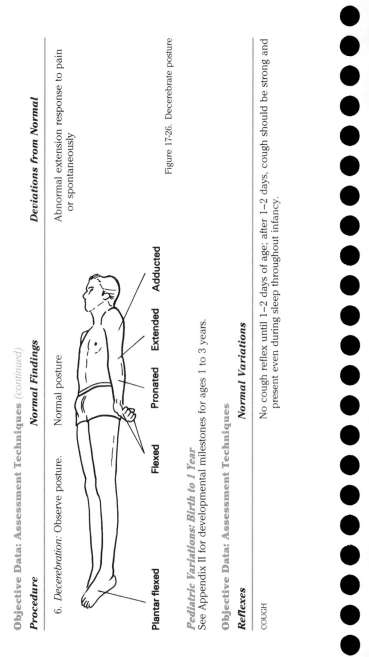

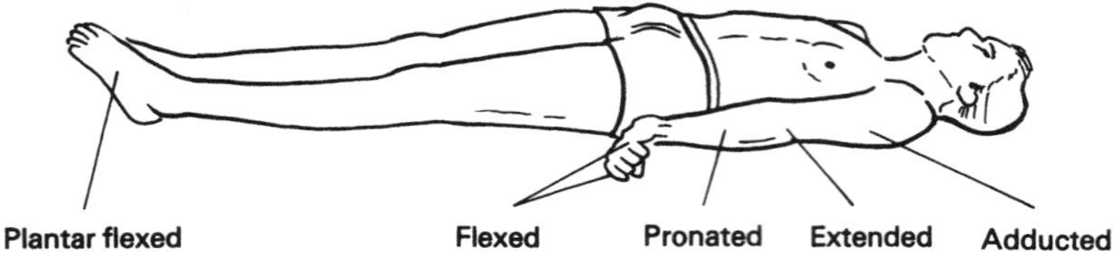

Plantar flexed Flexed Pronated Extended Adducted

Figure 17-26. Decerebrate posture

Pediatric Variations: Birth to 1 Year

See Appendix II for developmental milestones for ages 1 to 3 years.

Objective Data: Assessment Techniques

Reflexes	Normal Variations
COUGH	No cough reflex until 1–2 days of age; after 1–2 days, cough should be strong and present even during sleep throughout infancy.

ROOTING: Infant turns head toward side of face stroked.	Disappears at about 3–12 months
EXTENSION: When tongue is pressed or touched, infant forces tongue outward.	Disappears at about age 4 months
GRASP: Touch to palm of hand or soles of feet causes flexion of hands/toes.	Palmar grasp should disappear at about age 3 months.
BABINSKI REFLEX: Stroking outer sole of foot from heel to toe causes big toe to rise (dorsiflexion) and other toes to fan out.	Disappears after 1 year
MORO: Sudden jarring or change in equilibrium causes sudden extension and abduction of extremities, with thumb forming "C" shape; crying.	Disappears at about 3–4 months
STARTLE: Sudden noise causes abduction of arms, clenched hands.	Disappears at about 4 months

Reflexes	Normal Variations
CRAWLING: Infant on abdomen will make crawling movements with arms and legs.	Disappears at about age 6 weeks
DANCE: Infant held so sole of feet touch table will simulate walking movements.	Disappears at about 3–4 weeks
NECK RIGHTING: In supine infant, if head is turned to one side, shoulder and trunk will turn to that side.	Disappears around 10 months
ASYMMETRIC TONIC NECK: Infant's head quickly turns to one side, arm and leg on that side will extend, opposite leg and arm will flex.	Disappears at about 3–4 months

Geriatric Variations

- Generalized decreased and slowed reflexes

Possible Related Collaborative Problems

Potential complications:
Increased intracranial pressure
Meningitis
Paralysis
Spinal cord compression
Seizures

Teaching Tips for Selected Nursing Diagnosis

Nursing Diagnosis	***Teaching Tips***
Risk fo Injury related to seizure activity	Teach appropriate precautions and care, including the following: • Use of padded tongue blade, wallet, or cloth to maintain airway • Protection of client from harm during seizures • Positioning on side after seizure • Significance of drug maintenance

CHAPTER 18

Nutritional Assessment

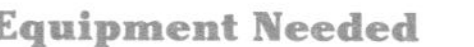

Equipment Needed

- Beam balance scale
- Metric measuring tape
- Skinfold calipers

I. Subjective Data: Focus Questions

Client's perception of his or her nutritional status, appetite, 3-day intake (fluid and foods), knowledge of nutrition, food preferences, food intolerances, food allergies, food practices related to culture or religion, who shops for food, food preparation, past or current use of health foods, vitamins or fad diets, activities of daily living, exercise, use of leisure time, recent weight loss or gains.

II. Objective Data: Assessment Techniques

Assessment of the client's nutritional status consists of an overall inspection of muscle mass, distribution of fat, and skeleton. The examiner must determine if abnormalities found during assessment of the skin, mouth, thyroid, heart, abdomen, lungs, and nervous system are related to alterations in nutrition. (Refer to Chapters 5, 6, 7, 10, 11, 14, and 17.)

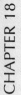

Procedure	***Normal Findings***	***Deviations from Normal***
A. General Inspection		
1. Observe the muscle mass over temporal areas, dorsum of hands, and spine for:		
Tone	Firm, developed	Flaccid, wasted, underdeveloped
Strength with voluntary movement	Strength equal bilaterally	Weak, sluggish
2. Observe body fat for distribution over waist, thighs, and triceps	Equal distribution; some fat under skin	Lack of fat under skin Increased bony prominences Emaciated Cachexic Abundant fatty tissue Abdominal ascites (due to fluid shift in protein)
3. Observe skeleton for posture	Erect, no malformations, smooth and coordinated gait	Poor posture, difficulty walking, bowed legs, knock-knees
4. Observe energy level	Energetic	Fatigued, irritable
5. Observe skin for color and texture	Pink, smooth, turgor present	Pale, rough, dry, flaky, petechiae, lacks subcutaneous fat, loss of turgor

II. Objective Data: Assessment Techniques *(continued)*

Procedure	Normal Findings	Deviations from Normal
6. Observe nails for color and texture	Nails firm; skin under nails pink	Pale, brittle, opaque, spoon shaped, ridged
7. Observe hair for texture	Lustrous and shiny	Brittle, dry
8. Observe lips for color and texture	Pink, smooth, moist	Swollen, puffy, lesions, fissures at corners of mouth
9. Observe tongue for color and texture	Deep red with papillae	Beefy red, smooth, swollen, atrophy or hypertrophy
10. Observe teeth for position and condition	Straight with no cavities	Missing, malpositioned, cavities
11. Observe gums for condition and color	Smooth, firm, and pink	Inflamed, spongy, swollen, red, bleed easily
12. Observe eyes for moisture, lesions	Clear, moist surfaces, transparent cornea	Pale or red eye; membranes, dry, increased vascularity, dull appearance of cornea
13. Observe reflexes	Reflexes normal	Loss of or decreased ankle and knee reflexes
14. Observe pulse and blood pressure	Normal heart rate and blood pressure for age	Tachycardia, hypertension, irregular pulse
B. Anthropometric Measurements		
1. Measure height by having client stand erect against wall without shoes. Record height in centimeters.		

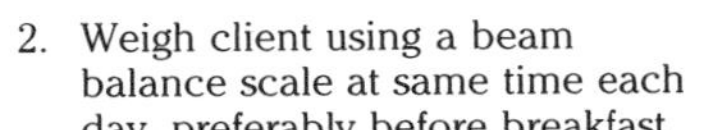

2. Weigh client using a beam balance scale at same time each day, preferably before breakfast.	Body weight within 10% of ideal range (compare findings to Appendix VI) or use following formula:	Body weight less than 10–20% ideal range (undernutrition) Body weight greater than 10% IBW (overweight) Body weight greater than 20% IBW (obesity)
Calculate ideal body weight (IBW) *or* Record weight in kilograms and compare to standardized height and weight table (Appendixes V and VI).	*Female IBW* = 100 lb for 5 ft + 5 lb for each inch >5 ft ± 10% for large or small frame. *Male IBW* = 106 lb for 5 ft + 6 lb for each inch >5 ft ± 10% for large or small frame $\%\text{IBW} = \frac{\text{actual weight}}{\text{ideal body weight}} \times 100$	
3. Measure midarm circumference (MAC) to determine skeletal muscle mass: a. Instruct client to hang upper arm in an independent position with elbow at 90° angle and palms up.	Refer to Table 18-1 for reference data, and compare to client's prior measurements.	MAC decreases with malnutrition and increases with fat and muscle hypertrophy.

Table 18-1. Midarm Circumference (cm)

Age (years)	*Percentile*		
	50th	***15th***	***5th***
Males			
18–24	30.7	27.6	25.7
25–34	32.0	28.9	27.0
35–44	32.7	29.5	27.8
45–54	32.0	28.9	26.7
55–64	31.7	28.2	25.6
65–74	30.7	27.3	25.3
Females			
18–24	26.4	23.5	22.1
25–34	27.8	24.8	23.3
35–44	29.2	25.8	24.1
45–54	30.3	26.6	24.3
55–64	30.2	26.1	23.9
65–74	29.9	26.2	23.8

(Source: Bishop CW, Bowen PE, and Ritchey SJ. (1981) American Journal of Clinical Nutrition 34:2530.)

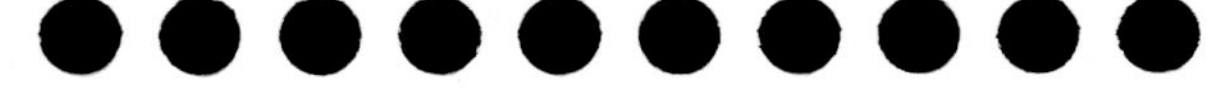

II. Objective Data: Assessment Techniques *(continued)*

Procedure	*Normal Findings*	*Deviations from Normal*
b. Find midpoint of nondominant arm halfway between the top of the acromion process and olecranon process (Fig. 18-1). Mark midpoint, and measure MAC while client flexes arm (Fig. 18-2).		
4. Measure triceps skinfold (TSF) to determine subcutaneous fat stores by: a. Instructing client to hang nondominant arm freely. b. Grasp skinfold and subcutaneous fat between thumb and forefinger 1 cm above midpoint mark.	Refer to Table 18-2 for reference data, and compare to client's prior measurements.	Refer to Table 18-2 for reference data, and compare to client's prior measurements.

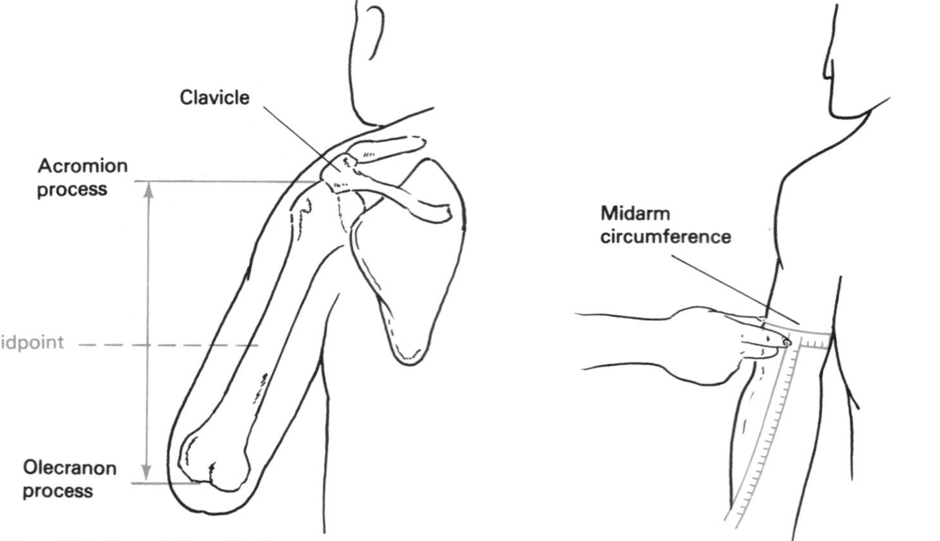

Figure 18-1. Determining midpoint to measure MAC.

Figure 18-2. Measuring midarm circumference.

Table 18-2. Triceps Skinfold (mm)

Age (years)	*Percentile*		
	50th	***15th***	***5th***
Males			
18–24	9.5	6.0	4.0
25–34	12.0	6.0	4.5
35–44	12.0	7.0	5.0
45–54	11.0	7.0	5.0
55–64	11.0	6.5	5.0
65–74	11.0	6.5	4.5
Females			
18–24	18.0	12.0	9.4
25–34	21.0	13.5	10.5
35–44	23.0	16.0	12.0
45–54	25.0	17.0	13.0
55–64	25.0	16.0	11.0
65–74	23.0	16.0	11.5

(Source: Bishop CW, Bowen PE, and Ritchey SJ. (1981) American Journal of Clinical Nutrition 34:2530.)

Procedure	Normal Findings	Deviations from Normal
Pull skin away from muscle, and apply calipers (Fig. 18-3). Read after 2–3 seconds. (Ask client to flex arm after you grasp skinfold. You still have the muscle if you feel a contraction.) *Note:* Three repeated measurements can be averaged for increased accuracy.		
5. Use the following formula to calculate the midarm muscle circumference: MAMC (cm) = MAC (cm) − [0.314 × TSF (cm)]	Refer to Table 18-3 for reference data, and compare to client's previous measurements.	Refer to Table 18-3 for reference data, and compare to client's previous measurements.

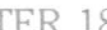

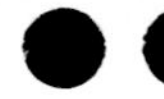

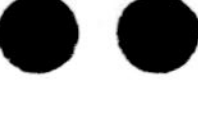

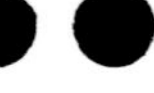

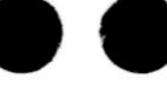

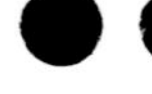

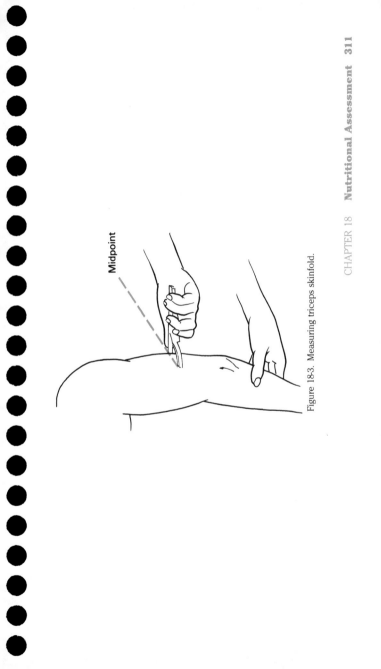

Figure 18-3. Measuring triceps skinfold.

Table 18-3. Midarm Muscle Circumference (cm)

Age (years)	Percentile 50th	15th	5th
Males			
18–24	27.2	25.0	23.5
25–34	28.0	25.8	24.2
35–44	28.7	26.2	25.0
45–54	28.1	25.6	24.0
55–64	27.9	25.4	22.8
65–74	26.9	24.3	22.5
Females			
18–24	20.6	18.8	17.7
25–34	21.4	19.3	18.3
35–44	22.0	19.7	18.5
45–54	22.2	19.9	18.8
55–64	22.6	20.1	18.6
65–74	22.5	20.0	18.6

(Source: Bishop CW, Bowen PE, and Ritchey SJ. (1981) American Journal of Clinical Nutrition 34:2530.)

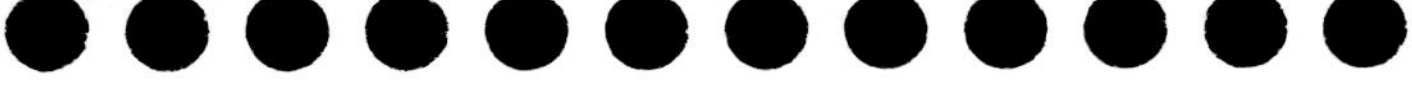

II. Objective Data: Assessment Techniques *(continued)*

Procedure	*Normal Findings*	*Deviations from Normal*
C. Assess client's dietary requirements and intake by asking client to keep 3-day diary of food and fluid intake.		
1. Calculate client's daily caloric requirements with following formula:	Meets caloric requirements	Consumes more or less than caloric requirements for age, height, body build, and weight
Multiply IBW in lb × cal/lb of IBW based on sex and activity level found in Table 18-4.		
Compare daily caloric requirements with client's daily consumption. (Refer to Appendix IX to estimate caloric intake.)		
2. Compare client's intake to USDA recommended food guidelines (Table 18-5). (Refer to Appendix VIII.)	Consumes 2 milks, 2 meats, 4 fruits or vegetables, and 4 grains per day	Consumes more or less than 2 milks, 2 meats, 4 fruits or vegetables, and 4 grains per day

Table 18-4. USDA Guidelines for Calculating Calorie Requirements (cal/lb IBW)

Activity	*Male*	*Female*
Sedentary	16	14
Moderate	21	18
Heavy	28	22

Based on activity level, multiply ideal body weight (IBW) in lb by appropriate number of calories/lb according to gender.

Table 18-5. USDA Food Guidelines

Food Guide Pyramid

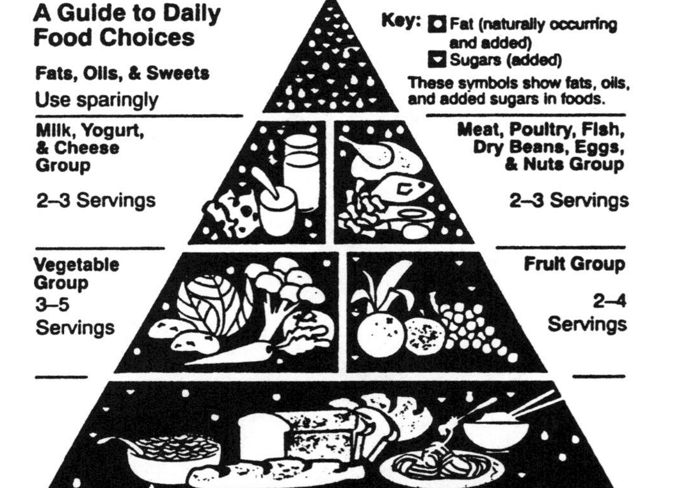
A Guide to Daily Food Choices
Fats, Oils, & Sweets
Use sparingly
Key: Fat (naturally occurring and added)
Sugars (added)
These symbols show fats, oils, and added sugars in foods.
Milk, Yogurt, & Cheese Group
2–3 Servings
Meat, Poultry, Fish, Dry Beans, Eggs, & Nuts Group
2–3 Servings
Vegetable Group
3–5 Servings
Fruit Group
2–4 Servings

Bread, Cereal, Rice, & Pasta Group 6–11 Servings

Pediatric Variations

Physiologic Growth Patterns

- Growth is most rapid during the first year of life.
- Birth weight doubles at age 4 to 6 months and triples by 1 year.
- Length increases 50% the first year of life.
- Teeth erupt first year of life.
- Growth decreases from ages 1 to 6 years, but biting, chewing, and swallowing abilities increase.
- Muscle mass and bone density increase from ages 1 to 6 years.
- There is a latent uneven period of growth from ages 1 to 12 years.
- Permanent teeth erupt at ages 6 to 12 years.
- School-aged children tolerate larger, less frequent meals.
- Nutritional needs increase during growth spurts (ages 10 to 15 years for girls and ages 12 to 19 years for boys).

Dietary Requirements

- Allow 1000 calories plus 100 more per each year of age (e.g., a 5 year old needs 1500 calories per day).
- Children need 3 milks, 2 meats, 4 fruits or vegetables, and 4 grains per day.
- Adolescents need 4 milks, 2 meats, 4 fruits or vegetables, and 4 grains per day.
- The American Academy of Pediatrics recommends infants be breast-fed the first year of life. Solid foods should not be introduced before ages 4 to 6 months.

Assessment Techniques

Infants: Use pediatric pan scale. Obtain weight, length, and head circumference. Identify type of feeding and iron source.

Children and adolescents: Weigh child and obtain height. Identify adequacy of meals and snacks and source of iron, calories, and protein.

Geriatric Variations

- Elderly clients may have atrophy on dorsum of hands even with good nutrition.
- Assess for poor-fitting dentures and decreased ability to taste.
- Elderly tend to eat less and more irregularly as they get older. This tends to increase with social isolation.
- Elderly have decreased peristalsis and nerve sensation, which may lead to constipation. Encourage fluids and dietary bulk to avoid laxative abuse.
- Caloric requirements decrease in response to a decreased basal metabolic rate, decreased activity, and change in body composition. A 10% decrease in calories is recommended for people ages 51 to 75 and a 20% to 25% decrease in calories for people over age 75.
- A decrease in mobility and vision may impair the ability to purchase and prepare food.
- Sensory taste losses may lead to anorexia.
- Fifty percent of elderly are thought to be economically deprived, which may affect nutrition when meats and milks are omitted from diet to save money.
- Drugs may alter appetite, taste, and digestion.
- Dietary recall may be difficult for the elderly.
- Skinfold measurements are often inaccurate due to changes in subcutaneous fat.

Cultural Variations

- Great variations may be seen in nutritional preferences, eating habits, and patterns of various groups (Andrews and Boyle, 1995; Giger and Davidhizar, 1991).
- Foods, beverages, and medications are classified as hot/cold by many Asians and Hispanics (e.g., yin/yang by Chinese); it is very important for these clients to seek a balanced consumption based on these theories.
- Many non-northern Europeans have some degree of lactose intolerance.*
- Classification of "food" and "non-food" items vary in cultures.
- Cultural or religious dietary rules or laws are of great importance to some groups (e.g., Orthodox Jews).
- Some groups may have diseases precipitated by certain foods or medications (e.g., G-6-PD deficiency; lactose deficiency).
- Some cultural food preferences are contraindicated in specific disease states (e.g., Japanese client with hypertension, who consumes high sodium soy sauce).

Possible Related Collaborative Problems

Hypoglycemia
Hyperglycemia
Electrolyte imbalance
Anemia

*Clients with lactose intolerance may be able to consume yogurt, buttermilk, fermented cheese, and acidophilus milk, or they may use products such as chewable tablets or liquid drops to act in place of the lactose enzyme.

Teaching Tips for Selected Nursing Diagnoses

Nursing Diagnoses	Teaching Tips
Adult Client	
NURSING DIAGNOSIS: Opportunity to enhance nutritional-metabolic pattern	Encourage proper oral hygiene. Teach nutritional guidelines: • Eat a variety of foods from the 5 food groups. • Strive to maintain a healthy weight. • Eat plenty of vegetables, fruits, and grains. • Choose diet low in fats, saturated fats, and cholesterol. • Encourage starches and fibers. • Avoid excessive sugar and salt. • Limit alcoholic intake (recommended by U.S. Department of Agriculture, U.S. Department of Health and Human Services, Nutrition and Your Health: Dietary Guidelines for Americans, 1990). Teach client how to get the most for his or her food dollar and how to read food labels, and teach ways to maintain nutrients in foods: • Buy frozen vegetables and ripe produce. • Encourage proper food storage and preparation to retain nutritional value. • Teach how to prepare low-fat foods: Suggest substituting applesauce or yogurt for butter when baking. Use bouillon or tomato juice instead of oil for sautéing. Use herbs and spices to replace the fat with flavor.

Nursing Diagnoses	Teaching Tips
NURSING DIAGNOSIS: Altered Nutrition: More than body requirements	Provide client with information on social support groups. Teach client self-assessment and rewarding techniques when proper nutrition is followed. Teach client how to calculate caloric intake and caloric expenditure and how to explore forms of exercise that meet client's needs. Assist client to replace frequent unhealthy snacking with nutritious snacks. Teach dietary guidelines and food choices for Americans recommended by the U.S. Department of Health and Human Services.
Pediatric Client	
NURSING DIAGNOSIS: Altered Nutrition: Potential for more than body requirements	Teach parents to avoid overfeeding infants. Encourage proper formula dilution. Teach avoidance of empty caloric foods. Discourage use of food for rewarding behavior.
NURSING DIAGNOSIS: Risk for Altered Nutrition: Less than body requirements	Teach parents to avoid restricting normal intake of fat. Teach that low-fat diets are dangerous to growing infants because fat is essential to metabolism of some vitamins and other substances and to hormone production associated with growth and development.

CHAPTER 19

Maternal Physical Assessment

Pregnancy produces changes in every body system. FIndings in a physical assessment that would be considered abnormal in the nonpregnant client may be a result of pregnancy and not an abnormal state. In this chapter the physical changes that occur in a woman as a result of pregnancy are identified as Normal Variations. Changes that are not a result of pregnancy or that represent an abnormal state during pregnancy are identified as Deviations from Normal.

For the sake of brevity, those systems described previously will not be repeated. Only variations of pregnancy will be noted. For procedures, the reader is referred to sections describing assessment of specific body systems.

During pregnancy, physical assessment should be performed every month for the first 28 weeks, every 2 weeks from week 28 to week 36, and then every week. More frequent examinations may be indicated for pregnancies at risk.

This chapter is divided into four sections; Prenatal Maternal Assessment, Prenatal Fetal Assessment, Intrapartal Maternal Assessment, and Postpartal Maternal Assessment.

Prenatal Maternal Assessment

Equipment Needed

See Chapters 4 through 14 for specific body system to be assessed.

I. Subjective Data: Focus Questions

A. *Past pregnancies:* Outcome of each? Number of living children? Complications? Length of labor? Years since last pregnancy?

B. *Current pregnancy:* Estimated due date. Confirmed by ultrasound? Problems during pregnancy? Cramping or bleeding? Planned pregnancy? Date of first prenatal visit? Prenatal education? Concurrent disease? Medications?

II. Objective Data: Systems Review

System	Normal Variations	Deviations from Normal
A. General physical survey		
1. Age	Ideal childbearing years: 16 to 35	Younger than 16 or older than 35: increased risk to mother and baby
2. Weight	Average weight gain: 25–35 lbs First trimester—2–4 lbs Second trimester—11 lbs (1 lb/wk) Third trimester—11 lbs (1 lb/wk)	Prepregnant weight <100 lb or >200 lb; sudden gain of more than 2 lb/wk; weight loss or failure to gain

II. Objective Data: Systems Review *(continued)*

System	*Normal Variations*	*Deviations from Normal*
3. Blood pressure	Range of 90–139/60–89; falls during second trimester; prepregnant level first and third trimesters	$\geq$140/90 or increase of 30 mm Hg above baseline systolic or 15 mm Hg above baseline diastolic taken with client in side-lying position
4. Pulse	60–90 beats/min; may increase 10–15 beats/min higher than prepregnant levels	Irregularities; persistently <60 or >100 at rest
5. Behavior	First trimester: tired, ambivalent Second trimester: introspective, energetic Third trimester: restless, preparing for baby, labile moods (father may experience some of these same behaviors)	Denial of pregnancy, withdrawal, depression, psychosis
B. Skin color	Linea nigra (Fig. 19-1); striae gravidarum (Fig. 19-1); chloasma (Fig. 19-2); spider nevi	Pale, yellow
C. Head and neck		
1. Nose	Nasal stuffiness, nosebleeds	Facial edema, headache
2. Eyes		Blurred vision, visual spots
3. Neck	Slight enlargement of thyroid	

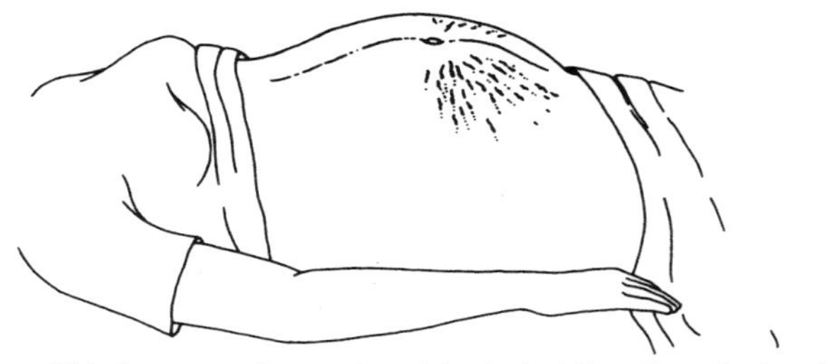

Figure 19-1. Pregnancy pigmentation: abdominal midline (linea nigra) and striae gravidarum. Dark-haired, brown skinned women are more prone to pregnancy pigmentation.

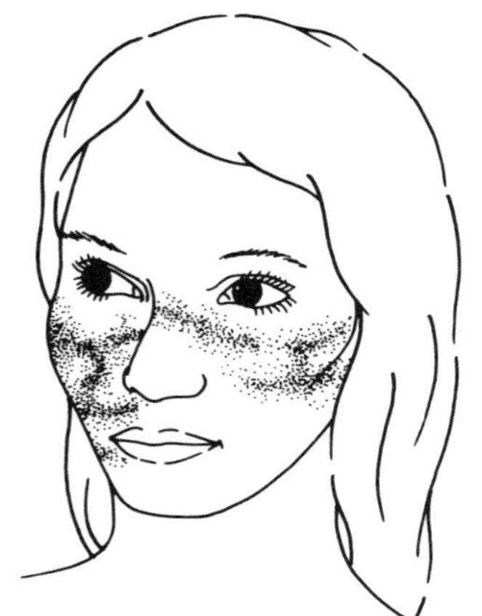

Figure 19-2. Marked chloasma of pregnancy.

II. Objective Data: Systems Review *(continued)*

System	*Normal Variations*	*Deviations from Normal*
D. Cardiovascular system		
1. Heart	Short systolic murmurs	Progressive dyspnea, palpitations, markedly decreased activity tolerance
2. Blood volume	Increases throughout pregnancy; peaks at 30% to 50% above prepregnant levels at 32–34 weeks	
E. Peripheral vascular system	Late pregnancy: dependent edema, varicose veins, supine hypotension	Perineal varicosities; calf pain; generalized edema; diminished pedal pulses
F. Respiratory system	Increased anteroposterior diameter; thoracic breathing; slight hyperventilation; shortness of breath in late pregnancy	Dyspnea
G. Breasts	Increased size and nodularity; tenderness; prominent vascularization; colostrum in third trimester; darkening of nipples and areola	Localized redness; localized pain and warmth
H. Gastrointestinal system	Nausea and vomiting, increased saliva, heartburn, bloating, constipation	Severe epigastric pain, severe nausea and vomiting

I. Genitourinary-reproductive systems	Urinary frequency in first and third trimesters; increased pigmentation of vulva and vagina; increased vaginal discharge	Flank pain, burning on urination, oliguria, proteinuria, purulent discharge, vaginal bleeding
J. Musculoskeletal system	Relaxation of pelvic joints: "waddling" gait; increased lumbar curve, backache; diastasis recti, leg cramps	
K. Neurological system	(No changes from normal)	Hyperactive reflexes, clonus

Prenatal Fetal Assessment

Equipment

- Bed or examination table
- Drape
- Pillow
- Paper centimeter tape measure
- Fetoscope or Doppler

I. Subjective Data: Focus Questions

Has the baby been active? First time movement felt?

II. Objective Data: Assessment Techniques

Procedure	Normal Findings	Deviations from Normal
A. *Inspection*		
With client in a supine position and head slightly elevated on a pillow, inspect the abdomen for shape and contour of fetus. (Time spent in the supine position should be minimal. This position puts the weight of the baby and uterus on the aorta and obstructs blood flow.)		
B. *Palpation*		
Using both hands, gently palpate the outline of the fetus and the top of the uterus (fundus). Using the centimeter tape, measure from the top of the symphysis pubis to the top of the uterine fundus (Fig. 19-3).		
Measure fundal height and multiply by $^8/_7$ (this equals weeks gestation; see Fig. 19-4).	Accurate within 4 weeks until 36 weeks. Obesity or extremes in height may alter findings.	Lag in progression; sudden increase in size
C. *Auscultation*		
With Doppler or fetoscope, listen for fetal heartbeat. Locate fundus; begin listening halfway between the fundus and the pubis. Work outward in widening circles until a beating sound is heard. Compare the beating with the maternal pulse. If it is different, count beats for a full minute.		
Auscultate fetal heart rate for the following:		
Presence	Audible at 15–20 weeks gestation with fetoscope; audible at 10–12 weeks gestation with Doppler	Absence after 20th week of gestation

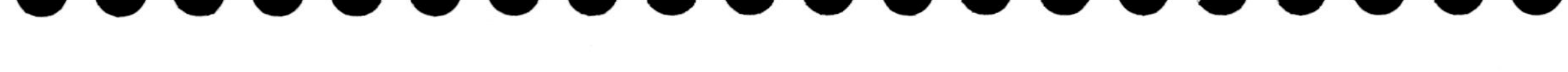

Rate	Very rapid initially; gradually slows to 120–160 beats/min at term; increase with fetal movement	Less than 120 beats/min; no change or decrease with movement
Rhythm	Irregular	A marked variance or variance less than 5 beats/min

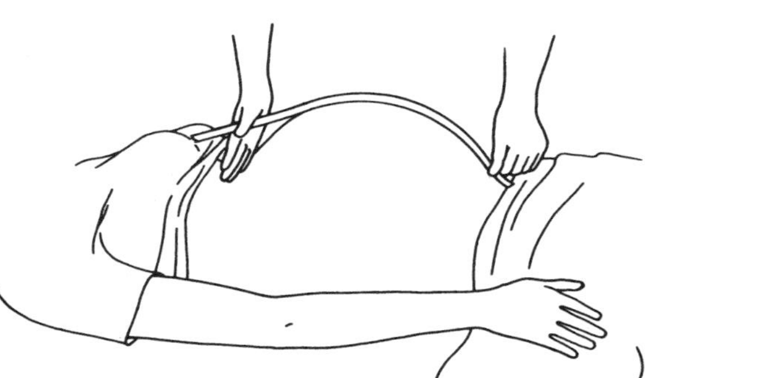

Figure 19-3. Measurement of fundal height from the symphysis.

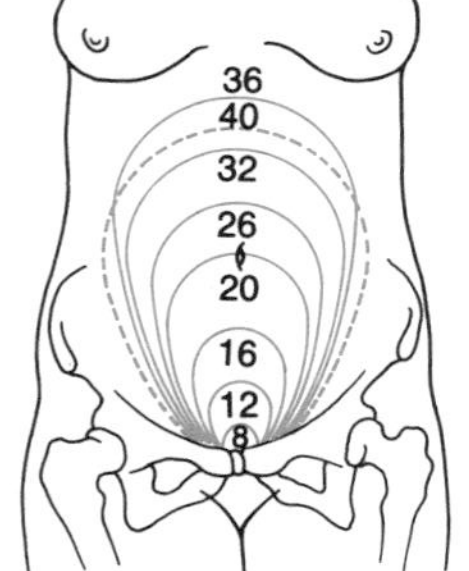

Figure 19-4. Approximate height of the fundus at various weeks of pregnancy.

Cultural Variations

- RH-negative blood is rare in nonwhite groups
- Dizygote twinning is higher in blacks than whites or Asians

Possible Related Collaborative Problems

Potential complications:

Bleeding disorder of pregnancy:
- Spontaneous abortion
- Placenta previa
- Abruptio placentae

Pregnancy-induced hypertension (PIH)

Dehydration

Gestational diabetes

Preexisting medical conditions:
- Hyperglycemia/hypoglycemia
- Hypertension
- Renal malfunctioning
- Cardiac conditions

Hyperemesis gravidum

Ectopic pregnancy

Teaching Tips for Selected Nursing Diagnoses

Nursing Diagnoses	Teaching Tips
NURSING DIAGNOSIS: Risk for ineffective management of therapeutic regimen during pregnancy	Inform client of normal variations during the prenatal period. Also inform client of those abnormal symptoms to be reported immediately. Encourage client to write down questions; provide time to discuss them. Instruct client on methods to cope with normal variations (e.g., nausea and vomiting). Encourage attendance at prenatal classes and appropriate reading material.

PRENATAL NURSING DIAGNOSIS: Risk for altered nutrition: Less than body requirements related to increased metabolism and fetal demands.	Diet should be selected from Basic Five Food Groups, with an additional 300 calories per day over recommended daily allowances. A balanced diet should provide all essential nutrients during pregnancy except folic acid and iron. These should be supplemented throughout pregnancy, because adequate amounts are closely related to fetal well-being and pregnancy outcome.
NURSING DIAGNOSIS: Body Image Disturbance related to effects of physical changes during pregnancy	An exercise program started early in pregnancy and continued throughout will help maintain muscle tone and facilitate a return to prepregnant size after delivery. Exercise has the added benefit of creating a feeling of well-being and satisfaction. Exercise programs should be approved by the obstetrician prior to initiation. In general, those activities practiced prior to pregnancy can be continued unless they have a potential of causing physical harm to mother and baby. Allow client to express her feelings about body changes, and reassure her that most changes are reversible or minimized after delivery. Emphasize positive changes.
NURSING DIAGNOSIS: Opportunity to enhance parenting	Beginning education on growth and development of fetus and infant early in pregnancy can provide an opportunity for prospective parents to anticipate and understand development and expected patterns of developmental skill mastery.
NURSING DIAGNOSIS: Opportunity to enhance infant nutrition	The decision to breast or bottle feed the infant is usually made during or prior to pregnancy. Providing factual information with an opportunity for questions and answers early in pregnancy will facilitate a decision best suited to the client's needs and lifestyle.

Intrapartal Maternal Assessment

During the intrapartal period, an initial physical assessment should be done on admission to the labor room, and findings should be compared to those of the prenatal period. The order of the assessment will vary based on presenting signs of labor.

Equipment Needed

- Bed with pillow
- Sterile examination glove
- Lubricant
- Electronic fetal monitor or Doppler
- Nitrazine paper
- Reflex hammer

I. Subjective Data: Focus Questions

Gravida? Para? Age? Estimated date of confinement (EDC)? When did contractions begin? Rupture of membranes? Color of fluids? Vaginal bleeding and amount? Frequency and duration of contractions? Prenatal care? Problems with this pregnancy? Duration and outcome of previous labors? Childbirth preparation? Blood type and Rh? Concurrent disease?

II. Objective Data: Assessment Techniques

Procedure	Normal Findings	Deviations from Normal

Abdominal Assessment

A. Inspection

Have client completely undress except for gown. Place in a supine position with head slightly elevated. Knees and hips should be flexed with feet resting on mattress. Examination with the client in this position should be performed as rapidly as possible to prevent supine hypotension or fetal compromise.

Inspect abdomen for the following:

Procedure	Normal Findings	Deviations from Normal
Size	Large variation; fundus just below xiphoid process	Small or large for gestational age
Shape	Fetal outline longitudinal	Fetal outline horizontal

B. Palpation

With client on back and head slightly elevated, place fingertips on fundus of uterus. During a contraction, the fundus becomes firm. Client should relate when she feels a contraction start and when it ends. Time seconds from beginning to end of contractions (duration). Calculate elapsed time from beginning of one contraction to beginning of another (frequency). Do this for several contractions in sequence to determine regularity. During contraction, gently push in on fundus with fingertips and note degree to which fundus indents (intensity). A large amount of subcutaneous tissue over the fundus may interfere with accurate assessment of intensity. Palpate several contractions in a row. To palpate bladder, gently push in on abdomen directly above symphysis pubis and release. Note degree of resistance met.

II. Objective Data: Assessment Techniques

Procedure	Normal Findings	Deviations from Normal
1. Palpate fundus for the following:		
a. Frequency of contractions	As labor progresses, contractions gradually get closer together, in a regular pattern progressing to every 2 to 3 minutes. May be less frequent during second stage.	Irregular pattern; more frequent than every 2 minutes
b. Duration of contractions	Gradually increases to 60–90 sec as labor progresses	No increase; greater than 90 seconds
c. Intensity of contractions	Gradually become stronger; fundus feels hard (rocklike); internal pressure monitor 40–60 mm Hg	No increase; greater than 60 mm Hg

Note: Contraction frequency and duration may be monitored with an electronic fetal monitor tocodynamometer. However, intensity can only be determined with an intrauterine pressure catheter.

Procedure	Normal Findings	Deviations from Normal
2. Palpate above symphysis pubis for the bladder.	Soft, spongy	Bouncy, full

C. Auscultation

Locate fetal heart rate (see prenatal section) and apply external fetal monitor ultrasound transducer or Doppler. Fetal heart rate (FHR) must be monitored every 5 minutes during the second stage of labor. For any questionable FHR, fetus at risk, or difficulty obtaining a fetal heart rate recording, an internal fetal electrode should be used for monitoring after membranes have ruptured.

Monitor fetal heart rate for the following:

Baseline rate (must be determined by a 10-minute strip)	120–160 bpm	<120 or >160 bpm for a 10-minute period
Baseline variability (measurable only with internal fetal electrode)	5–25 bpm	<5 bpm for longer than 20 minutes and not associated with maternal medication
Periodic changes	Periodic acceleration (increased FHR with fetal movement, stimulation, or contractions) Early onset deceleration (mirrors contraction and occurs in late first stage and second stage of labor)	Periodic decelerations (decreased FHR with contractions, repetitive variable decelerations, late decelerations; prolonged or slow return to baseline; associated loss of variability)

Procedure	Normal Findings	Deviations from Normal
Perineal Assessment		
A. Inspection		
With client in a supine position, have her rest her feet on the bed with knees and hips flexed. Instruct client to relax and separate knees. If discharge is noted, touch it with a strip of Nitrazine paper to check for ruptured bag of waters.		
1. Observe perineum for the following:		
a. Lesions	None	Vesicles, warts, open sores
b. Discharge	Bloody mucus; clear or milky fluid; amniotic fluid will turn Nitrazine paper blue	Bright red blood; purulent fluid; green or brown fluid Lubricant or blood may give a false-positive result with Nitrazine paper
c. Swelling	May be present in second stage of labor	Present before second stage of labor
2. Observe vaginal opening for the following:		
a. Shape	As fetal head descends, perineum flattens and bulges.	
b. Fetal parts	Occiput becomes visible during second stage of labor.	Fetal hand or foot; loop of umbilical cord

B. Palpation

Have client separate knees, and instruct her to relax perineum. Put on sterile examination glove, and lubricate index and middle fingers. Gently insert fingers into vagina and palpate cervix and fetal presenting part. Insert finger between cervix and presenting part, and rotate entire circumference of cervix. This examination should be performed on admission and thereafter only when behavior and contraction pattern indicate progression of labor.

1. Palpate cervix for the following:

a. Position	In early labor, cervix may be in posterior vaginal vault. It becomes more anterior as labor progresses.	
b. Effacement	Primipara: Effacement before dilatation Multipara: Effacement and dilatation simultaneous	Swelling of part or all of cervix
c. Dilatation (in cm)	Primipara: Average 1 cm/hr; may be slower in early phase Multipara: Average 1.5 cm/hr	Failure to progress with active labor longer than 24 hours; complete dilatation in less than 3 hours of labor

II. Objective Data: Assessment Techniques *(continued)*

Procedure	*Normal Findings*	*Deviations from Normal*
2. Palpate presenting part of the fetus for the following:		
a. Amniotic membrane	If intact, can be felt over presenting part; may rupture prior to or during labor	
b. Presentation	Cephalic; should feel skull, suture lines, and one or both fontanelles (Fig. 19-5); caput succedaneum may mask landmarks	Breech: soft tissue, anus, or testicles; other small parts such as hands, feet
c. Position	Cephalic; posterior fontanelle felt in anterior position, anterior fontanelle in posterior position	Anterior fontanelle in anterior position; fontanelles in transverse position
d. Station (Fig. 19-6)	Primipara: 0 station; gradually descends during second stage Multipara: May be—1 station or higher at onset of labor	Failure to descend to 0 station during first stage of labor; failure to descend during second stage with pushing longer than 2 hours
e. Umbilical cord	Not palpable	May feel loop or pulsations

Note: If painless, bright red vaginal bleeding occurs, vaginal examination should be omitted. If fetal gestational age is less than 34 weeks and membranes have ruptured with no evidence of labor, vaginal examination should be omitted.

A

B

C

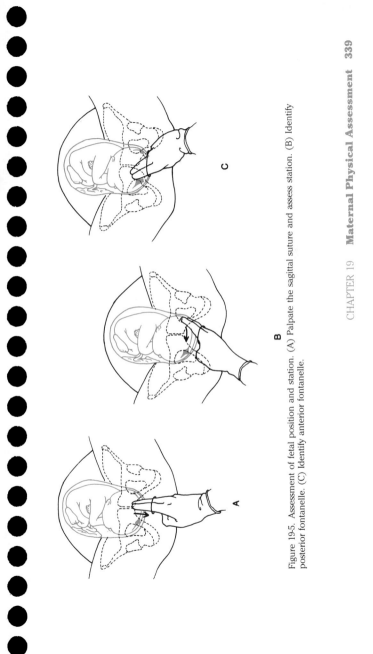

Figure 19-5. Assessment of fetal position and station. (A) Palpate the sagittal suture and assess station. (B) Identify posterior fontanelle. (C) Identify anterior fontanelle.

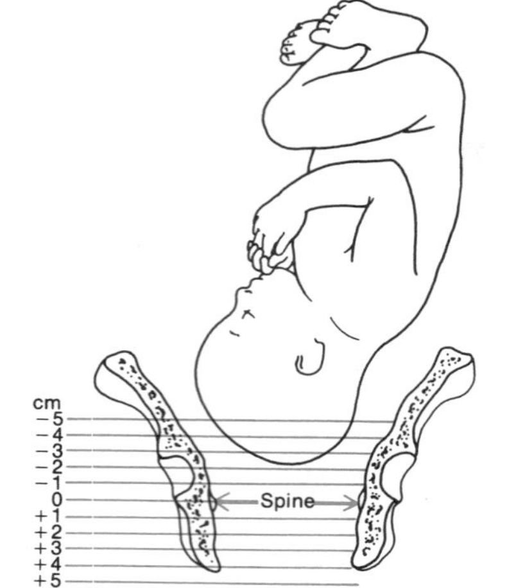

Figure 19-6. Measuring station of the fetal head while it is descending.

II. Objective Data: Assessment Techniques *(continued)*

Procedure	Normal Findings	Deviations from Normal
Peripheral Vascular Assessment		
A. Inspection		
With client in semi-Fowler's position, observe face, hands, legs, and feet.		
1. Observe face for the following:		
a. Color	Pink	Red, pale
b. Edema	None	Periorbital edema
2. Observe extremities for the following:		
a. Color	Pink	Pale, blue
b. Swelling	Dependent in ankles	Swelling in the tibia or hands, not relieved by elevating
B. Auscultation		
With client in a side-lying position, auscultate blood pressure between contractions.		
Auscultate BP every hour or more often as indicated	Prenatal level increased during contractions	$\geq$140/90 or increase of 30 mm Hg systolic or 15 mm Hg diastolic
C. Percussion		
Percuss extremities for reflexes and clonus.	See Chapter 3 for normal findings.	Hyperreflexia or clonus

II. Objective Data: Assessment Techniques *(continued)*

Procedure	Normal Findings	Deviations from Normal
Behavioral Assessment		
Observe behavior of client during all stages of labor. Observe for behavior changes:		
Early labor (1–4 cm)	Excited, happy	Irrational
Active labor (4–7 cm)	Cooperative; increased dependence on support person	Uncooperative, psychotic
Transition (7–10 cm)	Irritable, inner focused, hopeless	Confused

Possible Related Collaborative Problems

Potential complications:

- Preeclampsia/eclampsia
- Bleeding disorders:
  - Placenta previa
  - Abruptio placentae
  - Uterine rupture
- Fetal malpresentation
- Fetal malposition
- Hypertension
- Fetal distress
- Labor dystocia
- Cephalopelvic disproportion
- Premature labor

Teaching Tips for Selected Nursing Diagnoses

Nursing Diagnoses	*Teaching Tips*
NURSING DIAGNOSIS: Acute pain related to uterine contractions	Instruct and demonstrate relaxation techniques. Provide feedback on muscle relaxation. Offer encouragement and support. Provide comfort measures such as gentle massage; temperature control; clean, dry, and wrinkle-free linens; ice chips or lip lubricant. The laboring woman should be encouraged to assume varying positions of comfort and ambulate unless complications contraindicate this. Provide analgesics as needed.
NURSING DIAGNOSIS: Fear related to unfamiliar environment, pain, and concern for fetal well-being	Orient to surroundings. Provide short and simple explanation for all procedures and encourage questions. Provide evidence of fetal well-being (monitor data). Encourage support person to stay with client. Client should not be left alone during active labor.
NURSING DIAGNOSIS: Risk for fluid Volume Deficit related to increased muscle activity, increased respiratory rate, nausea and vomiting, and decreased gastric motility or absorption	Offer small amounts of fluids such as ice chips or popsicles. Avoid solid foods, which are difficult to digest and often promote vomiting. Medicate if vomiting persists. Monitor for dehydration or decreased placental perfusion. Administer IV fluids as indicated.

Postpartal Maternal Assessment

The postpartum period begins with the delivery of the placenta and lasts an average of 6 weeks, during which time all body systems return to prepregnant levels. Some changes are rapid, and others occur over time. During the first 24 hours many drastic changes occur, and frequent assessment is essential.

Changes occurring as an expected part of postpartum recovery are identified as Normal Findings. The reader is referred to Chapter 3 for a more detailed description of technique for assessing various body systems.

I. Subjective Data: Focus Questions

Problems during pregnancy? Labor: Induction, augmentation, length of labor? Gravida, para? Method of delivery? Size of baby? Anesthesia/analgesia? Concurrent disease?

II. Objective Data: Assessment Techniques

Procedure	***Normal Findings***	***Deviations from Normal***
Monitor the following:		
Temperature	100.4°F (38°C) in first 24 hours	Higher than 100.4°F in first 24 hours or 100.4°F and above on any 2 of the first 10 days postpartum

Blood pressure	No change from prepregnant levels	Pregnancy-induced hypertension (PIH) can occur up to 48 hours postpartum. Persistent elevation of blood pressure from PIH beyond 48 hrs.
Pulse	Bradycardia (50 to 70 bpm) for 6–10 days	Tachycardia. Preexisting hypertension may be difficult to control. Postural hypotension may occur when assuming the upright position after delivery.
Weight	Initial 10–12 lb loss; 10–20 lb loss in next 6–8 weeks	
Behavior		
First 2 to 3 days postpartum	Preoccupied with food and sleep; passive and dependent	Psychosis
After 2 to 3 days postpartum	Increased interest in control of body functions, mothering skills; gradually includes others into social circle; transient depression, let down feeling, cries easily	Failure to assume maternal role; prolonged depression; unrealistic expectations of newborn

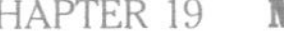

II. Objective Data: Assessment Techniques *(continued)*

Procedure	***Normal Findings***	***Deviations from Normal***
Breast Assessment		
A. Inspection		
With client in supine or semi-Fowler's position, inspect breasts.		
1. Nonnursing mother		
a. Size	May be enlarged initially; will gradually return to prepregnant size	Full; engorged
b. Shape	May sag	
c. Color	May have striae	Localized redness, tenderness
2. Nursing mother		
a. Size	Enlarged	
b. Texture	Increased nodularity	Heat, localized pain
c. Nipples	Everted, tender	Blisters, cracked, bleeding
d. Discharge	Colostrum; thin milk, may leak between feedings	Purulent
B. Palpation		
Gently palpate all quadrants of each breast.		
1. Nonnursing mother		
a. Tenderness	Soft	Full, tender
b. Texture	Nodular	Lumps, masses

2. Nursing mother		
a. Tenderness	Full, slightly tender	Painful
b. Texture	Small lumps	Hardened area, most often in upper, outer quadrant

Abdominal Assessment

A. Inspection

Place client in a supine position with knees extended and head slightly elevated on a pillow. Inspect abdomen for the following:

Size	Uterus visible, outlined unless obese; gradually recedes to prepregnant size with exercise (Fig. 19-7)	Distention
Color	Striae dark red or purple; recede to silvery or white and become smaller	Yellow, pale
Texture	Loose and flabby	Dry, cracked

B. Palpation

Have client empty bladder and assume supine position. Place one hand over lower abdomen above symphysis pubis to support uterus. With the fingertips of the other hand, locate the fundus. Start in the midline, slightly above the umbilicus, and press in and down. Work fingers gradually down toward the symphysis pubis until the fundus of the uterus is located. It should feel like a firm, round ball, similar to a grapefruit. Measure the distance above or below the umbilicus in finger breadths (Fig. 19-8). If the uterus is not firm, gently massage until firm; then gently push down on fundus and observe for expression of clots from the vagina.

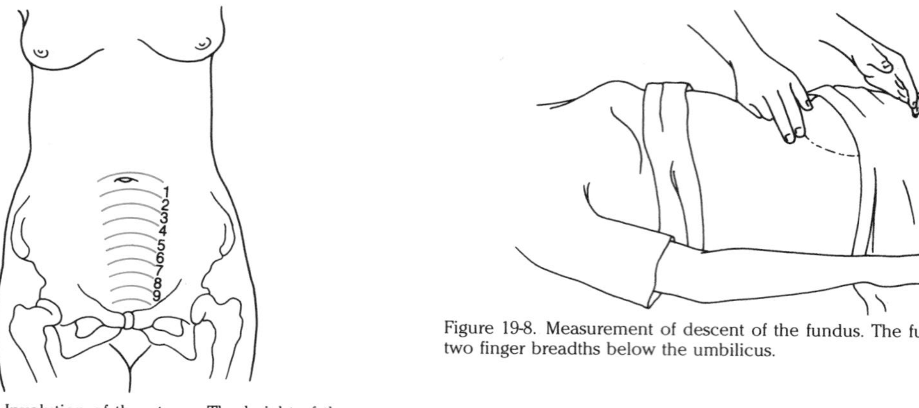

Figure 19-7. Involution of the uterus. The height of the fundus decreases about one finger breadth (approximately 1 cm) each day.

Figure 19-8. Measurement of descent of the fundus. The fundus is located two finger breadths below the umbilicus.

II. Objective Data: Assessment Techniques *(continued)*

Procedure	***Normal Findings***	***Deviations from Normal***
Palpate fundus for the following:		
Location	Midline	Deviated to left or right
Consistency	Firm; boggy to firm with massage; smooth surface	Boggy; does not stay firm after massage; lumpy
Height	Halfway between umbilicus and symphysis immediately after delivery; within 12 hours, at the umbilicus or 1 cm above; descends 1 cm/day	More than 1 cm above umbilicus; failure to descend
Expression of clots	Small clots or increased flow with massage	Large clots; continuous trickle of blood with firm fundus

II. Objective Data: Assessment Techniques *(continued)*

Procedure	Normal Findings	Deviations from Normal
Assessment of Face and Extremities		
A. Inspection		
To inspect the face and extremities, the supine position is preferred. Adequate light must be available.		
1. Inspect face for the following:		
a. Color	Petechiae after prolonged second stage of labor	Pale
b. Edema	None	Periorbital
2. Inspect extremities for the following:		
a. Color	Pink; red tones visible under dark pigmentation	Dusky, mottled
b. Edema	Slight pedal	Pitting edema, edema of hands
B. Palpation		
With legs extended, gently palpate calves. Place one hand on knee, and gently dorsiflex each foot. Palpate for the following:		
Tenderness	May have generalized muscle tenderness	Localized tenderness or pain
Texture	Smooth	Knots or lumps in calf
Homans' sign	Negative (no pain)	Positive (pain in calf)

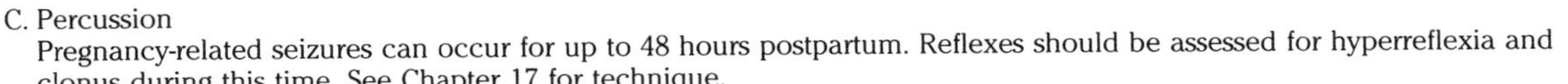

C. Percussion

Pregnancy-related seizures can occur for up to 48 hours postpartum. Reflexes should be assessed for hyperreflexia and clonus during this time. See Chapter 17 for technique.

Bladder Assessment

A. Inspection

Have client void within 4 hours after delivery or sooner if there are bleeding problems during the immediate postpartum period. Inspect voiding for

Amount	200 cc or more each voiding; diuresis of greater than 2000 cc in first 24 hours	Less than 100 cc per voiding; unable to void
Color	Yellow, clear; may be mixed with lochia	Dark, cloudy, bloody

B. Palpation

Have client empty bladder and assume supine position. Palpate for bladder above the symphysis pubis. If unable to void within 4 hours after delivery or if bladder is full, empty bladder with a catheter.

Palpate bladder	Nonpalpable	Spongy mass in lower abdomen

Procedure	*Normal Findings*	*Deviations from Normal*
Assessment of Perineum		
A. Inspection Have client turn to side and flex upper leg. Place one hand on upper buttock and gently separate so perineum is visible. Inspect perineum for the following:		
Approximation of episiotomy	Skin edges meet	Skin edges gap
Color	Pink to red	Purple, mottled
Swelling	Generalized swelling for 12–24 hours	Localized swelling with increased pain
Lochia	1–3 days: dark red; few small clots may increase during breast feeding Days 3–10: pinkish red Days 10–20: creamy yellow 4 to 8 peri pads in 1 day, gradually decreasing in amount	Purulent, large clots; return to dark red after several days; more than 8 peri pads per day or saturated pad in 1 hour
Odor	None; musky scent	Foul odor
Hemorrhoids	Small, nontender	Swollen, painful

Possible Related Collaborative Problems

Potential complications:

- Hemorrhage:
  - Uterine atony
  - Hematoma
  - Cervical/vaginal lacerations
- Urinary retention
- Breast engorgement/abscess
- Preeclampsia/eclampsia
- Retained placenta
- Infections
- Exacerbation of preexisting medical conditions:
  - Heart conditions
  - Hypertension
  - Hyperglycemia
  - Hypoglycemia

Teaching Tips for Selected Nursing Diagnoses

Nursing Diagnoses	***Teaching Tips***
NURSING DIAGNOSIS: Sleep Pattern Disturbance related to fatigue and increased need for sleep	All teaching sessions should be brief and reinforced with written information about infant care and self-care (e.g., care of breasts). Encourage mother to sleep when baby sleeps. Advise mother to avoid strenuous activities until 6-week postpartum physical examination. Enlist help of other family members.
NURSING DIAGNOSIS: Opportunity to enhance infant care and self-care	Demonstrate infant care and allow time for mother to practice. A follow-up phone call or home visit can assist in evaluation and reinforcement of information taught. Include fathers whenever possible.

Teaching Tips for Selected Nursing Diagnoses

Nursing Diagnoses	Teaching Tips
NURSING DIAGNOSIS: Family Coping: Potential for growth related to addition of family member and role changes	Discuss plans for incorporating new member into family. Offer suggestions to decrease sibling jealousy. Explore plans for infant care, division of labor, and changes in activities of daily living.
NURSING DIAGNOSIS: Opportunity to enhance parenting	Discuss normal growth and development of infant; emphasize things infant can do. Provide early and continued contact of infant and parents to maximize bonding. Teach parents skills needed to meet infant's physical and psychological needs.
NURSING DIAGNOSIS: Altered Parenting related to inadequate skills, unrealistic expectation of infant, stress, lack of adequate support	Be aware of risk factors for child abuse/neglect that may be evident during postpartal period. Explore resources available to parents, and make appropriate referrals for follow-up or support groups.
NURSING DIAGNOSIS: Ineffective Breastfeeding related to lack of knowledge	Clarify misconceptions, and provide instructions or proper technique. Assist with first feedings and problems such as soreness or difficulty grasping, etc.
NURSING DIAGNOSIS: Ineffective Infant Feeding Pattern	May use nipple with larger hole. Hold infant in upright position during feeding. Burp often (after every $\frac{1}{2}$ ounce). Needs frequent feedings with careful monitoring of intake and weight gain. May need to teach parents gavage feedings. If so, infant will attempt to nurse at each feeding and be gavage-fed remaining formula.

NURSING DIAGNOSIS:
Interrupted Breastfeeding

To continue breast milk supply mother should pump breasts at intervals similar to infant feeding patterns. Milk letdown is optimal immediately after infant contact. Mother should be relaxed and have privacy. If possible, both breasts should be emptied simultaneously. Increased fluid consumption is needed for milk production. To terminate breastfeeding mother should avoid any stimulation of breasts. Encourage well-supporting bra. Painful engorgement may be alleviated with analgesics and intermittent ice packs to breasts.

CHAPTER 20

Initial Newborn Physical Assessment

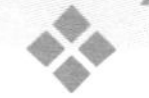

Equipment Needed

- Gloves
- Stethoscope
- Tape measure

I. Subjective Data: Focus Questions

Prenatal history: Gravida? Para? Estimated date of confinement (EDC)? Gestational age? Maternal history? Risk factors? Prenatal exposure to drugs? Complications? Blood type? Maternal testing?

Labor and delivery history: Date, time, type of delivery? Prolonged labor? Narcotics? Time of rupture of membranes? Intrapartum complications? Shoulder dystocia?

Postpartum history: Apgar scores? Respiratory effort? Resuscitation efforts? Medications? Procedures performed? Evidence of injury? Void? Stool?

Social: Parent interaction? Significant others? Cultural variations? Type of infant feeding? Male circumcision requested?

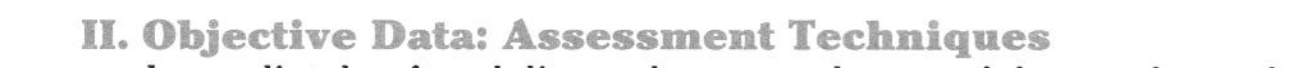

II. Objective Data: Assessment Techniques

Immediately after delivery the general state of the newborn should be evaluated while the infant is in supine position under a radiant warmer with the temperature probe attached to the abdomen. Apgar scores (Table 20-1) are assigned at 1 and 5 minutes after delivery.

Procedure	*Normal Findings*	*Deviations from Normal*
Apgar Score Assessment		
A. Auscultate apical pulse	>100	<100 or absent
B. Inspect chest/abdomen for respiratory effort	Crying	Absent, slow, irregular respirations
C. Stroke back or soles of feet	Crying	Grimace, no response
D. Inspect muscle tone by extending legs/arms. Observe degree of flexion and resistance in extremities	Extremities flexed, active movement	Moderate degree of flexion, limp
E. Inspect body/extremities for skin color	Full body pink, extremities acrocyanosis	Cyanosis, pale
F. Determine Total Apgar Score at 1 and 5 minutes after birth (see Table 20-1)	8–10	<8

After the Apgar Score has been assigned, a thorough assessment is performed on the newborn: vital signs and measurements, physical examination assessments, and gestational age assessment are performed.

Table 20-1. Apgar Score

	Scores 0	*Scores 1*	*Scores 2*
Heart rate	Absent	<100 beats/min	>100 beats/min
Respiratory rate	Absent	Slow, irregular	Good lusty cry
Reflex Irritability	No response	Grimace, some motion	Cry, cough
Muscle tone	Flaccid, limp	Flexion of extremities	Active flexion
Color	Cyanotic, pale	Pink body, acrocyanosis	Pink body/extremities

II. Objective Data: Assessment Techniques *(continued)*

Procedure	*Normal Findings*	*Deviations from Normal*
Assessment of Vital Signs and Measurements		
A. Monitor axillary temperature	(36.4° to 37.2°C) 97.5° to 99°F	(<36.4° or >37.2°C) <97.5° or >99°F
B. Inspect and auscultate breath sounds. Monitor respiratory rate	Easy, nonlabored, clear bilaterally 30–60 breaths/min	Labored, nasal flaring, rhonchi, rales, retractions, grunting <30 or >60 breaths/min
C. Auscultate apical pulse	Regular 120–160 beats/min (100 sleeping, 180 crying.)	Irregular <100 or >180 beats/min
D. Weigh newborn (unclothed) using a newborn scale	2500–4000 g	<2500 g >4000 g
E. Measure length (see Fig. 4-2)	44–55 cm	<44 cm >55 cm
F. Measure head circumference (see Fig. 4-2)	33–35.5 cm	<32 cm >37 cm
G. Measure chest circumference (see Fig. 4-2)	30–33 cm (1–2 cm < head)	<29 cm >34 cm

Procedure	Normal Findings	Deviations from Normal
Assessment of Gestational Age		
The newborn's gestational age is examined within 4 hours after birth to identify any potential age-related problems that may occur within the next few hours after birth. The newborn's neuromuscular and physical maturity is examined. After examination, boxes on the New Ballard Scoring Tool (Figs. 20-1 & 20-2) that most closely describe and depict the newborn's neuromuscular and physical maturity are marked and scores are assigned to assess gestational age.		
Neuromuscular Maturity (see Fig. 20-1)		
Assess each of the following with the newborn in the supine position:		
A. *Posture:* With newborn undisturbed	Arms/legs flexed	Arms/legs limp, extended away from body
B. *Square window:* Bend wrist toward ventral forearm until resistance is met. Measure angle (see Fig. 20-3)	0–30°	>30°
C. *Arm recoil:* Bilaterally flex elbows up with hands next to shoulders and hold approximately 5 seconds. Extend arms down next to side, release. Observe elbow angle and recoil	Elbow angle <90°, rapid recoil to flexed state	Elbow angle >110°, delayed recoil

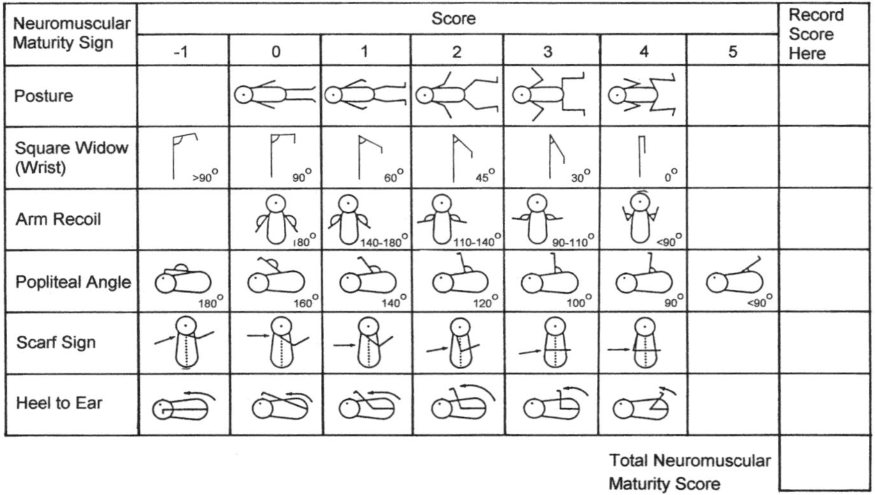

Neuromuscular Maturity Sign	Score							Record Score Here
	-1	0	1	2	3	4	5	
Posture								
Square Widow (Wrist)	>90°	90°	60°	45°	30°	0°		
Arm Recoil		180°	140-180°	110-140°	90-110°	<90°		
Popliteal Angle	180°	160°	140°	120°	100°	90°	<90°	
Scarf Sign								
Heel to Ear								
							Total Neuromuscular Maturity Score	

Figure 20-1. Neuromuscular maturity for the maturational assessment of gestational age (New Ballard Score).

Physical Maturity Sign	-1	0	1	2	3	4	5	Record Score Here
Skin	sticky, friable, transparent	gelatinous, red, translucent	smooth, pink, visible veins	superficial peeling &/or rash, few veins	cracking pale areas rare veins	parchment, deep cracking, no vessels	leathery, cracked, wrinkled	
Lanugo	none	sparse	abundant	thinning	bald areas	mostly bald		
Plantar Surface	heel-toe 40-50 mm: -1 <40mm: -2	>50 mm no crease	faint red marks	anterior transverse crease only	creases ant. 2/3	creases over entire sole		
Breast	imperceptible	barely perceptible	flat areola, no bud	Stippled areola 1-2 mm bud	raised areola 3-4 mm bud	full areola 5-10 mm bud		
Eye/Ear	lids fused loosely: -1 tightly: -2	lids open, pinna flat, stays folded	sl. curved pinna; soft; slow recoil	well-curved pinna; soft but ready recoil	formed & firm instant recoil	thick cartilage, ear stiff		
Genitals (Male)	scrotum flat smooth	scrotum empty, faint rugae	testes in upper canal, rare rugae	testes descending, few rugae	testes down, good rugae	testes pendulous, deep rugae		
Genitals (Female)	clitoris prominent & labia flat	prominent clitoris & small labia minora	prominent clitoris & enlarging minora	majora & minora equally prominent	majora large minora small	majora cover clitoris & minora		
							Total Physical Maturity Score	

Score

Neuromuscular______

Physical__________

Total____________

Maturity Rating

Score	Weeks
-10	20
-5	22
0	26
5	26
10	28
15	30
20	32
30	36
35	38
40	40
45	42
50	44

Gestational Age (weeks)

By Dates__________

By Ultrasound_______

By Exam__________

Figure 20-2. Physical maturity and maturity rating scale for the maturational assessment of gestational age (New Ballard Score).

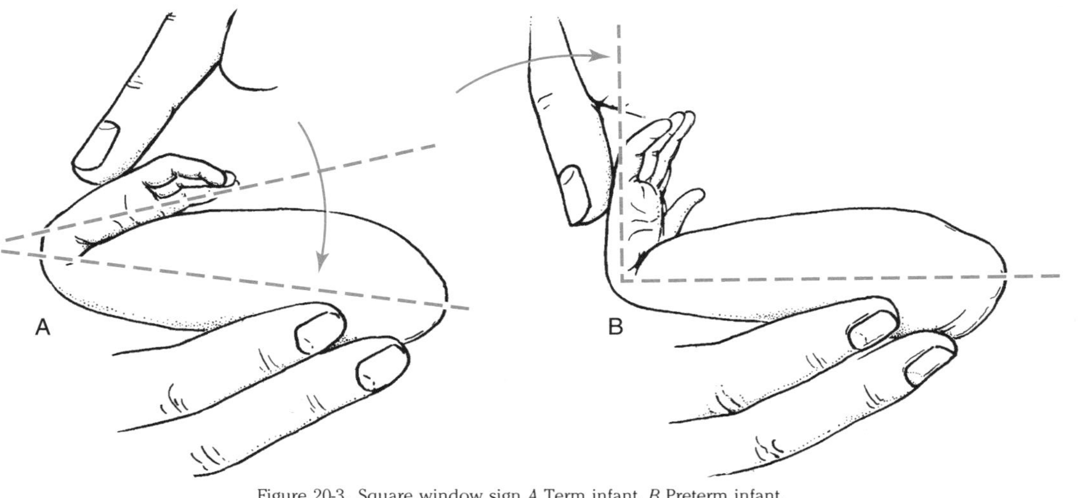

Figure 20-3. Square window sign *A* Term infant. *B* Preterm infant.

II. Objective Data: Assessment Techniques *(continued)*

Procedure	*Normal Findings*	*Deviations from Normal*
D. *Popliteal angle:* Flex thigh on top of abdomen. Push behind ankle and extend lower leg up towards head until resistance is met. Measure angle behind knee	<100°	>100°
E. *Scarf sign:* Lift arm across chest towards opposite shoulder until resistance is met. Note location of elbow in relation to middle of chest (see Fig. 20-4)	Elbow position less than midline of chest	Elbow position midline of chest or greater, toward opposite shoulder
F. *Heel to ear:* Pull leg toward ear on same side, keeping buttocks flat on bed. Inspect popliteal angle and proximity of heel to ear (see Fig. 20-1)	Popliteal angle <90°, heel distal from ear	Popliteal angle >90°, heel proximal to ear
Physical Maturity (see Fig. 20-2)		
A. Observe skin	Parchment, few or no vessels on abdomen, cracking in ankle area especially	Translucent, visible veins, rash, leathery, wrinkled

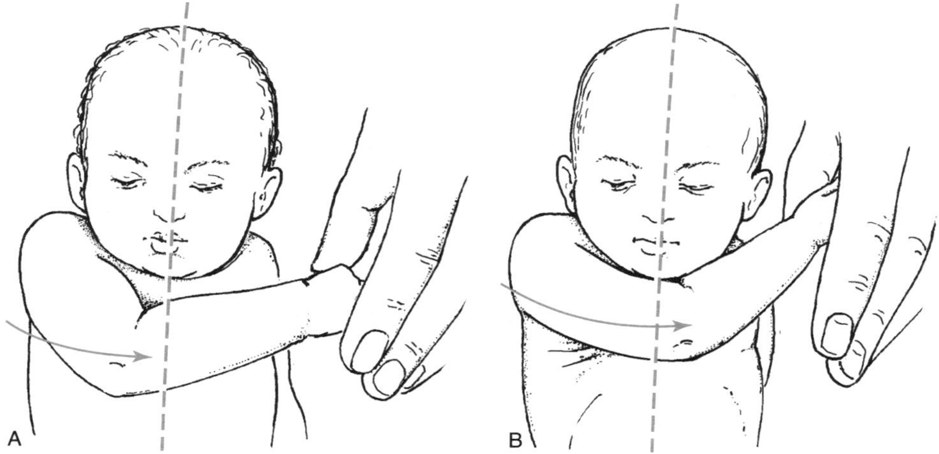

A

B

Figure 20-4. Scarf sign. *A* Term infant. *B* Preterm infant.

II. Objective Data: Assessment Techniques *(continued)*

Procedure	*Normal Findings*	*Deviations from Normal*
B. Inspect for lanugo	Thinning, balding on back/shoulders/ knees	Fine hair on face, abundant
C. Inspect plantar surface of feet for creases	Creases on anterior $\frac{2}{3}$ or entire sole	Anterior transverse crease on sole only, no creases
D. Inspect and palpate breast bud tissue with middle finger and forefinger. Measure bud in millimeters	Raised areola, full areola	Absence of bud tissue, bud <3 mm
E. Observe ear cartilage in upper pinna for curving. Fold pinna down toward side of head and release. Observe recoil of ear	Pinna well curved, cartilage formed, instant recoil	Pinna slightly curved, slow recoil
F. Genitals:		
Male: Observe scrotum for rugae and palpate position of testes	Deep rugae. Testes positioned down in scrotal sac	Decreased presence of rugae. Testes positioned in upper inguinal canal.
Female: Observe labia majora, labia minora and clitoris	Labia majora covers labia minora and clitoris	Labia majora and labia minora equally prominent, clitoris prominent
Score Rating		
A. On Figs. 20-1 and 20-2 mark the boxes that most closely represent each observation. Add the total	35–45	<35 or >45

scores from both tables and plot on the left column of the Maturity Rating Chart found in Fig. 20-2.		
B. This score corresponds to the number in weeks on its right on the Maturity Rating scale. Circle the weeks	Gestational age 38–42 weeks	Gestational age <38 or >42 weeks
C. Using gestational weeks assessed, plot length, weight, and head circumference on Figs. 20-5, 20-6, 20-7, 20-8, respectively	Tenth through the ninetieth percentile is appropriate for gestational age (AGA)	Less than the tenth percentile (small for gestational age), greater than the ninetieth percentile (large for gestational age)

In addition to the Apgar Assessment and the Gestational Age Assessment, the nurse also performs a thorough head-to-toe assessment. The head-to-toe assessment is reviewed at the end of each chapter under Pediatric Variations.

Physical Assessment

Assess each of the following systems:

Respiratory	30–60 breaths/min. Unlabored, chest/abdominal movement synchronized, clear bilaterally, transient rales, nose appears normal with patent nares bilaterally, nose breathers	<30 or >60 breaths/min. Retractions, nasal flaring, grunting, tachypnea, see-saw movement, apnea, decreased breath sounds

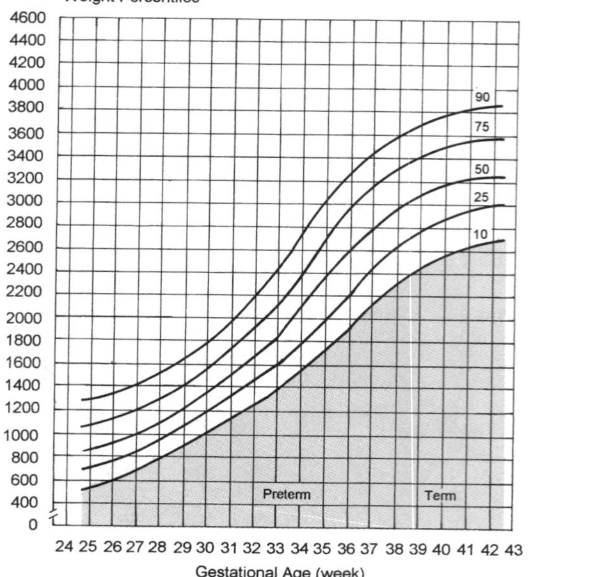

Figure 20-5. Weight percentiles for newborn infants.

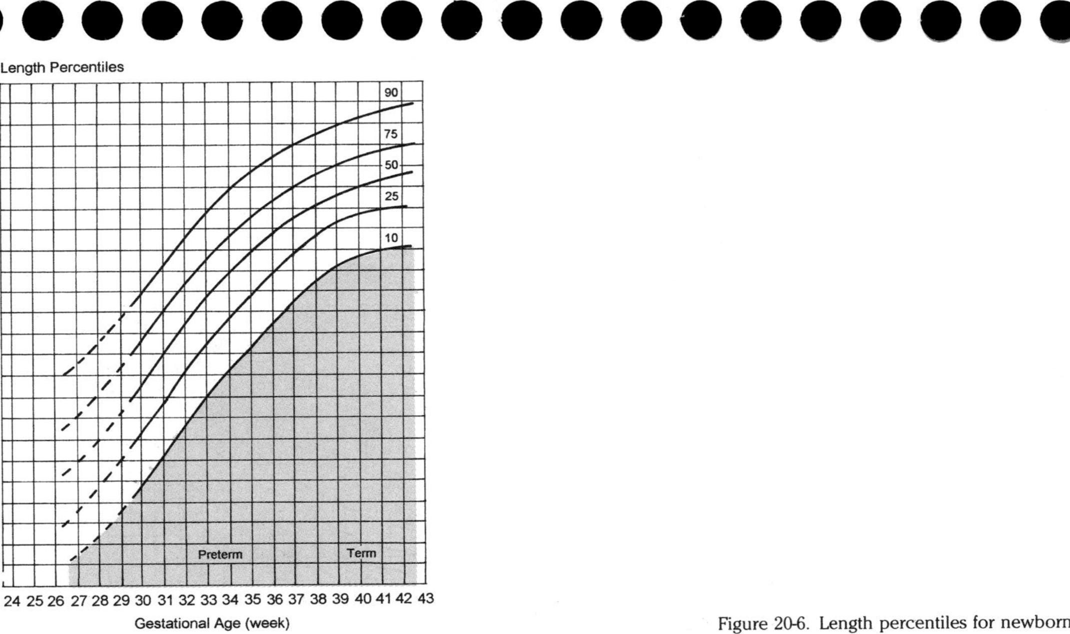

Figure 20-6. Length percentiles for newborn infants.

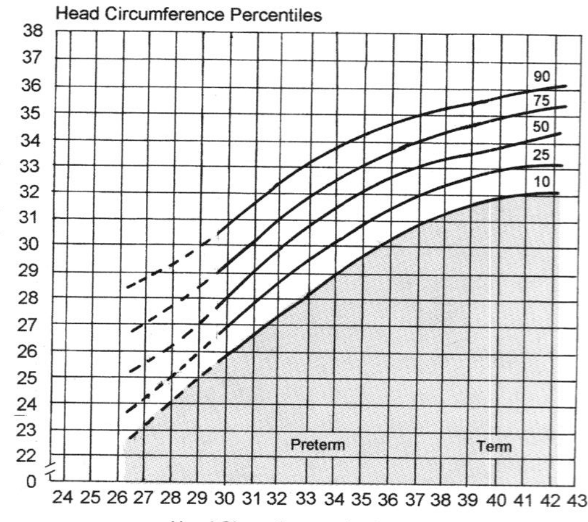

Figure 20-7. Head circumference percentiles for newborn infants.

Classification of Infant*	Weight	Length	Head Circ.
Large for Gestational Age (LGA) (> 90th percentile)			
Appropiate for Gestational Age (AGA) (10th to 90th percentile)			
Small for Gestational Age (SGA) (< 10th percentile)			

* Place an "x" in the appropriate box (LGA, AGA, or SGA) for weight, for length, and for head circumference.

Figure 20-8. Classification of infant for gestational age.

II. Objective Data: Assessment Techniques *(continued)*

Procedure	*Normal Findings*	*Deviations from Normal*
Cardiovascular	120–160 beats/min. Regular rhythm. Color pink, acrocyanosis. Capillary refill <2 sec. Brachial/femoral pulses present, equal bilaterally	<110 or >180 beats/min. Weak pulse, tachycardia, bradycardia, persistent murmur, cyanosis, unequal pulses
Neurological	Alert when awake. Normal, lusty cry. Reflexes: See Neurological Assessment Chapter 17	Asymmetrical/weak/absent response with stimulation
Sensory	Ears symmetrical, well formed, parallel to outer canthus of eye, infant responds to sound. Eyes symmetrical, alert, clear sclera; iris slate grey or brown; infant follows objects to midline. Eyelids transient edema, absence of tears	Ears: preauricle dimple or tag, low-set. Eyes: unequal pupils, purulent discharge
Musculoskeletal	Tone flexed, extremities resist when extended and return to flexed state when released	Limp, flaccid, poor tone

Head	Anterior fontanelle diamond shape, 3–4 cm × 2–3 cm, soft, flat. Posterior fontanelle triangular shape, 1–2 cm. Head round with mild-moderate molding. Sutures palpable, overriding. A common variation is *caput succedaneum*. Symmetry in face	Cephalhematoma, hydrocephalus, bulging fontanelle, microcephaly
Neck/Clavicles	Neck moves freely. Infant attempts to control head when hyper-extended, holds head midline position. Clavicles symmetrical/intact	Webbing of neck, abnormal masses, limp. Crepitus when clavicle palpated along with decreased movement in arm of that side
Extremities	5 fingers/toes each extremity. No webbing, normal palmar creases, bilateral movement with full ROM in arms/legs	Polydactyl, syndactyl, absent digits
	Legs: equal length, bilateral gluteal/thigh creases, no hip click, normal position of feet	Positive Ortolani's Maneuver (see Fig. 16-8). Unequal thigh/gluteal creases
Vertebral column	No openings, straight spine, no curves	Opening in spinal column, pilonidal dimple

II. Objective Data: Assessment Techniques *(continued)*

Procedure	*Normal Findings*	*Deviations from Normal*
Gastrointestinal	Oral mucosa/lips pink, palate intact. Epstein pearls	Cyanosis, white patches on oral mucosae, abnormal fusion of lip/palate
	Retains feedings	Excessive salivation, unable to tolerate feedings
	Patent anus, meconium passed within 24–48 hours after birth	No passage of meconium
	Abdomen shape cylindrical, round, soft; bowel sounds present 30–60 minutes after birth, liver palpable 1–2 cm below costal margin.	Sunken/distended, masses palpable
	Umbilical cord white, drying. Three vessels present in cord	Abnormal insertion of umbilical cord, discolored cord. Two vessels present in cord
Genitourinary	Void within first 24 hours after birth	No urinary output beyond 48 hours after birth
Male	Testes descended within scrotal sac, meatus at tip of penis	Testes found in inguinal canal, scrotal sac edematous, meatus positioned above or below tip of penis
	Circumcision: site dry, minimal swelling and drainage	Bright red active bleeding at circumcision site

Female	Labia majora covers labia minora, vaginal discharge	Edema, tags present
Integumentary	Pink, warm/dry smooth, soft; good turgor, peeling hands/feet. Nails extend to end of fingers or beyond, well formed. *Common variations:* Acrocyanosis, harlequin color change, *vernix caseosa* in creases or absent, lanugo sparse, veins rarely visible, milia over nose/chin. *Pigmentation: erythema toxicum,* mongolian spots common in dark-skinned newborns over dorsal area and buttocks. Stork bites, ecchymosis secondary to application of forcep marks	Minimal adipose tissue, poor turgor, generalized cracking or peeling of skin, lacerations, lesions, meconium stained/ yellow vernix/skin. Jaundice within 24 hours after birth, cyanosis, generalized edema, pallor, hemangiomas, *nevus flammeus, nevus vascularis,* Café-au-lait spots, vesicles, pustules

Possible Related Collaborative Problems

Potential complications:
Ineffective airway clearance
Ineffective breathing pattern
Ineffective thermoregulation
Altered nutrition
Infection
- Circumcision
- nosocomial
- bacterial

Injury
- elevated bilirubin levels

Teaching Tips for Selected Nursing Diagnoses

Nursing Diagnoses	***Teaching Tips***
Ineffective Breathing Pattern (transient alteration in lung expansion)	Monitor respiratory status q 30 min $\times 4$ until stable, then per protocol. Auscultate breath sounds per protocol. Promote oxygenation and fluid drainage by placing infant on side; use postural drainage with head of bed slightly lower than body. Have suction equipment ready for use.

Ineffective Thermoregulation (cool environment, decrease in body fat)	Assess temp q 30 min ×4, then per protocol. Maintain temperature at 97.6–99.2°F. Keep infant temperature probe attached properly to skin to ensure reading probe accurately. Monitor for signs and symptoms of cold stress. Keep infant warm/dry. Postpone bath until temperature is stable. Apply cap to head and extra blankets to infant if temperature <97.6. Teach parents mechanisms of heat loss: radiation, convection, conduction, evaporation. Teach techniques used to prevent cold stress and to maintain/increase infant temperature (i.e., dress, cap, blanket wrap, cuddle, etc.). Teach parents correct procedure in taking newborn axillary temperature, reading thermometer, interpreting results.

Appendices

Appendix I

Nursing Assessment Form Based on Functional Health Patterns

Client Profile

Name ______________ Birthdate ______________ Sex ________

Ethnic origin ______________ Religion ______________

Medical diagnoses ______________

Present treatment ______________

Past treatments ______________

Past hospitalizations ______________

Current Medications

Name	*Dose*	*Purpose*	*Problems*

Subjective

Health Perception-Health Management Pattern

Reason for seeking health care ______________________
____
____

Health rating 1 Poor 2 Fair 3 Excellent

Perception of illness ______________________________
____

Effect of illness on ADLs ___________________________

Use of alcohol ___________________________________

tobacco ___________________________________

drugs _____________________________________

Special health habits _______________________________
____

Last immunizations ________________________________

Compliance with treatments __________________________
____

Objective

Appearance ______________________________________

Grooming ____

Posture ____

Expressions ______________________________________

Ht ____________ Wt ____________

P ____________ R ____________ T ____________

(oral, axil., rectal)

BP sitting R ____________ L ____________

standing R ____________ L ____________

Nutritional-Metabolic Pattern

Daily Food and Fluid Intake

B.F. ______

Lunch ______

Supper ______

Snacks ______

Food intolerances ______

Difficulty chewing ______

Dysphagia ______

Sore gums ______

Sore tongue ______

N and V ______

Abd. pains ______

Antacids ______

Laxatives ______

Skin condition ______

Hair condition ______

Nail condition ______

Ideal wt. ______ Difficulty gaining ______

losing ______

Skin: Color ______

Lesions ______ Texture ______

Temp ______ Moisture ______

Turgor ______

Hair: Color ______

Amt. ______ Texture ______

Scalp lesions ______ Dry ______

Nails: Color ______

Shape ______ Condition ______

Texture ______ Tenderness ______

Oral Mucosa: ______ Teeth No. ______

Condition ______

Lesions ______

Gums ______ Tongue ______

Subjective

Nutritional-Metabolic Pattern (cont'd.)

Cold/heat intolerances ______

Voice changes ______

Difficulty with nervousness ______

Elimination Pattern

Bowel habits

Frequency ______ Color ______ Pain ______

Consistency ______ Laxatives ______

Enemas ______ Suppositories ______

Ileostomy ______ Colostomy ______

Bladder habits

Frequency ______ Amt. ______ Color ______

Pain ______ Hematuria ______

Incontinence ______ Nocturia ______

Retention ______ Infections ______

Catheter ______ Type ______

Objective

Abdomen

Contour ______

Lesions ______ Umbilicus ______

Striae ______ Veins ______

Bowel sounds char. ______

Frequency ______

Size of liver dullness ______

Masses palpated ______

Liver palpated ______

Spleen palpated ______

Rectum

Rashes ______

Lesions ______ Tenderness ______

Activity-Exercise Pattern

Daily Activities

Hygiene ______

Cooking ______

Shopping ______

Housework ______

Yard work ______

Eating times ______

Dyspnea ______ Palpations ______

Chest pain ______ Stiffness ______

Weakness ______ Aching ______

Leisure activities ______

Exercise routine ______

Occupation ______

Effect of illness on activities ______

______

Musculoskeletal

Gait ______ Posture ______

Extremity swelling ______

Symmetry ______ ROM ______

Crepitus ______ Tone ______

Strength ______

Respiratory

Thorax shape ______

Symmetry ______ Retractions ______

Tenderness ______

Diaphragmatic level ______

Breath sounds ______

Adventitious sounds ______

Cardiovascular

Jugular venous pressure ______

Pulsations ______ Heaves ______

Lifts ______

PMI ______ S_1 ______ S_2 ______

S_3 ______ S_4 ______ Murmurs ______

Subjective

Sleep-Rest Pattern

Sleep time ______ Quality ______

Difficulty falling asleep ______

Difficulty remaining asleep ______

Sleep aids ______

Sleep medications ______

Sexuality-Reproduction Pattern

Female Menstruation

Date began ______ Last cycle ______

Length ______

Problems ______

______

______

Objective

Peripheral Vascular Pulses

Carotids ______ Radial ______

Ulnar ______ Brachial ______

Popliteal ______ Femoral ______

Pedal ______ Posterior tibial ______

Bruits ______

Appearance ______

Yawning ______ Irritability ______

Short attention span ______

Breasts

SBE ______ When ______

Shape ______ Symmetry ______

Nipples ______ Discharge ______

Masses ______ Lymph nodes ______

Female: Menstruation (cont'd.)

Gravida ______ Para ______ Abortions ______

Current pregnancy ____________________

Infertility ____________________

Male-Female

Contraception used ____________________

____

Undesirable side-effects ____________________

Problems with sexual activities ____________________

____

____

Effect of illness on sexuality ____________________

____

____

Sexually transmitted diseases ____________________

____

Pain ______ Burning ______

Discomfort during intercourse ____________________

Male Genitalia

Testicular exam ______ When ______

Masses ______ Swelling ______

Texture ______

Penile exam ______

Masses ______ Growths ______

Lesions ______ Discharge ______

Foreskin retraction ____________________

Urethral opening ____________________

Inguinal masses ____________________

Lymph nodes ____________________

Female Genitalia

Labia ______ Color ______

Swelling ______ Symmetry ______

Urethral opening ______

Discharge ____________________

Vaginal opening ____________________

Lesions ______ Discharge ______

Hymen ______ Inflammation ______

Subjective

Sensory-Perceptual Pattern

Perceptions of: Vision ____________________
Hearing __________ Taste __________
Smell __________ Sensation __________
Pain ____________________
Aids for vision ____________________
Aids for hearing ____________________

Objective

Visual Acuity: OD __________ OS __________
OU __________ Visual fields __________
EOMs ____________________
PERRLA ____________________
Fundoscopic Exam: Red reflex __________
Optic disc __________ Macula __________
Arterioles/venules ____________________
Hearing: Weber __________ Rinne __________
Ext. canal ____________________
Tympanic membrane ____________________
Sensations: Superficial __________ Deep pressure __________
2 point discrimination __________
Cranial Nerves
I. Olfactory ____________________
II. Optic ____________________
V. Trigeminal ____________________
III, IV, VI. Oculomotor, Trochlear, Abducens __________
VII. Facial __________ Acoustic __________

Subjective

Cognitive Pattern

Understanding of illness ______

Understanding of treatments ______

Ability to express self ______

Ability to recall:

Remote ______

Recent ______

Ability to make decisions ______

Expression of feelings ______

Objective

Behavior ______

Speech ______ Vocabulary ______

Mood ______

Thought processes ______

Orientation: Person ______

Time ______ Place ______

Attention ______ Information ______

Vocabulary ______

Abstract reasoning ______

Similarities ______ Judgment ______

Sensory perception and coordination ______

Subjective

Role-Relationship Pattern

Role in family ______________________________

Responsibility ______________________________

Work role ______________________________

Social role ______________________________

Level of satisfaction ______________________________

Effect of illness on roles ______________________________

____

Self-Perception–Self-Concept Pattern

Identity ______________________________

Perception of abilities ______________________________

Body image ______________________________

Coping-Stress Tolerance Pattern

Stressors ______________________________

Coping methods ______________________________

Support systems ______________________________

Objective

Communication between family members ______________________________

Family visits ______________ length ______________

Draw Family Genogram.

Subjective

Value-Belief Pattern

Values ______________________

Goals ______________________

Source of hope/strength ______________________

Significant religious person ______________________

Religious practices ______________________

Relationship with God ______________________

Objective

Presence of religious articles ______________________

Religious activities ______________________

____

Visits from clergy ______________________

Appendix II

Developmental Information—Age 1 Month to 18 Years

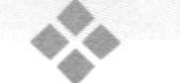

Age	*Physical Development*	*Language (Cognitive) Development (based on Piaget)*	*Psychosocial Development (based on Erikson)*	*Nurse's Approach to Assessment*
Overview of birth to 1 year		*Sensorimotor stage of development*	*Developmental task: trust vs. mistrust.* Learns to trust and to anticipate satisfaction. Sends cues to mother/caretaker. Begins understanding self as separate from others (body image).	Involve caretaker in assessment, e.g., allow him or her to hold child in lap for parts of examination.
1 to 2 months	Lifts chin and chest off bed. Holds extremities in flexion and moves at random; weak neck	Can discriminate between various sensations and prefers certain ones. Follows moving objects with eyes.	Begins to bond with mother during alert periods.	Conserve infant's body heat. Assess while asleep or quiet. Place infant on table or in

	muscles. Activity varies between quiet sleep to drowsiness to alert activity.			caretaker's arms. Give bottle if awake.
3 to 4 months	Head and back control developing. Holds rattle. Looks at own hands. Infant reflexes begin to disappear. Able to sit propped. Props self on forearm in prone position. Rolls from side to back and vice versa and from back to abdomen. Takes objects to mouth. Drools with eruption of lower teeth.	Responds to parent. Social smile. Begins to vocalize; coos, babbles. Locates sounds by turning head, looking.	Learns to signal displeasure. Shows excitement with whole body. Begins to discriminate strangers. Squeals.	Speak softly to infant. Use brightly colored toys, bells, rattles to elicit necessary responses and to distract. Assess ears, mouth, nose last. Assess lungs and heart when quiet.
5 to 8 months	Begins to develop teeth. Birth weight doubled. Grasps objects. Sits unsupported.	Begins to imitate sounds, two-syllable words (dada, mama). Responds to own name.	Increased fear of strangers. Definite likes/dislikes. Responds to "no."	Place on caretaker's lap (same as above).

Age	*Physical Development*	*Language (Cognitive) Development (based on Piaget)*	*Psychosocial Development (based on Erikson)*	*Nurse's Approach to Assessment*
9 to 12 months	Birth weight tripled. Anterior fontanel nearly closed. Learns to pull in order to stand, creep, and crawl.	Says two words besides "dada, mama." Understands simple commands. Imitates animal sounds.	Looks for hidden objects. Unceasing determination to move about. Clings to mother. Shows emotion. Plays peek-a-boo and pat-a-cake.	
1 to 3 years	Begins to walk and run well. Drinks from cup, feeds self. Develops fine motor control. Climbs. Begin self-toileting. Kneels without support. Steady growth in height/weight. Adult height will be approximately double the height at age 2. Dresses self by age 3.	*Preoperational stage of development.* Has poor time sense. Increasing verbal ability. Formulates sentences of 4 to 5 words by age 3. Talks to self and others. Has misconceptions about cause and effect. Interested in pictures. *Fears:* • Loss/separation from parents—peak • Dark • Machines/equipment • Intrusive procedures • Bedtime	*Developmental task: autonomy vs. shame and doubt.* Establishes self-control, decision making, independence (autonomy). Extremely curious and prefers to do things himself. Demonstrates independence through negativism. Very egocentric;	Be flexible. Begin assessment with play period to establish rapport. Be honest. Praise for cooperation. Begin slowly; speak to child. Involve caretaker/parent in holding on exam table. Let child hold security object. Allow child to play with stethoscope, tongue blade, flashlight before using on child if

		Speaks to dolls and animals. Increasing attention span. Knows own sex by age 3.	believes he or she controls the world. Attempts to please parents. Participates in parallel play; able to share some toys by age 3.	possible. Assess face, mouth, eyes, ears last. May need to restrain when lying prone. If resistant, save that part of the assessment for later.
4 to 6 years	Growth slows. Locomotion skills increase and coordination improves. Tricycle/bicycle riding. Throws ball but difficulty catching. Constantly active, increasing dexterity. Eruption of permanent teeth. Skips, hops, jumps rope.	Preoperational/thought stage of development continues. Language skills flourish. Generates many questions, e.g., How, Why, What? Simple problem solving. Uses fantasy to understand and problem solve. *Fears:* • Mutilation • Castration • Dark • Unknown • Inanimate • Unfamiliar objects Causality related to proximity of events. Enjoys mimicking and imitating adults.	*Developmental tasks: initiative vs. guilt.* Attempts to establish self like his or her parents, but independent. Explores environment on own initiative. Boasts, brags, has feelings of indestructibility. Family is primary social group. Peers increasingly important. Assumes sex roles. Aggressive, very curious. Enjoys	Establish rapport through talking and play. Introduce self to child. Have parent present but direct conversation to child. Games such as "follow the leader" and "Simon says" can be used to elicit necessary behaviors. Explain each assessment in simple language. Ask for child's help and use flattery. Use pictures, models, or items he or

Age	Physical Development	Language (Cognitive) Development (based on Piaget)	Psychosocial Development (based on Erikson)	Nurse's Approach to Assessment
			activities such as sports, cooking, shopping. Cooperative play. Likes rules. May stretch the truth and tell large stories.	she can see or touch. Reserve genital examination for last; drape accordingly.
6 to 11 years	Moves constantly. Physical play prevalent; sports, swimming, skating, etc. Increased smoothness of movement. Grows at rate of 2 inches/7 lbs a year. Eyes/hands well coordinated.	*Concrete operations stage of development.* Organized thought; memory concepts more complicated. Reads, reasons better. Focuses on concrete understanding. *Fears:* • Mutilation • Death • Immobility • Rejection • Failure	*Developmental task: industry vs. inferiority.* Learns to include values and skills of school, neighborhood, peers. Peer relationships important. Focuses more on reality, less on fantasy. Family is main base of security and identity. Sensitive to reactions of others. Seeks approval and	Explain all procedures and impact on body. Encourage questioning and active participation in care. Be direct about explanation of procedures, based on what child will hear, see, smell, and feel. (In addition, explain body part involved, and use anatomical names and pictures to explain step by step.)

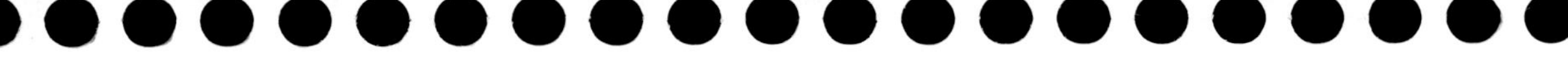

			recognition. Enthusiastic, noisy, imaginative, desires to explore. Likes to complete a task. Enjoys helping others.	Be honest. Reassure child that he or she is liked. Provide privacy. Involve parents, but give child choice as to whether parent will stay during exam. Reason and explain. Allow child some choice as to direction of assessment. May be able to proceed as if assessing adult. Praise cooperation.
12 to 18 years	Well developed. Rapid physical growth (early adolescence: maximum growth). Secondary sex characteristics. (See Chapter 15, Genitourinary-Reproductive	*Formal operations stage of development.* Abstract reasoning, problem solving. Understanding of multiple cause-and-effect relationships. May plan for future career. *Fears:* • Mutilation • Disruption of body image	*Developmental task: identity vs. role confusion.* Predominant values are those of peer group. Early adolescence: outgoing and enthusiastic.	Respect privacy. Accept expression of feelings. Direct discussions of care and condition to child. Ask for child's opinions and encourage questions. Allow input into

Age	*Physical Development*	*Language (Cognitive) Development (based on Piaget)*	*Psychosocial Development (based on Erikson)*	*Nurse's Approach to Assessment*
	Assessment.)	• Rejection by peers	Emotions are extreme, with mood swings. Seeking self-identity; sexual identity. Wants privacy and independence. Develops interests not shared with family. Concern with physical self. Explores adult roles.	decisions. Be flexible with routines. Explain all procedures/ treatments. Encourage continuance of peer relationships. Listen actively. Identify impact of illness on body image, future, and level of functioning. Correct misconceptions. Involve parent in assessment only if child requests presence.

Appendix III

Recommended Childhood Immunization Schedule United States—January 1995

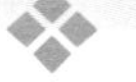

Vaccines are listed under the routinely recommended ages. Shaded bars indicate range of acceptable ages for vaccination.

Age → ***Vaccine ↓***	***Birth***	***2 mos***	***4 mos***	***6 mos***	***12[5] mos***	***15 mos***	***18 mos***	***4–6 yrs***	***11–12 yrs***	***14–16 yrs***
Hepatitis B[1]	HB-1									
		HB-2		HB-3						
Diphtheria, Tetanus, Pertussis[2]		DTP	DTP	DTP	DTP or DTaP at 15+ m			DTP or DtaP	Td	
H. influenzae type b[3]		Hib	Hib	Hib	Hib					

Polio	OPV	OPV	OPV	OPV
Measles, Mumps, Rubella[4]			MMR	MMR or MMR

[1] Infants born to HBsAg-negative mothers should receive the second dose of hepatitis B vaccine between 1 and 4 months of age, provided at least 1 month has elapsed since receipt of the first dose. The third dose is recommended between 6 and 18 months of age.

Infants born to HBsAg-positive mothers should receive immunoprophylaxis for hepatitis B with 0.5 ml Hepatitis B Immune Globulin (HBIG) within 12 hours of birth, and 0.5 ml of either Merck Sharp & Dohme vaccine (Recombivax HB) or of SmithKline Beecham vaccine (Engerix-B) at a separate site. In these infants, the second dose of vaccine is recommended at 1 month of age and the third dose at 6 months of age. All pregnant women should be screened for HBsAg in an early prenatal visit.

[2] The fourth dose of DTP may be administered as early as 12 months of age, provided at least 6 months have elapsed since DTP3. Combined DTP-Hib products may be used when these two vaccines are to be administered simultaneously. DTaP (diphtheria and tetanus toxoids and acellular pertussis vaccine) is licensed for use for the 4th and/or 5th dose of DTP vaccine in children 15 months of age or older and may be preferred for these doses in children in this age group.

[3] *Three H. influenzae* type b conjugate vaccines are available for use in infants: HbOC [HibTITER] (Lederle Praxis); PRP-T [ActHIB; OmniHIB] (Pasteur Mérieux, distributed by SmithKline Beecham; Connaught); and PRP-OMP [PedvaxHIB] (Merck Sharp & Dohme). Children who have received PRP-OMP at 2 and 4 months of age do not require a dose at 6 months of age. After the primary infant Hib conjugate vaccine series is completed, any licensed Hib conjugate vaccine may be used as a booster dose at 12–15 months.

[4] The second dose of MMR vaccine should be administered EITHER at 4–6 years of age OR at 11–12 years of age.

[5] Vaccines recommended in the second year of life (12–15 months of age) may be given at either one or two visits.

Approved by the Advisory Committee on Immunization Practices (ACIP), the American Academy of Pediatrics, and the American Academy of Family Physicians (AAFP).

Appendix IV

Psychosocial Development Tasks of the Young Adult, Mature Adult, and Aging Adult

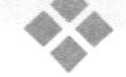

Young Adult Developmental Task: Intimacy vs. Isolation

Behavior to Assess:

Accepts self: physically, cognitively, and emotionally
Establishes independence from parental home
Expresses love responsibly, emotionally, and sexually
Establishes an intimate bond with another human being
Finds a social friendship group
Becomes involved as part of a community
Establishes a philosophy of living and life
Begins a profession or a life's work that provides a means of contribution
Learns to solve problems of life that accompany independence from parental home

Mature Adult Developmental Task: Generativity vs. Stagnation

Behavior to Assess:

Establishes/maintains healthful life patterns
Discovers self as a life-mate for another person
Derives satisfaction from contributing to growth and development of others

Establishes an abiding intimacy
Helps children grow and mature
Maintains a stable home
Finds pleasure in an established work or profession
Takes pride in self and family accomplishments and contributions
Contributes to the community to support its growth and development
Adjusts to physical changes of aging
Develops deeper, sustained friendships
Integrates leisure with work life
Develops a philosophy of life that includes an understanding of mortality
Prepares for eventual retirement
Supports aging parents/relatives

Aging Adult Developmental Task: Ego Integrity vs. Despair

Behavior to Assess:

Adjusts to changing physical self
Recognizes changes present as a result of aging, in relationships and activities
Maintains relationships with children, grandchildren, other relatives
Continues interests outside self and home
Completes transition from retirement at work to satisfying alternative activities
Establishes relationships with others his or her own age
Adjusts to deaths of relatives, spouse, and friends
Maintains maximum level of physical functioning through diet, exercise, and personal care
Finds meaning in past life and faces inevitable mortality of self and significant others
Integrates philosophical or religious values into understanding of self to promote comfort
Reviews accomplishments and recognizes meaningful contributions he or she has made to community and relatives

Appendix V

Height-Weight-Head Circumference Charts for Children

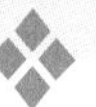

BOYS: BIRTH TO 36 MONTHS
PHYSICAL GROWTH
NCHS PERCENTILES*

NAME ______________________ RECORD # __________

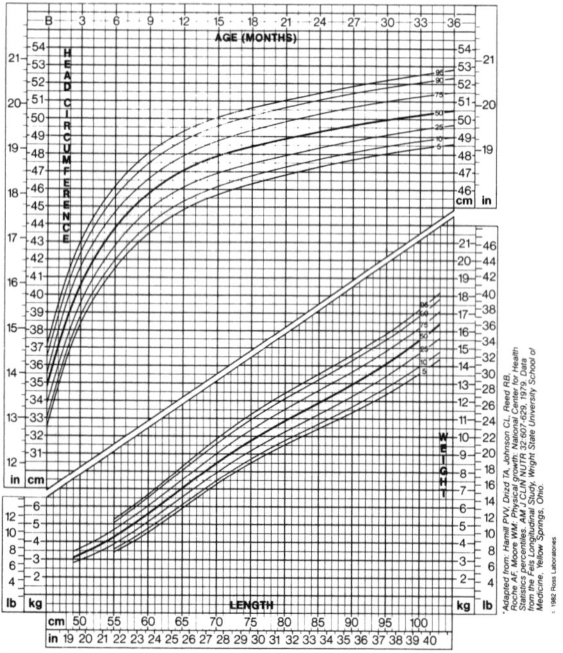

AGE (MONTHS): B 3 6 9 12 15 18 21 24 27 30 33 36

HEAD CIRCUMFERENCE (cm): 31–54; (in): 12–21

WEIGHT (kg): 2–21; (lb): 4–46

LENGTH (cm): 50 55 60 65 70 75 80 85 90 95 100
(in): 19 20 21 22 23 24 25 26 27 28 29 30 31 32 33 34 35 36 37 38 39 40

Percentiles: 5, 10, 25, 50, 75, 90, 95

*Adapted from: Hamill PVV, Drizd TA, Johnson CL, Reed RB, Roche AF, Moore WM: Physical growth: National Center for Health Statistics percentiles. AM J CLIN NUTR 32:607-629, 1979. Data from the Fels Longitudinal Study, Wright State University School of Medicine, Yellow Springs, Ohio.

DATE	AGE	LENGTH	WEIGHT	HEAD CIRC	COMMENT

SIMILAC® WITH IRON
Infant Formula

ISOMIL®
Soy Protein Formula with Iron

Used and reprinted with permission of Ross Laboratories

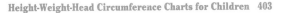

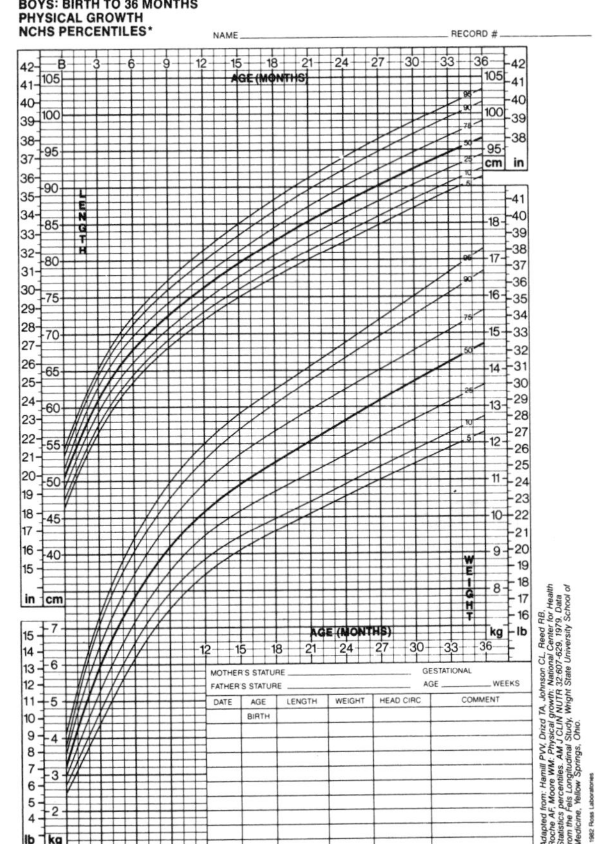
BOYS: BIRTH TO 36 MONTHS
PHYSICAL GROWTH
NCHS PERCENTILES*
NAME
RECORD #
AGE (MONTHS)
LENGTH
WEIGHT
in
cm
kg
lb
MOTHER'S STATURE
FATHER'S STATURE
GESTATIONAL AGE
WEEKS
DATE
AGE
LENGTH
WEIGHT
HEAD CIRC
COMMENT
BIRTH
*Adapted from: Hamill PVV, Drizd TA, Johnson CL, Reed RB, Roche AF, Moore WM: Physical growth: National Center for Health Statistics percentiles. AM J CLIN NUTR 32:607-629, 1979. Data from the Fels Longitudinal Study, Wright State University School of Medicine, Yellow Springs, Ohio.
© 1982 Ross Laboratories

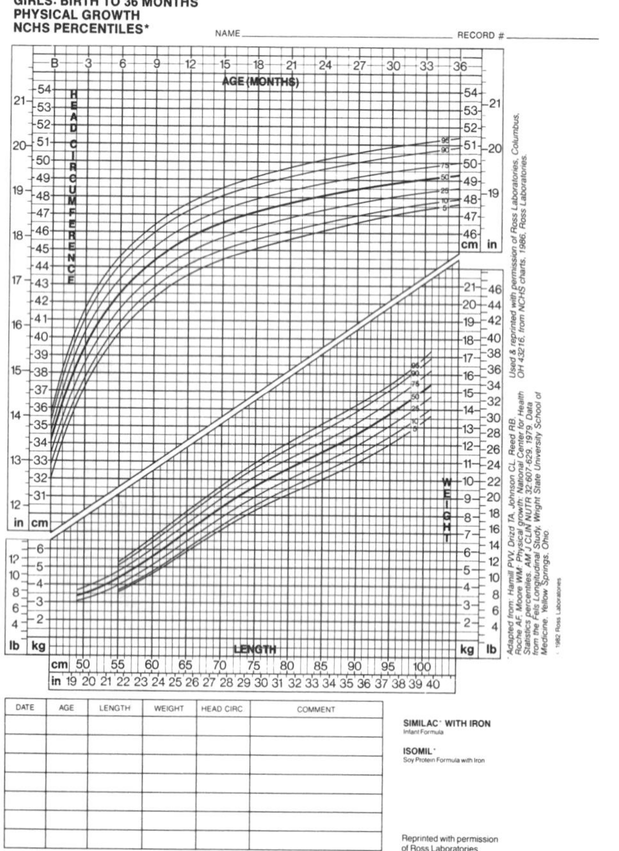
GIRLS: BIRTH TO 36 MONTHS
PHYSICAL GROWTH
NCHS PERCENTILES*
NAME
RECORD #
AGE (MONTHS)
B 3 6 9 12 15 18 21 24 27 30 33 36
HEAD CIRCUMFERENCE
WEIGHT
LENGTH
cm 50 55 60 65 70 75 80 85 90 95 100
in 19 20 21 22 23 24 25 26 27 28 29 30 31 32 33 34 35 36 37 38 39 40
in cm
lb kg
cm in
kg lb
95 90 75 50 25 10 5
*Adapted from: Hamill PVV, Drizd TA, Johnson CL, Reed RB, Roche AF, Moore WM: Physical growth: National Center for Health Statistics percentiles. AM J CLIN NUTR 32:607-629, 1979. Data from the Fels Longitudinal Study, Wright State University School of Medicine, Yellow Springs, Ohio.
Used & reprinted with permission of Ross Laboratories, Columbus, OH 43216, from NCHS charts, 1986, Ross Laboratories.
© 1982 Ross Laboratories
DATE
AGE
LENGTH
WEIGHT
HEAD CIRC
COMMENT
SIMILAC® WITH IRON
Infant Formula
ISOMIL®
Soy Protein Formula with Iron
Reprinted with permission of Ross Laboratories

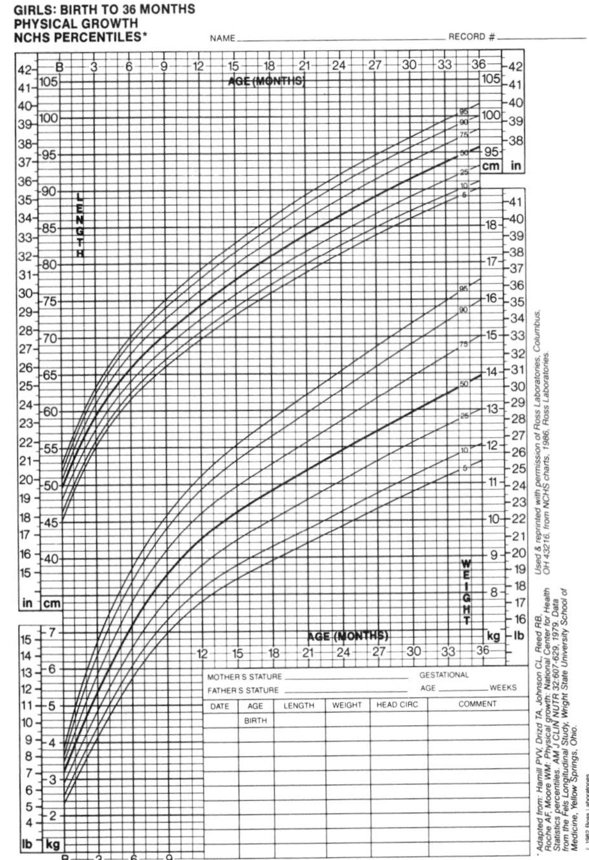

Used and reprinted with permission of Ross Laboratories

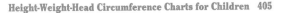

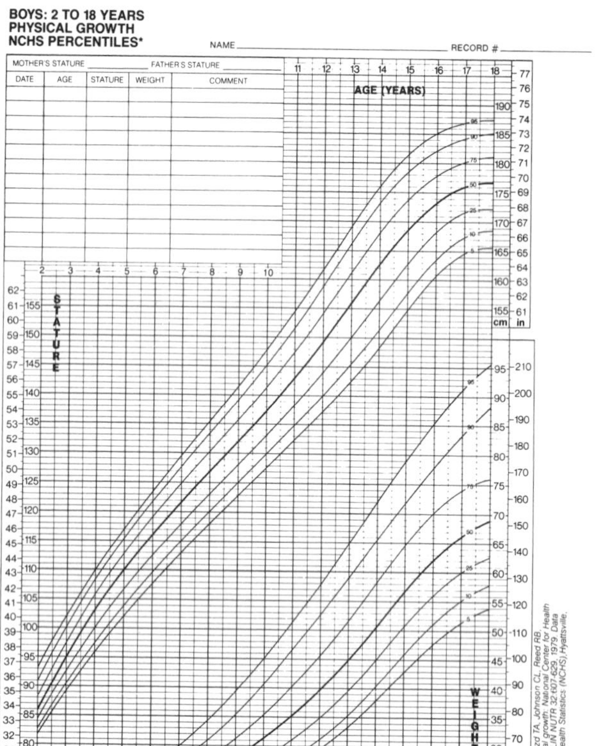

Used and reprinted with permission of Ross Laboratories

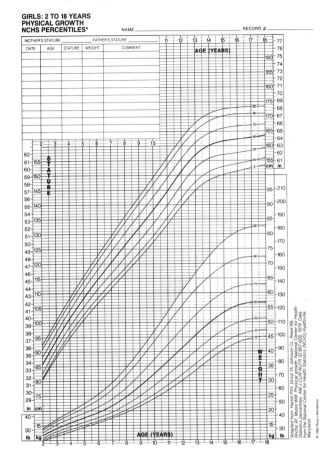

GIRLS: 2 TO 18 YEARS
PHYSICAL GROWTH
NCHS PERCENTILES*

NAME ______________________ RECORD # __________

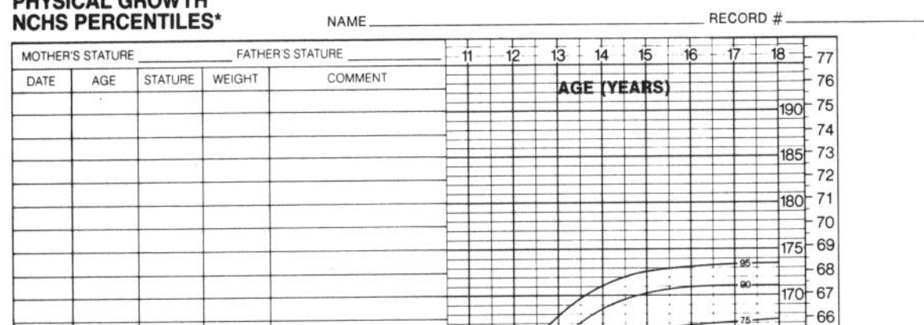

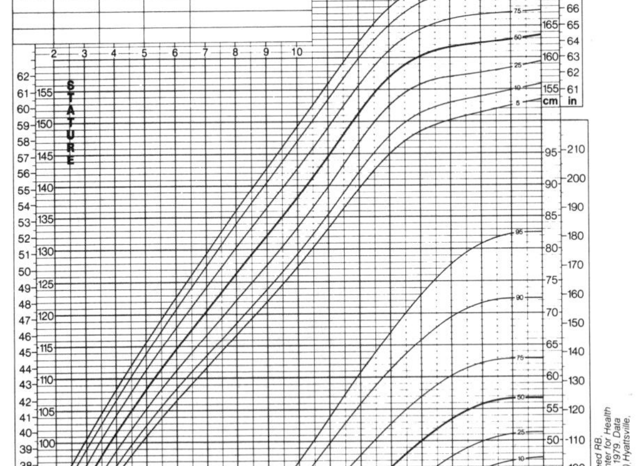

*Adapted from: Hamill PVV, Drizd TA, Johnson CL, Reed RB, Roche AF, Moore WM: Physical growth: National Center for Health Statistics percentiles. AM J CLIN NUTR 32:607-629, 1979. Data from the National Center for Health Statistics (NCHS), Hyattsville, Maryland.

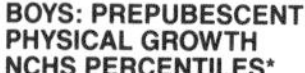

BOYS: PREPUBESCENT PHYSICAL GROWTH NCHS PERCENTILES*

NAME ______________________ RECORD # ______________

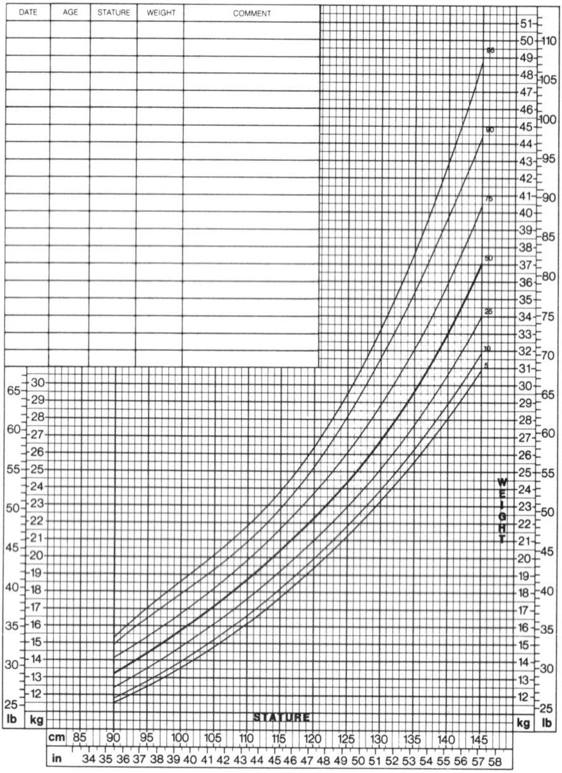

DATE
AGE
STATURE
WEIGHT
COMMENT
STATURE
WEIGHT
cm
in
kg
lb
5
10
25
50
75
90
95

*Adapted from: Hamill PVV, Drizd TA, Johnson CL, Reed RB, Roche AF, Moore WM: Physical growth: National Center for Health Statistics percentiles. AM J CLIN NUTR 32:607-629, 1979. Data from the National Center for Health Statistics (NCHS), Hyattsville, Maryland.

Used and reprinted with permission of Ross Laboratories

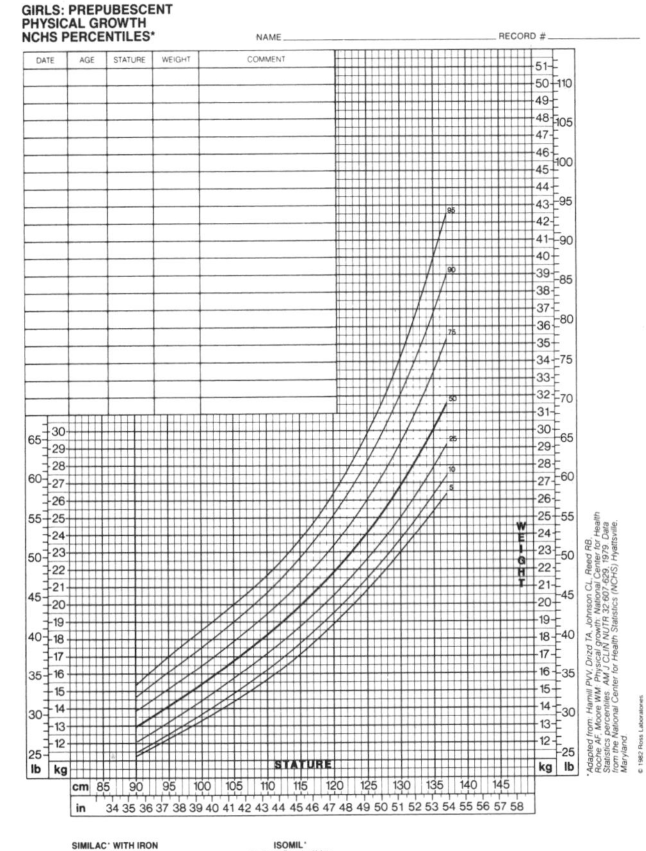

*Adapted from: Hamill PVV, Drizd TA, Johnson CL, Reed RB, Roche AF, Moore WM: Physical growth: National Center for Health Statistics percentiles. AM J CLIN NUTR 32:607-629, 1979. Data from the National Center for Health Statistics (NCHS) Hyattsville, Maryland.

SIMILAC® WITH IRON
Infant Formula

ISOMIL®
Soy Protein Formula with Iron

Appendix VI

Height and Weight Tables for Adults

Weights for Men*
(according to frame, ages 25–59)

***(in shoes)*†**

Feet	*Inches*	***Small Frame***	***Medium Frame***	***Large Frame***
5	*2*	*128–134*	*131–141*	*138–150*
5	*3*	*130–136*	*133–143*	*140–153*
5	*4*	*132–138*	*135–145*	*142–156*
5	*5*	*134–140*	*137–148*	*144–160*
5	*6*	*136–142*	*139–151*	*146–164*
5	*7*	*138–145*	*142–154*	*149–168*

5	8	140–148	145–157	152–172
5	9	142–151	148–160	155–176
5	10	144–154	151–163	158–180
5	11	146–157	154–166	161–184
6	0	149–160	157–170	164–188
6	1	152–164	160–174	168–192
6	2	155–168	164–178	172–197
6	3	158–172	167–182	176–202
6	4	162–176	171–187	181–207

*Weight in pounds (in indoor clothing weighing 5 pounds).

†Shoes with 1-inch heels.

(Data from Build study, 1979, Society of Actuaries and Association of Life Insurance Medical Directors of America, 1980. Copyright 1983 Metropolitan Life Insurance Company.)

Weights for Women*
(according to frame, ages 25–59)

Height (in shoes)†				
Feet	**Inches**	**Small Frame**	**Medium Frame**	**Large Frame**
4	10	102–111	109–121	118–131
4	11	103–113	111–123	120–134
5	0	104–114	113–126	122–137
5	1	106–118	115–129	125–140
5	2	108–121	118–132	128–143
5	3	111–123	121–135	131–147
5	4	114–127	124–138	134–151
5	5	117–130	127–141	137–155
5	6	120–133	130–144	140–159
5	7	123–136	133–147	143–163

5	*8*	*126–139*	*136–150*	*146–167*
5	*9*	*129–142*	*139–153*	*149–170*
5	*10*	*132–145*	*142–153*	*152–173*
5	*11*	*135–148*	*142–156*	*155–176*
6	*0*	*138–151*	*145–159*	*158–179*

**Weight in pounds (in indoor clothing weighing 5 pounds).*

†Shoes with 1-inch heels.

(Data from Build study, 1979, Society of Actuaries and Association of Life Insurance Medical Directors of America, 1980. Copyright 1983 Metropolitan Life Insurance Company.)

Appendix VII

Rosenbaum Pocket Vision Screener

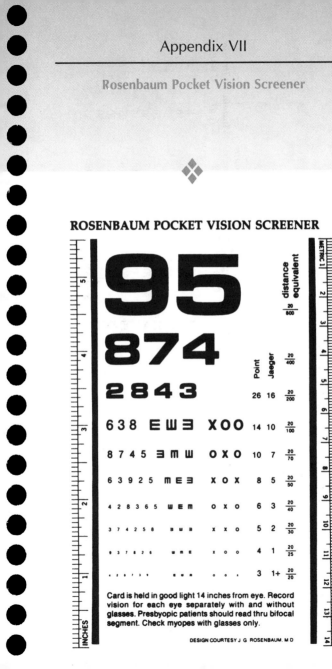

ROSENBAUM POCKET VISION SCREENER

			Point	Jaeger	distance equivalent
95					20/800
874					20/400
2843			26	16	20/200
638	E Ш Ǝ	X O O	14	10	20/100
8 7 4 5	Ǝ m Ш	O X O	10	7	20/70
6 3 9 2 5	m E Ǝ	X O X	8	5	20/50
4 2 8 3 6 5	Ш E m	O X O	6	3	20/40
3 7 4 2 5 8	Ǝ Ш Ǝ	X X O	5	2	20/30
9 3 7 8 2 6	Ш m E	X O O	4	1	20/25
			3	1+	20/20

Card is held in good light 14 inches from eye. Record vision for each eye separately with and without glasses. Presbyopic patients should read thru bifocal segment. Check myopes with glasses only.

DESIGN COURTESY J. G. ROSENBAUM, M.D.

Appendix VIII

Recommended Daily Dietary Allowances*

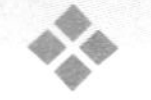

		Weight†		*Height†*			*Fat-Soluble Vitamins*				
Category	***Age***	***(kg)***	***(lb)***	***(cm)***	***(in)***	***Protein (g)***	***Vitamin A (µg RE)‡***	***Vitamin D (µg)§***	***Vitamin E (mg α-TE)¶***	***Vitamin K (µg)***	***Vitamin C (mg)***
Infants	0.0–0.5	6	13	60	24	13	375	7.5	3	5	30
	0.5–1.0	9	20	71	28	14	375	10	4	10	35
Children	1–3	13	29	90	35	16	400	10	6	15	40
	4–6	20	44	112	44	24	500	10	7	20	45
	7–10	28	62	132	52	28	700	10	7	30	45
Males	11–14	45	99	157	62	45	1000	10	10	45	50
	15–18	66	145	176	69	59	1000	10	10	65	60
	19–24	72	160	177	70	58	1000	10	10	70	60
	25–50	79	174	176	70	63	1000	5	10	80	60
	51+	77	170	173	68	63	1000	5	10	80	60

Females	11–14	46	101	157	62	46	800	10	8	45	50
	15–18	55	120	163	64	44	800	10	8	55	60
	19–24	58	128	164	65	46	800	10	8	60	60
	25–50	63	138	163	64	50	800	5	8	65	60
	51+	65	143	160	63	50	800	5	8	65	60
Pregnant						60	800	10	10	65	70
Lactating											
1st 6 months						65	1300	10	12	65	95
2nd 6 months						62	1200	10	11	65	90

*Designed for the maintenance of good nutrition of practically all healthy people in the United States. The allowances, expressed as average daily intakes over time are intended to provide for individual variations among most normal persons as they live in the United States under usual environmental stresses. Diets should be based on a variety of common foods to provide other nutrients for which human requirements have been less well defined.

†Weights and heights of reference adults are actual medians for the U.S. population of the designated age, as reported by NHANES II. The use of these figures does not imply that the height-to-weight ratios are ideal.

‡Retinol equivalents. 1 RE = 1 μg retinol or 6 μg B-carotene.

§As cholecalciferol. 10 μg cholecalciferol = 400 IU of vitamin D.

¶α-Tocopherol equivalents. 1 mg d-α-tocopherol = 1 α-TE.

‖1 NE (niacin equivalent) is equal to 1 mg of niacin or 60 mg of dietary tryptophan.

(Subcommittee on the Tenth Edition of the RDAs. Recommended dietary allowances. 10th ed. Washington, DC: National Academy Press, 1989.)

Water-Soluble Vitamins						*Minerals*						
Thiamin (mg)	**Riboflavin (mg)**	**Niacin (mg NE)**‖	**Vitamin B_6 (mg)**	**Folate (µg)**	**Vitamin B_{12} (µg)**	**Calcium (mg)**	**Phosphorus (mg)**	**Magnesium (mg)**	**Iron (mg)**	**Zinc (mg)**	**Iodine (µg)**	**Selenium (µg)**
0.3	0.4	5	0.3	25	0.3	400	300	40	6	5	40	10
0.4	0.5	6	0.6	35	0.5	600	500	60	10	5	50	15
0.7	0.8	9	1.0	50	0.7	800	800	80	10	10	70	20
0.9	1.1	12	1.1	75	1.0	800	800	120	10	10	90	20
1.0	1.2	13	1.4	100	1.4	800	800	170	10	10	120	30
1.3	1.5	17	1.7	150	2.0	1200	1200	270	12	15	150	40
1.5	1.8	20	2.0	200	2.0	1200	1200	400	12	15	150	50
1.5	1.7	19	2.0	200	2.0	1200	1200	350	10	15	150	70
1.5	1.7	19	2.0	200	2.0	800	800	350	10	15	150	70
1.2	1.4	15	2.0	200	2.0	800	800	350	10	15	150	70
1.1	1.3	15	1.4	150	2.0	1200	1200	280	15	12	150	45
1.1	1.3	15	1.5	180	2.0	1200	1200	300	15	12	150	50
1.1	1.3	15	1.6	180	2.0	1200	1200	280	15	12	150	55
1.1	1.3	15	1.6	180	2.0	800	800	280	15	12	150	55
1.0	1.2	13	1.6	180	2.0	800	800	280	10	12	150	55
1.5	1.6	17	2.2	400	2.2	1200	1200	320	30	15	175	65
1.6	1.8	20	2.1	280	2.6	1200	1200	355	15	19	200	75
1.6	1.7	20	2.1	260	2.6	1200	1200	340	15	16	200	75

Appendix IX

Protein and Calorie Counter

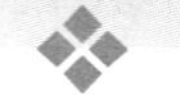

	Serving Size	*Grams of Protein*	*Calories*
Butter	1 pat	Trace	36
Margarine	1 pat	Trace	36
Cooking/salad oil (Corn)	1 tablespoon	-0-	119
Salad Dressings			
French	1 tablespoon	0.1	66
Italian	1 tablespoon	Trace	83
Mayonnaise	1 tablespoon	0.2	101
Sugar	1 teaspoon	-0-	15
Syrups			
Molasses (light)	1 fl oz	-0-	103
Maple	1 tablespoon	-0-	33
Table blends (cane and maple)	1 tablespoon	-0-	33
Candy			
Caramels	1 oz	1.1	113
Chocolate (sweet)	1 oz	1.2	144
Fudge (chocolate)	1 oz	0.8	113

Toppings/spreads			
Whipped cream	1 tablespoon	0.3	53
Sour cream	1 tablespoon	0.0	72
Cream cheese	1 tablespoon	1.1	52
Jelly	1 tablespoon	Trace	49
Jam	1 tablespoon	0.1	54
Honey	1 tablespoon	0.1	64
High Protein Foods			
Beef (cooked)			
Chuck steak	1 piece (3 oz)	20.6	320
Rump roast	1 piece (3 oz)	21.2	269
Lean ground beef	1 patty (4 oz)	23.4	202
Pork (cooked)			
Bacon	2 slices	3.8	86
Ham	2 pieces (3 oz)	19.6	318
Pork chop	1 (2.7 oz)	19.3	305
Chicken (cooked)			
Light	1/2 breast	25.7	160
Dark	1 drumstick	12.2	88
Fish (cooked)			
Flounder	1 fillet (3 oz)	30.0	202
Tuna (packed in oil)	1 can (6 1/2 oz)	44.5	530

	Serving Size	*Grams of Protein*	*Calories*
Cheese			
Cheddar	1 slice	6.0	96
Cottage	1 oz	3.9	30
American	1 slice	3.0	48
Eggs (hard cooked)	1 large	6.5	82
Milk products			
Whole milk	1 cup	8.5	159
Evaporated milk	1 cup	17.6	345
Half and Half	1 cup	7.7	324
Nonfat instant (powder)	1 cup	24.3	244
Ice cream	1 cup	6.0	257
Others			
Dried beans (great northern)	1 cup	14.0	212
Dried peas	1 cup	16.0	230
Peanut butter	1 tablespoon	4.0	94

Nutritive Value of American Foods in Common Units, U.S.D.A. Handbook No. 456. 11/88.

Appendix X

Selected Laboratory Values for Adults and Children

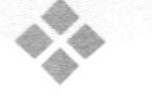

Determination	Reference Range: Conventional Units	Reference Range: SI Units	Clinical Significance
Bleeding time	2–8 min	2–8 min	Prolonged in thrombocytopenia, defective platelet function, and aspirin therapy
Partial thromboplastin time (activated)	20–45 sec		Prolonged in deficiency of fibrinogen, factors II, V, VII, IX, X, XI, and XII, and in heparin therapy
Prothrombin consumption	Over 20 sec		Impaired in deficiency of factors VIII, IX, and X
Prothrombin time	9.5–12 sec		Prolonged by deficiency of factors I, II, V, VII, and X, fat malabsorption, severe liver disease, coumarin-anticoagulant therapy
Erythrocyte count	*Males:* 4,600,000–6,200,000/mm^3	4.6–6.2 × 10^{12}/L	Increased in severe diarrhea and dehydration, polycythemia, acute poisoning, pulmonary fibrosis

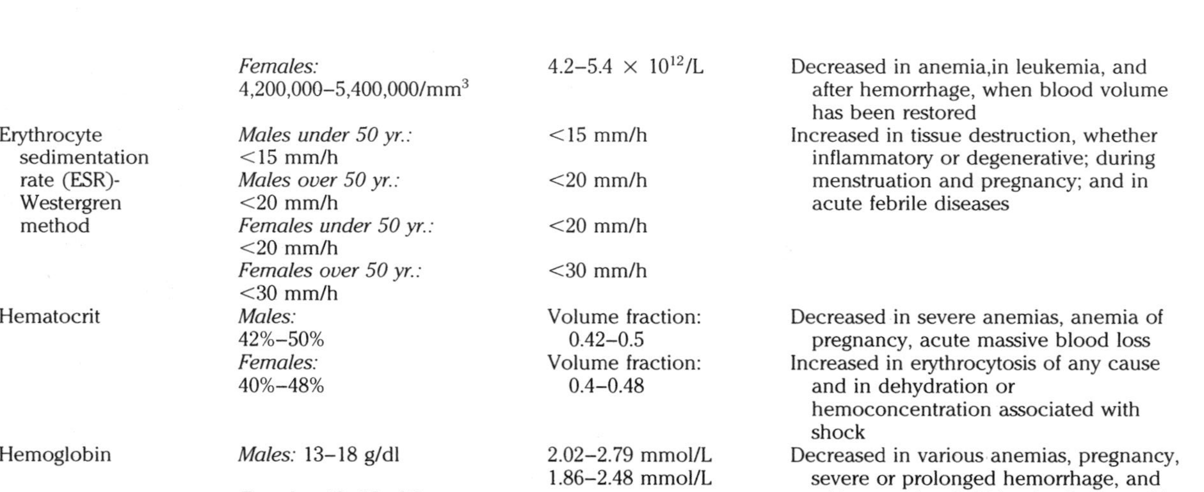

	Females: 4,200,000–5,400,000/mm^3	4.2–5.4 × 10^{12}/L	Decreased in anemia,in leukemia, and after hemorrhage, when blood volume has been restored
Erythrocyte sedimentation rate (ESR)-Westergren method	*Males under 50 yr.:* <15 mm/h	<15 mm/h	Increased in tissue destruction, whether inflammatory or degenerative; during menstruation and pregnancy; and in acute febrile diseases
	Males over 50 yr.: <20 mm/h	<20 mm/h	
	Females under 50 yr.: <20 mm/h	<20 mm/h	
	Females over 50 yr.: <30 mm/h	<30 mm/h	
Hematocrit	*Males:* 42%–50%	Volume fraction: 0.42–0.5	Decreased in severe anemias, anemia of pregnancy, acute massive blood loss
	Females: 40%–48%	Volume fraction: 0.4–0.48	Increased in erythrocytosis of any cause and in dehydration or hemoconcentration associated with shock
Hemoglobin	*Males:* 13–18 g/dl	2.02–2.79 mmol/L	Decreased in various anemias, pregnancy, severe or prolonged hemorrhage, and with excessive fluid intake. Increased in polycythemia, chronic obstructive pulmonary disease
	Females: 12–16 g/dl	1.86–2.48 mmol/L	

Determination	Normal Adult Reference Range		Clinical Significance	
	Conventional Units	**SI Units**	**Increased**	**Decreased**
Bilirubin	*Total:* 0.1–1.2 mg/d	1.7–20.5 μmol/L	Hemolytic anemia (indirect)	
	Direct: 0.1–0.2 mg/dl	1.7–3.4 μmol/L	Biliary obstruction and disease	
	Indirect: 0.1–1 mg/dl	1.7–17.1 μmol/L	Hepatocellular damage (hepatitis) Pernicious anemia Hemolytic disease of newborn	
Blood gases *Oxygen, arterial (whole blood):*				
Partial pressure (Pa_{O_2})	95–100 mm Hg	12.64–13.30 kPa	Polycythemia	Anemia
Saturation (Sa_{O_2})	94%–100%	*Volume fraction:* 0.94–1	Anhydremia	Cardiac decompensation Chronic obstructive pulmonary disease

Carbon dioxide, arterial (whole blood):				
Partial pressure ($Paco_2$)	35–45 mm Hg	4.66–5.99 kPa	Respiratory acidosis Metabolic alkalosis	Respiratory alkalosis Metabolic acidosis
pH (whole blood arterial)	7.35–7.45	7.35–7.45	Vomiting Hyperpnea Fever Intestinal obstruction	Uremia Diabetic acidosis Hemorrhage Nephritis
Calcium	8.5–10.5 mg/dl	2.125–2.625 mmol/L	Tumor or hyperplasia of parathyroid Hypervitaminosis D Multiple myeloma Nephritis with uremia Malignant tumors Sarcoidosis Hyperthyroidism Skeletal immobilization Excess calcium intake: milk-alkali syndrome	Hypoparathyroidism Diarrhea Celiac disease Vitamin D deficiency Acute pancreatitis Nephrosis After parathyroidectomy

Determination	Normal Adult Reference Range		Clinical Significance	
	Conventional Units	***SI Units***	***Increased***	***Decreased***
Chloride	95–105 mEq/L	95–105 mmol/L	Nephrosis Nephritis Urinary obstruction Cardiac decompensation Anemia	Diabetes Diarrhea Vomiting Pneumonia Heavy metal poisoning Cushing's syndrome Burns Intestinal obstruction Febrile conditions
Cholesterol	150–200 mg/dl	3.9–5.2 mmol/L	Lipemia Obstructive jaundice Diabetes Hypothyroidism	Pernicious anemia Hemolytic anemia Hyperthyroidism Severe infection Terminal states of debilitating disease
Creatinine	0.7–1.4 mg/dl	62–124 μmol/L	Nephritis Chronic renal disease	Kidney diseases
Glucose	*Fasting:* 60–110 mg/dl	3.3–6.05 mmol/L	Diabetes Nephritis	Hyperinsulinism Hyperthryoidism

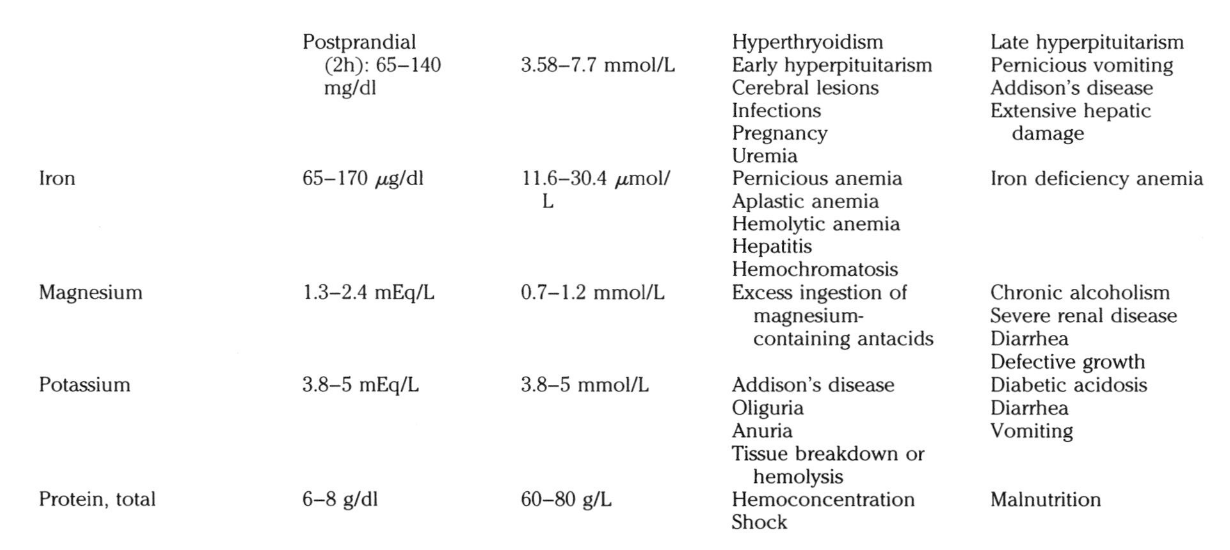

	Postprandial (2h): 65–140 mg/dl	3.58–7.7 mmol/L	Hyperthryoidism Early hyperpituitarism Cerebral lesions Infections Pregnancy Uremia	Late hyperpituitarism Pernicious vomiting Addison's disease Extensive hepatic damage
Iron	65–170 μg/dl	11.6–30.4 μmol/L	Pernicious anemia Aplastic anemia Hemolytic anemia Hepatitis Hemochromatosis	Iron deficiency anemia
Magnesium	1.3–2.4 mEq/L	0.7–1.2 mmol/L	Excess ingestion of magnesium-containing antacids	Chronic alcoholism Severe renal disease Diarrhea Defective growth
Potassium	3.8–5 mEq/L	3.8–5 mmol/L	Addison's disease Oliguria Anuria Tissue breakdown or hemolysis	Diabetic acidosis Diarrhea Vomiting
Protein, total	6–8 g/dl	60–80 g/L	Hemoconcentration Shock	Malnutrition

Determination	Normal Adult Reference Range: Conventional Units	Normal Adult Reference Range: SI Units	Clinical Significance: Increased	Clinical Significance: Decreased
Albumin *Globulin*	3.5–5 gm/dl 1.5–3 gm/dl	35–50 g/L 15–30 g/L	Multiple myeloma (globulin fraction) Chronic infections (globulin fraction) Liver disease (globulin)	Hemorrhage Loss of plasma from burns Proteinuria
Sodium	135–145 mEq/L	135–145 mmol/L	Hemoconcentration Nephritis Pyloric obstruction	Alkali deficit Addison's disease Myxedema
Thyroid-stimulating hormone (TSH)—RIA		0.3–5 m/IU/L	Hypothyroidism	Hyperthryoidism
Thyroid-binding globulin	10–26 μg/dl	100–260 μg/L	Hypothyroidism Pregnancy Estrogen therapy Oral contraceptives Genetic and idiopathic	Androgens and anabolic steroids Nephrotic syndrome Marked hypoproteinemia Hepatic disease

Urea nitrogen (BUN)	10–20 mg/dl	3.6–7.2 mmol/L	Acute glomerulonephritis Obstructive uropathy Mercury poisoning Nephrotic syndrome	Severe hepatic failure Pregnancy
Uric acid	2.5–8 mg/dl	0.15–0.5 mmol/L	Gouty arthritis Acute leukemia Lymphomas treated by chemotherapy Toxemia of pregnancy	Xanthinuria Defective tubular reabsorption

(Adapted from Suddarth: Lippincott's Manual of Nursing Practice, 5th ed, p 1535–1549. Philadelphia, JB Lippincott, 1992.)

Appendix XI

Sample Adult Nursing Health History and Physical Assessment

Health History

A. Client Profile

S.L. is a 72-year-old white female, born on a small farm in southern Missouri. Appears younger than stated age. English speaking, with a German ethnic origin. High school graduate and presently retired. Lives in a one-bedroom apartment on first floor. Drives own car. Seeks health care in local community hospital 4 miles from home. Major reason for seeking health care is for routine checkup—has not had one for 8 years. Understands that she has noninsulin-dependent diabetes mellitus (NIDDM—Type II), which is controlled with 1800 ADA diet and moderate amount of exercise. Also has "mild rheumatoid arthritic" pains in right hip and finger joints in early AMS; relieved with exercise, warm baths, and ASA.

Treatments/medications:

1. Prescribed: none
2. OTC
   a. ASA gr × prn for "arthritis aches." Takes about 2 × per month. Denies nausea, abd. pains, or evidence of bleeding while taking.
   b. Mylanta prn for "gas pains."
   c. Dulcolax supp. 3 ×/week for past 4 years.
   d. Multivitamin 1 qd, for past 4 years.

Past Illnesses/Hospitalizations:

1. Appendectomy age 18.
2. Left arm fracture age 20.
3. Cholecystectomy age 56, performed for complaint of gas pains after eating fatty foods. Satisfied with care received at local hospital.

Allergies:

Denies food, drug, and environmental allergies.

B. Developmental History

Developmental Level: Integrity vs. Despair

Describes childhood as a very happy time for her. Becomes excited and smiles as she relates stories of her childhood on the farm. States she was an average child and ran and played like all the others. Companions were brothers and sisters. Has been married for 55 years. Describes relationship with husband as close and sharing. Owned and operated a restaurant for 30 years with husband and was a waitress at another store after they retired from their own. Lived in a large house until 1976. Currently lives in a one-bedroom apartment. Active in church and society. Volunteers at community functions. She and her husband are active in their church. States she enjoys being retired and lives a "comfortable" life. Does not voice financial concerns. Has begun to write will and distribute personal heirlooms to son and grandchildren. States she is not afraid of death and wishes to have the "business part taken care of" in order to enjoy the rest of her life together with her husband.

C. Health Perception—Health Management Pattern

1. Client's rating of health:
   Scale: 10-best; 1-worst
   5 years ago: 10
   Now: 8
   5 years from now: 6
   Sees health deterioration as normal aging process and states, "I feel really good when I look at a lot of people my age with all their problems and the medicine they take."
2. Health does not interfere with self-care or other desired activities of daily living. Unaware of signs and symptoms and TX of hyperglycemia and hypoglycemia. Denies use of alcohol, tobacco, and drugs.
3. Client seeks health care only in emergencies. Last medical exam September 1984. Keeps active and feels well. Feels life-style and faith "keeps her going." Does not check own blood sugar or do breast-self-exams.

D. Nutritional—Metabolic Pattern

States she is on regular diet as follows: Eats breakfast of whole wheat toast, one boiled egg, orange juice, and decaf. coffee at 7 A.M. Eats lunch at noon. Today had tuna, lettuce salad, apple, and milk. Eats light supper around 6 P.M. Typical dinner includes small serving broiled meat, green vegetables, piece of fruit, and glass of milk. Tries not to snack but will have fruit if she feels the urge. Drinks two 8-oz glasses of water a day. Drinks decaf. coffee—no tea or colas. Voices no dislikes or food intolerances.

Wears dentures. Last dental exam Oct. 1984. Denies problems with proper fit, eating, chewing, swallowing, sore throat, sore tongue, or colds. Complains of "canker sore" if she eats strawberries. Denies n/v, abd. pain, or excessive gas. Complains of dyspepsia approx. 2 ×/month, relieved by Mylanta. Does not associate this with time she takes ASA.

Describes skin and scalp as dry. Uses lotions frequently. Denies easy bruising, pruritus, or nonhealing sores. Nails are hard and brittle. Hair is fine and soft.

Current weight: 120# Height: 5′4″

Previous weight 150 lb 10 years ago. Desires to maintain current weight.
Weight fluctuates ±5#/month. Client states, "I've always had to watch what I eat because I gain so easily." Denies intolerance to heat or cold, or voice changes.

E. Elimination Pattern

Bowel Habits: Soft, formed, med. brown bm every third day after Dulcolax supp. States she becomes constipated without use of laxative. Denies mucus, bloody or tarry stools. States discomfort with bms starting in Sept. 1984. When having to strain with bms, felt "some kind of mass" prolapsing from rectum. Consulted her doctor, who explained to her "it was a piece of my colon slipping out." No surgical treatment or exercises prescribed. Gently reinserts tissue when this happens. Denies rectal bleeding, change in color, consistency, or habits.

Bladder Habits: Voids 4–5 ×/day, clear yellow urine. Denies current problems with dysuria, hematuria, polyuria, hesitancy, incontinence, or nocturia. Complaint of urgency during the colder months with no increase in frequency. Had polyuria and polydipsia prior to diagnosis of D.M. Developed UTI age 60, at which time she sought medical advice and was diagnosed with diabetes mellitus.

F. Activity—Exercise Pattern

1. ADLs on an average day: Arises at 6 A.M. Eats breakfast and does housekeeping. In early afternoon goes to the community center to eat lunch, quilt, and visit. Goes home around 2 P.M. Walks about 4 blocks with a friend every day. Cleans own house daily for one 2-hr period (incl.

dusting, vacuuming, washing). Denies palpitations, chest pain, sob, fatigue, wheezing, claudication, cramps, stiffness, or joint pain or swelling with activity. Walking relieves ache in hips and makes her feel good. After walking, returns home and relaxes with crafts and visiting with husband. During evenings attends church-related activities. Expresses satisfaction with activity and believes she functions above the level of the average person her age.

2. Hygiene: Showers and washes hair every day.
3. Occupational activities: Retired from being a cook and waitress. Volunteers to cook for church group. Occasionally has lower back pains when carrying large amounts of food or when carrying large trays.

G. Sexuality—Reproduction Pattern

Menstrual History: Age of menarche: approx. 12 yr; age of menopause: 50 yr. States "going through my change of life wasn't difficult for me physically or emotionally." Described menstrual period as regular, lasting 4 days with moderate flow. Denies postmenopausal spotting at this time.

Obstetric History: Gravida I, Para I. No complications with pregnancy or childbirth.

Contraception: Never used any form.

Sexual Activities: Sexually active. States, "My husband and I have good relations." Denies pain, discomfort, or postcoital bleeding.

Special Problems: Denies history of any sexually transmitted diseases. Denies problem with vaginal itching. Last Pap smear: negative in 1976.

H. Sleep—Rest Pattern

Goes to bed at 10 P.M. Denies difficulty falling asleep or sleeping. Feels well rested when she arises at 6 A.M. Never used sleep medications. Denies orthopnea and nocturnal dyspnea. Enjoys reading 1–2 pages of bible history each evening.

I. Sensory—Perceptual Pattern

1. Vision: Has worn glasses "all of my life." Cannot recall age at which they were prescribed. Prescription change from bifocals to trifocals August 1984. Complains of blurred vision without glasses. Denies diplopia, itching, excessive tearing, discharge, redness, or trauma to eyes.
2. Hearing: Believes she is "a little slow to grasp, and I think it may be because of my hearing." Does not wear hearing aid. Cannot recall last hearing test. Denies tinnitus, pain, discharge, or trauma to ears. Does not ask for questions to be repeated when asked at normal voice tone and level.
3. Smell: Denies difficulty with smell, pain, postnasal drip, sneezing, or frequent nosebleeds.
4. Touch: States "occasionally my feet feel numb"; subsides on own.
5. Taste: No difficulty tasting foods.

J. Cognitive Pattern

Speech clear without slur or stutter. Follows verbal cues. Expresses ideas and feelings clearly and concisely. States she has had a gradual loss of memory over past 5–6 years. Believes long-term memory is better than short-term. She can recall past weekly events but has trouble recalling dates, times, and places of events. Learns best by writing information down and then reviewing it. Makes major decisions jointly with husband after prayer.

Health History *(continued)*

K. Role—Relationship Pattern

Client has been married 55 years. Describes relationship as the best part of her life right now. Only son lives in Minnesota, and they visit 1–2 times a year. Is very fond of three grandchildren. Expresses desire to visit more often but states, "He has his own life and family now." Communicates once a month by phone. Explains her relationship with other members of the church and community groups as friendly and "family-like." Lives with husband in first-floor apartment. Has casual relationship with apartment neighbors—friendly but distant. Was the fourth of five children. See family genogram.

L. Self-Perception–Self-Concept Pattern

Describes self as a normal person. Talkative, outgoing, and likes to be around people but hates noisy environments. Happy with the person she has become and states, "I can definitely live with myself." States a weakness is that she worries about "little things" more now than she used to and tends to be irritated more easily. Cannot place specific onset of these feelings. Feels good about self-control of diabetes.

M. Coping–Stress Tolerance Pattern

States husband's high blood pressure has never been a source of stress to her. Shares confidences with husband and with a few close friends. Most stressful time in life was losing two brothers and a sister, all in 1982. States with the support of husband and church she handled it "better than most people would have." States she prays and eats when under stress. Cannot identify any major stresses that have occurred in the last year.

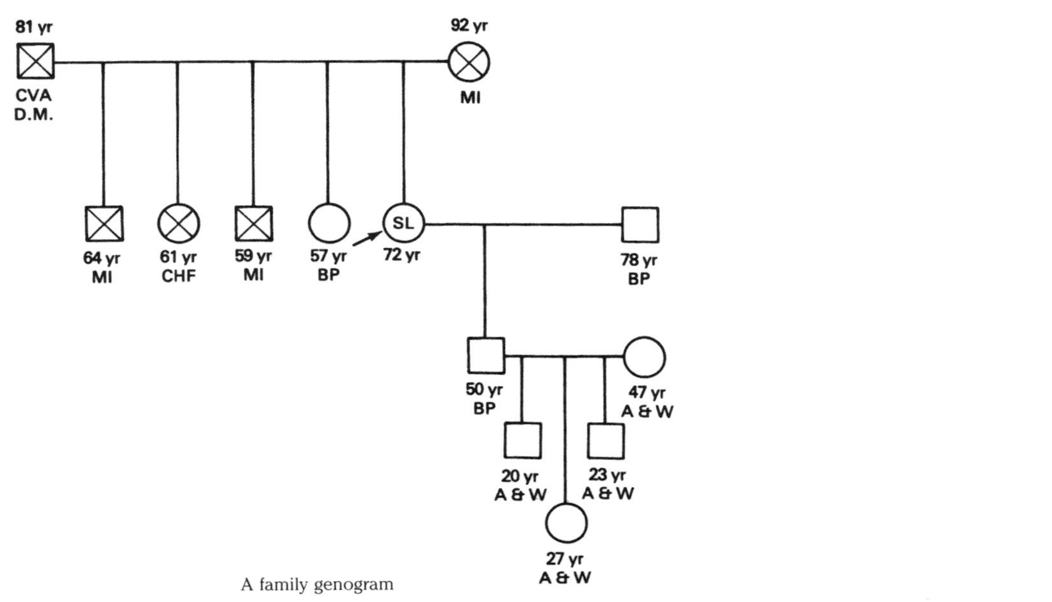

A family genogram

Health History *(continued)*

N. Value—Belief Pattern

Religious preference is Lutheran. Values relationship with husband, family, and God. Enjoys helping others in the church and community. Believes God is loving, supportive, and forgiving. Places God as first priority in life. States prayer is extremely important to her and practices it daily. States this personalizes her relationship with God. Has been Lutheran all her life and states she and her husband share in church activities together.

Physical Assessment

A. General Physical Survey

Ht: 5′4″ Wt: 120# Radial pulse: 71 Resp: 16 B/P: R arm—120/72, L arm—120/70 Temp: 98.6
Client alert and cooperative. Sitting comfortably on table with arms crossed and shoulders slightly slouched forward. Smiling with mild anxiety. Dress is neat and clean. Walks steadily with posture slightly stooped.

B. Assessment of Skin, Hair, and Nails

1. *Skin:* pale pink, warm and dry to touch. Skinfold returns to place after 1 second when lifted over clavicle. Tan "age spots" on posterior hands bilaterally in clusters of 4–5 and evenly distributed over lower extremities. 3-cm nodule with 2-mm macule in center noted in right axilla; indurated, nontender, and nonmobile. No evidence of vascular or purpuric lesions. No edema.

2. *Hair:* chin-length, gray, straight, clean, styled, med. textured, evenly distributed on head. No scalp lesions or flaking. Fine blond hair evenly distributed over arms bilaterally and sparsely on legs bilaterally. No hair noted on axilla or on chest, back, or face.
3. *Nails:* Fingernails med. length, and thickness, clear. Splinter hemorrhages noted on right thumb near fingertip in midline. No clubbing or Beau's lines.

C. Assessment of Head and Neck

Head symmetrically rounded, neck nontender with full ROM. Neck symmetrical without masses, scars, pulsations. Lymph nodes nonpalpable. Trachea in midline. Thyroid nonpalpable. Carotid arteries equally strong without bruits. Identifies light and deep touch to various parts of face.

CN V: Identifies light touch and sharp touch to forehead, cheek, and chin. Bilateral corneal reflex intact. Masseter muscles contract equally and bilaterally. Jaw jerk +1.

CN VII: Identifies sugar and salt on ant. 2/3s tongue. Smiles, frowns, shows teeth, blows out cheeks, and raises eyebrows as instructed.

D. Assessment of Eye

Eyes 2 cm apart without protrusion. Eyebrows sparse with = distribution. No scaliness noted. Lids pink without ptosis, edema, or lesions, and freely closeable bilaterally. Lacrimal apparatus nonedematous. Sclera white without increased vascularity or lesions noted. Palpebral and bulbar conjunctiva slightly reddened without lesions noted. Iris uniformly blue. PERRLA, EOMs intact bilaterally. Peripheral vision = to examiner's.

Visual acuity: With glasses off vision is blurred at 14″ away, but can identify number of fingers held up. With glasses on reads newspaper print at 14″.

Physical Assessment *(continued)*

Fundoscopic exam: Red reflex present bilaterally. Optic disk round with well-defined margins. Physiologic cup occupies disc. Arterioles smaller than venules. No A-V nicking, no hemorrhages, or exudates noted. Macula not seen. (CN II, III, IV, and VI intact.)

E. Assessment of Ear

L auricle without deformity, lumps, or lesions. R auricle with tag at top of pinna. Auricles and mastoid processes nontender. Bilateral auditory canals contain moderate amount dark brown cerumen. Tympanic membrane difficult to view due to wax.

Whisper test: Client identifies one out of two words in four attempts. Weber test: No lateralization of sound to either ear. Rinne test: AC is greater than BC both ears (CN VIII).

F. Assessment of Nose and Sinuses

External structure without deformity, asymmetry, or inflammation. Nares patent. Turbinates and middle meatus pale pink, without swelling, exudate, lesions, or bleeding. Nasal septum midline without bleeding, perforation, or deviation. Frontal and maxillary sinuses nontender. Identifies smell of coffee and soap (CN I).

G. Assessment of Mouth and Pharynx

Lips moist with peach lipstick. No lesions or ulcerations. Buccal mucosa pink and moist without discoloration or increased pigmentation. No ulcers or nodules. Upper and lower dentures secure. Gums pink and moist without inflammation, bleeding, or discoloration. Hard and soft palates smooth without lesions or masses. Tongue midline when protruded without fasciculations (CN XII intact), lesions, or masses. No lesions, discolorations, or ulcerations on floor of mouth, oral mucosa, or gums. Gag reflex intact, and client identifies sugar and salt on posterior of tongue. Uvula in midline and elevates on phonation. (CN IX and X intact.) Tonsils present without exudate, edema, ulcers, or enlargement.

H. Assessment of Heart

No pulsations visible. No heaves, lifts, or vibrations. PMI: 5th ICS to LMCL. Clear, brief heart sounds throughout. Physiologic S_2. No gallops, murmurs, or rubs. AP = 72/min and regular.

I. Assessment of Peripheral Vascular System

Arms: Equal in size and symmetry bilaterally; pale pink; warm and dry to touch without edema, bruising, or lesions noted. Radial pulses = in rate and amplitude; and strong. Allen's test: Right = 2-sec refill, left = 2-sec refill. Brachial pulses strong, equal, and even. Epitrochlear nodes nonpalpable.

Legs: Legs large in size and bilaterally symmetrical. Skin intact, pale pink; warm and dry to touch without edema, bruising, lesions, or increased vascularity. Superficial inguinal, horizontal, and vertical lymph nodes nonpalpable. Femoral pulses strong and equal without bruits. Popliteal pulse nonpalpable with client supine or prone. Dorsalis pedal and posterior tibial pulses strong and equal. No edema palpable. Homans' neg bilaterally. No retrograde filling noted when client stands. Toenails thick and yellowed. Special maneuver for arterial insufficiency: feet regain color after 4 seconds and veins refilled in 5 sec.

Physical Assessment *(continued)*

J. Assessment of Thorax and Lungs

Skin pale pink without scars, pulsations, or lesions. No hair noted. Thorax expands evenly bilaterally without retractions or bulging. Slope of ribs = 40°. No use of auxiliary respiratory muscles and no nasal flaring. Mild kyphosis. Respirations even, unlabored, and regular (16/min). No cough noted. No tenderness, crepitus, or masses. Tactile fremitus decreases below T5 bilaterally posteriorly, and 4th ICS anteriorly bilaterally. Thorax resonance throughout. Diaphragmatic excursion: Left—On inspiration diaphragm descends to T11, and on expiration diaphragm ascends to T9. Right—On inspiration diaphragm descends to T12, and on expiration diaphragm ascends to T9. Vesicular breath sounds heard in all lung fields. No rales, rhonchi, friction rubs, whispered pectoriloquy, bronchophony, or egophony noted.

K. Assessment of Breasts

Breasts moderate in size, round and symmetrical bilaterally. Skin pale pink with light brown areola. No dimpling or retraction. Free movement in all positions. Engorged vein noted running across UOQ to areola in right breast. Nipples inverted bilaterally. No discharge expressed. No thickening or tenderness noted. 2 cm, hard, immobile round mass noted in left breast in LOQ. Client denies ever noticing this. Nontender to palpation. Lymph nodes nonpalpable. Client does not know how to do SBE.

L. Assessment of Abdomen

Abdomen rounded, symmetrical without masses, lesions, pulsations, or peristalsis noted. Abdomen free of hair, bruising, and increased vasculature. Healed with appendectomy scar. Umbilicus in midline, without herniation, swelling or discoloration. Bowel sounds low pitched and gurgling at 22/min × 4 quads. Aortic, renal, and iliac arteries auscultated without bruit. No venous hums or friction rubs auscultated over liver or spleen. Tympany percussed over all 4 quads. 8 cm. liver span percussed in R MCL. Area of dullness percussed at 9th ICS in left post axillary line. No tenderness or masses noted with light and deep palpation in all 4 quadrants. Liver and spleen nonpalpable.

M. Genitourinary Assessment

No bulging or masses in inguinal area. 1-cm nodule palpated in R groin. Labia pink with decreased elasticity and vaginal secretions. No bulging of vaginal wall, purulent foul drainage, or lesions. Skene's gland not visible. Anal area pink with small amount of hair. Rectal mucosa bulges with straining.

N. Musculoskeletal Assessment

Posture slightly stooped with mild kyphosis. Gait steady, smooth, and coordinated with even base. Limited ROM of lateral flexion and extension of spine. Paravertebrals equal in size and strength. Shrugs shoulders and moves head to right and left against resistance (CN XI intact); upper extremities and lower extremities with full ROM. Muscles moderately firm bilaterally. No deviations, inflammations, or bony deformities. Small callus on left heel. Moves upper and lower extremities freely against gravity and against resistance. Rheumatoid nodule noted on dorsal surface of left hand.

O. Neurological Assessment

Mental Status: Pleasant and friendly. Appropriately dressed for weather with matching colors and patterns. Clothes neat and clean. Facial expressions symmetrical and correlate with mood and topic discussed. Speech clear and appropriate. Follows through with train of thought. Carefully chooses words to convey feelings and ideas. Oriented to person, place, time, and events. Remains attentive and able to focus on exam during entire interaction. Short-term memory intact, long-term memory before 1980 unclear—especially cannot recall dates and sequencing of events. General information questions answered correctly 100% of the time. Vocabulary suitable to educational level. Explains proverb accurately. Gives semi-abstract answers and enjoys joking. Is able to identify similarities 5 seconds after asked. Answers to judgment questions in realistic manner.

Physical Assessment *(continued)*

Cranial Nerves: I–XII intact (integrated throughout exam).

Cerebellar and Motor Function: Alternates finger to nose with eyes closed; occasionally tends to hit opposite side of nose. Rapidly opposes fingers to thumb bilaterally without difficulty. Alternates pronation and supination of hands rapidly without difficulty. Heel to shin intact bilaterally. Romberg: Minimal swaying. Tandem walk: Steady. No involuntary movements noted.

Sensory Status: Superficial light and deep touch sensation intact on arms, legs, neck, chest, and back. Position sense of toes and fingers intact bilaterally. Identifies point localization correctly. Identifies coin placed in hand and number written on back correctly.

Two-Point Discrimination (in mm)	***Right***	***Left***
Fingertips	6	6
Dorsal hand	15	15
Chest	45	49
Forearm	39	35
Back	45	45
Upper arm	40	45

Reflexes	***Right***	***Left***
Biceps	2+	2+
Triceps	2+	2+
Patellar	3+	3+
Achilles	2+	2+
Abdominal	1+	1+
Babinski	neg	neg

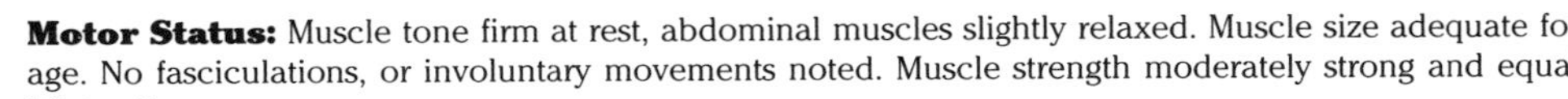

Motor Status: Muscle tone firm at rest, abdominal muscles slightly relaxed. Muscle size adequate for age. No fasciculations, or involuntary movements noted. Muscle strength moderately strong and equal bilaterally.

Client's Strengths

- Positive attitude and outlook on life
- Motivation to comply with prescribed diet
- Strong support systems: Husband and spiritual beliefs
- No physical limitations

Nursing Diagnoses

- Altered health seeking behavior related to lack of knowledge concerning importance of regular medical checkups, re: lesion in UOQ of left breast not seen by physician, no Pap smear, and no follow-up with diabetes.
- Acute right hip pain.
- Constipation related to lack of bowel routine and laxative overuse.
- Knowledge deficit: Signs and symptoms and treatment of hyperglycemia/hypoglycemia.
- Knowledge deficit: Management and causes of constipation.
- Knowledge deficit: SBE technique.

Collaborative Problems

- Potential complication: Hyperglycemia, hypoglycemia
- Potential complication: Hypertension

Appendix XII

Sample Pediatric Nursing Health History and Physical Assessment

Health History

A. Client Profile

R.B. is an active 9-year-old Caucasian male with a diagnosis of insulin-dependent diabetes mellitus for the past year. He lives in a large southeastern metropolitan community with his mother and 6-year-old sister. R.B.'s parents divorced 2 months ago. The adjustment without his father in the home has been difficult for R.B. His mother reports increased episodes of misconduct and lower grades at school. R.B. typically likes school and has received A's and B's but is now obtaining B's and C's. R.B. is currently receiving 5 units of regular insulin with 10 units of NPH insulin in the morning and 2 units of regular insulin with 5 units of NPH insulin in the evening. He tests his blood prior to each injection and at bedtime with assistance from his mother. He is on a 2500 calorie ADA diet. Food treats are allowed with appropriate diet modification once monthly. Immunization history is up-to-date.

Past Illnesses/Hospitalizations:

1. Tonsillectomy—age 5.
2. Medical diagnosis of IDDM—age 8.

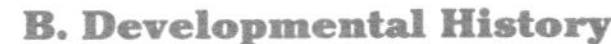

B. Developmental History

Erikson's Stage of Industry vs. Inferiority: R.B. describes his school experiences with enthusiasm, particularly enjoying math and science classes. He plays on a basketball team with classmates. Now he is experiencing some difficulty concentrating, stating he is having frequent headaches.

Piaget's Stage of Concrete Operations: R.B. is able to tell time and maintain a set schedule. He organizes objects based on multiple characteristics.

Freud's Stage of Latency: R.B. prefers to participate in games and activities with members of his same sex.

C. Health—Perception and Health-Management Pattern

Client's rating of health:
Scale: 10-best; 1-worst
1 year ago: 6; Now: 9.
Mother's rating of health:
1 year ago: 5; Now: 7.
Since R.B. was diagnosed with diabetes just 1 year ago, he and his mother are congruent with one another when indicating his status was lower then than it is now. Mother still believes his health state could improve, as she believes he is keeping "his feelings inside" and is "being stubborn" about taking his insulin on time and maintaining his prescribed diet. R.B. participates in self-care to regulate his diabetes but relies on his mother on school mornings and during more hurried times.

Health History *(continued)*

He goes for a routine evaluation of his blood sugar and Hgb A(1)C (glycosylated hemoglobin) values every 3 months, which usually average 110 mg/dl and 8%, respectively. On this visit, glucose was 453 mg/dl and Hgb A(1)C was 10%.

D. Nutritional–Metabolic Pattern

R.B.'s diet is maintained using the ADA exchange lists, including a mid-morning, mid-afternoon, and bedtime snack. He had lost 12 pounds at the time of initial diagnosis and was experiencing epigastric pain and vomiting. Mrs. B. is concerned since R.B.'s weight is 64 pounds now, placing him slightly under the 50th percentile for age. Although R.B. denies skipping injections or eating lunches or snacks high in carbohydrates, Mrs. B. cannot understand this episode of hyperglycemia. Mother states she "may not have been as careful with meals the past few weeks." Height is 52 inches, also in the 50th percentile for age. There are no episodes of poor wound healing or lesions on skin surfaces.

Prior to this hospitalization, R.B. vomited 3 ×'s last evening, and mother noted a "fruity smell" to his breath.

E. Elimination Pattern

Bladder: Voids 6–7 ×/day. Currently, was up to 10–12 ×/day. Denies enuresis, burning, or dysuria. Reports urine to be clear yellow.

Bowel: Denies constipation, bleeding, or pain upon defecation. Has daily bowel movement; moderate, formed, brown stool.

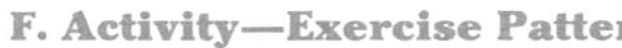

F. Activity—Exercise Pattern

Has physical education class for 50 minutes every morning on school days, prior to A.M. snack. Rides his bicycle most days after school with friends. Has basketball practice 3 days a week. Mother has provided a trampoline to use in the home on days of inclement weather.

G. Sexuality Pattern

Has normal prepubescent sexual development. Is beginning to inquire about the female gender and "having babies."

H. Sleep—Rest Pattern

Typically bedtime is at 9 P.M., except for special outings or when spending the night with a friend. Arises at 6:30 A.M. each morning to test blood, receive insulin, and have breakfast.

I. Sensory—Perceptual Pattern

Vision: Wears corrective lens for myopia, particularly for seeing the blackboard at school. Hearing, smell, touch, and taste perceptions WNL.

J. Cognitive Pattern

Has increasing development of reasoning and logical thought processes. Mother states he is "mechanically inclined" and enjoys putting models together and building projects. Is inquisitive about his environment and new experiences. Verbalizes ideas more easily when separate from mother.

Health History *(continued)*

K. Role—Relationship Pattern

Exhibits sibling rivalry with younger sister. Misses father, who lives 50 miles away and whom he sees only every other weekend. Has a close relationship with mother but states "she is telling me what to do all the time now." Visits maternal and paternal grandparents frequently. Maternal grandmother also has IDDM.

L. Self-Perception–Self-Concept Pattern

Does not see himself as being "different" from his friends. Participates in similar activities with peers and is "accepted" by them. Believes he has to be more "organized" than his friends because he has to eat, take insulin, and test his blood at certain times. Explains to classmates what to do if he becomes hypoglycemic.

M. Coping–Stress Tolerance Pattern

Describes "being lonely" since his father left. Although he is close to his mother and sister, he and his father did "guy things together," like working on the car and going fishing.

N. Value—Belief Pattern

Religious affiliation of the family is Roman Catholic. R.B. attends Mass on Sunday with his mother and younger sister. He practices denominational rituals. Both parents emphasize the importance of God and prayer.

Physical Assessment

A. General Appearance, Vital Signs, and Laboratory Findings

A well-nourished male child in no obvious pain or discomfort, resting quietly with mother present. Hygiene and attire are neat and clean. Responds to questions appropriately but is somewhat withdrawn. Verbalizes more openly when mother leaves room.

Temperature: 99.4 Apical Pulse: 94 Respirations: 20 B/P: 103/58

BUN: 22 mg/dl Glucose: 453 mg/dl Potassium: 5.4 mmol/L Hemoglobin: 13.7 g/dl Hematocrit: 41% Urine s.g. 1.028 Ketones: present ABGs: pH 7.26 Base excess (−6) mmol/L.

B. Assessment of Skin, Hair, and Nails

Skin: Warm, pink, dry; face flushed. No evidence of skin tenting over sternum, abdomen, or extremities. Capillary refill less than 2 seconds. Small abrasion approximately 2 cm × 2 cm over left patella, healing.

Hair: Evenly distributed brown in color, neatly combed. No evidence of dryness, lesions, or nits.

Nails: Nail biting noted; cuticles frayed.

C. Assessment of Head and Neck

Head symmetrical and normocephalic with full ROM. Neck mobile without tenderness, excessive pulsations, masses, or nuchal rigidity. Trachea midline; thyroid nonpalpable. Carotid arteries +2, without bruits. Small cervical nodes palpable, mobile, and nontender.

CN V (Trigeminal): Moves jaw from side to side; masseter and temporal muscles clenched and released; corneal reflex present; identifies pinprick to forehead, cheeks, jaw.

CN VII (Facial): Smiles, frowns, puffs out cheeks symmetrically; tastes salt, lemon, and artificial sweetener on anterior $^{2}/_{3}$s tongue.

D. Assessment of Eye

No hypertelorism, ptosis, redness, or drainage. Full ROM of EOMs in six cardinal fields (CN III, IV, VI) Sclera white; palpebral and bulbar conjunctiva pink and moist. Iris dark brown, clear. PERRLA.

Visual acuity: Snellen, 20/30 (CN II).

Fundoscopic exam: Red reflex present bilaterally. Optic disk round, with smooth margins. Venules larger than arterioles, without dilatation or hemorrhages.

E. Assessment of Ear

Left and right pinna in line with orbital line. Auricles and mastoid processes without masses, tenderness, or erythema. No drainage from either external auditory meatus. Tympanic membranes pearly gray; light reflex observed. Weber test has equal sound to both ears. Rinne test: AC > BC bilaterally (CN VIII Acoustic intact).

F. Assessment of Nose and Sinuses

Nares patent, without deformity, erythema, or tenderness to external or internal structures. Septum without deviations; turbinates and meatal openings pink. No tenderness of the supraorbital, infraorbital, and maxillary areas (CN I Olfactory intact).

G. Assessment of Mouth and Pharynx

Oral mucosa pink and sticky with acetone odor present. Lips cracked and dry. No dental caries; two small fillings in lower right molars. Gums, hard and soft palate, and tongue pink with no ulcerations or masses. Tonsils removed. Elevation of palate upon saying "ah," tongue midline without fasciculations; tastes salt and sweetener on posterior of tongue, gag reflex present (CN IX Glossopharyngeal, CN X Vagus, and CN XII Hypoglossal intact).

H. Assessment of Heart and Peripheral Vasculature

Normal sinus rhythm and rate at 94/min. PMI at the 5th ICS, slightly medial to the left MCL. Heart sounds clear with no murmurs present. Peripheral pulses strong, +2.

I. Assessment of Thorax and Lungs

Thorax oval with transverse diameter > AP diameter. Symmetrical respiratory excursion without distress or retractions. No cysts, supernummary nipples, masses, or tenderness. Clear vesicular sounds auscultated over anterior and posterior lung fields.

Physical Assessment *(continued)*

J. Assessment of Abdomen

Abdomen soft, round, and nondistended, without discoloration, hernias or lesions. Umbilicus midline. Bowel sounds low pitched, metallic at 28/min, heard in all four quadrants. Lower edge of liver percussed at right costal margin.

K. Genitourinary and Anal Assessment

Normal circumcised prepubescent (Tanner's Stage 1) male genitalia. Meatal opening at tip of penis, with no redness or discharge. Scrotal rugae present; testes descended into scrotal sac. No hydrocele, hernias, masses, or inguinal nodes palpable. Anal tissue pink.

L. Musculoskeletal Assessment

Symmetrical, free-moving gait. Strong muscle tone, with hand grips equal bilaterally. Syndactyly or polydactyly absent. No kyphosis, lordosis, or scoliosis. Full ROM of extremities with no joint swelling, redness, or tenderness. Shrugs shoulders against mild resistance (CN XI Accessory intact).

M. Neurological Assessment

Alert, oriented, and cooperative child; capable of counting backward from 20 to 1 in clear, distinct voice. Cranial nerves (I–XII) intact. Touches index fingers to nose repetitively upon request. Romberg's test negative. DTRs (triceps, biceps, brachioradialis, patellar, Achilles) all +2. Babinski reflex negative.

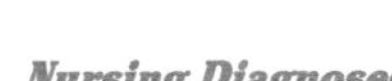

Nursing Diagnoses

Altered Nutrition: Less than body requirements related to:

1. Current gastrointestinal upset
2. Hyperglycemia secondary to diabetes mellitus
3. Possible irregularity with ADA meal planning since recent stress of parents' divorce.

Fluid Volume Deficit related to osmotic diuresis secondary to elevated glucose levels
Grieving related to absence of father in the home setting since parental divorce

Appendix XIII

Assessment of Family Functional Health Patterns

The nurse obtains data about the family's functional health patterns by interviewing the family as a group or by interviewing one or two family members who are reliable historians and seem knowledgeable of their family's health patterns. If data reveals a particular problem with an individual family member, the nurse can then focus attention on obtaining more data from that individual.

I. Family Profile

The purpose of the family profile is to obtain biographical family data (age, sex, and current health status of each family member). A genogram may be used to illustrate this information. See pgs. 27, 439 for examples.

II. Health Perception—Health Management Pattern

Subjective Data

- Describe your family's general health during the past few years.
- Has your family been able to participate in its usual activities (work, school, sports)?
- Describe what your family does to try to stay healthy (diet, exercise, etc.).
- From whom does your family seek health care? When?

- Describe how your family checks their health status (i.e., eye exams, dental exams, breast exams, testicular exams, medical checkups).
- Describe any behaviors in your family that are considered unhealthy.
- Who cares for family members who are or who become ill?

Objective Data

1. Observe the appearance of family members.
2. Observe the home (hazards and safety devices, storage facilities, cooking facilities).

III. Nutritional Metabolic Pattern

Subjective Data

- Describe typical breakfast, lunch, supper, and snacks that you eat as a family.
- What type of drinks do you usually have during the day and at night?
- How would you describe your family's appetite in general?
- How often does your family seek dental care? Are there any dental problems in your family?
- Does anyone in your family have skin rashes or problems with sores healing? Explain.
- Who usually prepares the family meals? Who shops for groceries?

Objective Data

1. Observe kitchen appliances, availability of food, and types of foods kept in the home, if possible.
2. Observe preparation of a family meal, if possible.
3. Observe family members for obvious signs of malnutrition or obesity.

IV. Elimination Pattern

Subjective Data
- Are laxatives used in your family? Explain.
- Are there problems with disposing of waste or garbage?
- Describe any recycling you do.
- Does your family have pets (indoor or outdoor)? How are their wastes disposed?
- Do you have problems with insects in your home? Explain.

Objective Data
1. Observe bathroom facilities.
2. Inspect home for insects.
3. Observe garbage and waste disposals.

V. Activity—Exercise Pattern

Subjective Data:
- Describe how your family exercises. Frequency?
- How does your family relax?
- What does your family do for enjoyment?
- Describe a typical day of activities in your family (work, school, play, games, meals, hobbies, house cleaning, yard work, cooking, exercise).

Objective Guidelines

1. Observe the pace of family activities.
2. Observe any exercise equipment kept in home.

VI. Sleep—Rest Pattern

Subjective Data

- When does your family generally go to bed and awaken? Do family members go to bed and arise at different times? Explain.
- Does your family seem to get enough time to sleep? to rest and relax?
- Do any family members work at night? How does this affect other family members?

Objective Data

1. Observe sleeping areas.
2. Observe temperament and energy level of family members.

VII. Sensory—Perceptual Pattern

Subjective Data

- Are there any hearing or visual problems that affect your family members?
- Are there any deficits in a family member's ability to taste and smell that affects how food is prepared for the family?
- Does pain seem to be a family problem? Explain. How is this managed?
- What is the usual form of pain relief used by family members?

VII. Sensory—Perceptual Pattern (continued)

Objective Data

1. Observe any visual or hearing aids used by family members.
2. Observe medications kept on hand to relieve pain.

VIII. Cognitive Pattern

Subjective Data

- Who makes the major family decisions? How?
- Describe the highest educational level of all family members.
- Does your family understand any illnesses and treatments that affect any of your family members?
- How does your family enjoy learning? (i.e., reading, watching TV, attending classes, etc.)
- Are there any problems with memory in the family? Explain.

Objective Data

1. Observe language spoken by all family members.
2. Observe use of words (vocabulary level), ability to grasp ideas, and express self.
3. Are family decisions present or future oriented? Observe family decision making strategies.
4. Observe school attended by children.

IX. *Self-Perception–Self-Concept Pattern*

Subjective Data

- Describe the general mood of your family (i.e., sad, happy, eager, depressed, anxious, relaxed)
- Do you consider yourselves to be a close family? How do you spend time together? Is this time satisfying?
- Do family members share any common goals? Explain.
- What does the family enjoy doing most together?
- How does your family deal with disagreements?
- How does your family express their affection, feelings, and/or concerns? Are they allowed to do so freely? Explain.
- Does your family seem to discuss problems that affect individual members?
- How does your family deal with change?

Objective Data

1. Observe family discussions.
2. Observe mood and temperament of family.
3. Observe how family members deal with conflict.
4. How do family members show concern and consideration for each other's needs and desires?

X. Role-Relationship Pattern

Subjective Data
- Describe how your family members support each other, show affection, and express concerns.
- Describe any problems with relationships between family members.
- Describe your family resources (financial, community support systems, family support systems).
- How active is your family in your neighborhood and/or community?
- Explain family responsibilities for various household chores (washing, cooking, driving, lawn maintenance, etc.).
- Explain how discipline is used in your family. How are family members rewarded? Describe any aggression and/or violence that occurs in your family.

Objective Data
1. Observe family interaction patterns (verbal and nonverbal).
2. Explore which family members take responsibility for managing and leading family activities.
3. Observe living space and ownership of rooms by family members.

XI. Sexuality—Reproductive Pattern

Subjective Data

If appropriate: Are sexual partners within home satisfied with sexual relationship and activities? Describe any problems.
- Are contraceptives used?
- Is family planning used? How?
- Are parents comfortable answering questions and explaining topics related to sexuality to their children?

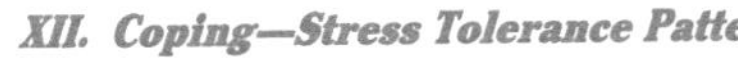

XII. Coping—Stress Tolerance Pattern

Subjective Data

- What major changes have occurred in your family during the last year? (e.g., divorce, marriage, family members leaving home, new members coming into home, death, illness, births, accidents, change in finances and/or occupation).
- How does your family *cope* with major stressors (i.e., exercise, discussion, prayer, drugs, alcohol, violence)?
- Who in the family copes best with stressors?
- Who has the most difficult time coping with stress?
- Who outside the family (i.e., friends, church, support groups) seems to help your family most during difficult times?

Objective Data

1. Observe affect and pace of family interactions.

XIII. Value—Belief Pattern

Subjective Data

- What does your family consider to be most important in life?
- What does your family want from life?
- What rules does your family hold most important?

- Is religion important in the family? What religion are family members? What religious practices are important to the family? Is a relationship with God important to the family?
- What does your family look forward to in the future?
- From where does the family's hope and strength come?

Objective Data

1. Observe family rituals and/or traditions.
2. Observe pictures and other articles (religious or other) in home.
3. Listen to general topics discussed in home by family members.
4. Observe the type of television programs viewed by family members and the type of music to which family members listen.

Appendix XIV

Nursing Diagnoses (Wellness, Risk, and Actual) Grouped According to Functional Health Patterns

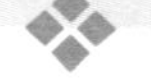

1. Health Perception Management Pattern

Wellness Diagnoses
Health Seeking Behaviors
Effective Management of Therapeutic Regimen

Risk Diagnoses
Risk for Injury
Risk for Suffocation
Risk for Poisoning
Risk for Trauma
Risk for Perioperative Positioning Injury

Actual Diagnosis
Energy Field Disturbance
Altered Growth and Development
Altered Health Maintenance
Ineffective Management of Therapeutic Regimen: Individual
Ineffective Management of Therapeutic Regimen: Family
Ineffective Management of Therapeutic Regimen: Community
Noncompliance

2. Nutritional Metabolic Pattern

Wellness Diagnoses
Effective Breastfeeding
*Opportunity to enhance nutritional metabolic pattern
*Opportunity to enhance skin integrity

(* Not on current NANDA list)
All other diagnosis are used with permission from the North American Nursing Diagnosis Association.

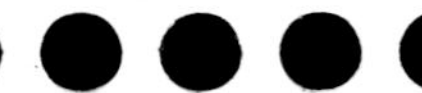
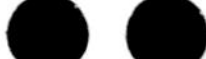

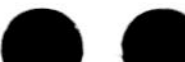
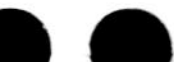
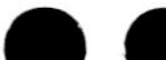

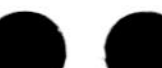

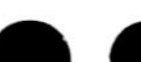

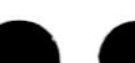

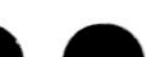

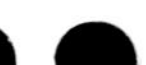

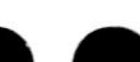

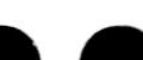
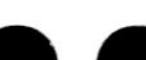
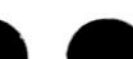

Risk Diagnoses

Risk for Altered Body Temperature
- Hypothermia
- Hyperthermia

Risk for Infection
*Risk for altered nutrition: more than body requirements
*Risk for altered nutrition: Less than body requirements
Risk for Aspiration

Actual Diagnoses

Decreased Adaptive Capacity: Intracranial
Ineffective Thermoregulation
Fluid Volume Deficit
Fluid Volume Excess
Altered Nutrition: Less than body requirements
Altered Nutrition: More than body requirements
Ineffective Breastfeeding
Interrupted Breastfeeding
Ineffective Infant Feeding Pattern
Impaired Swallowing
Altered Protection
Impaired Tissue Integrity
Altered Oral Mucous Membrane
Impaired Skin Integrity

3. Elimination Pattern

Wellness Diagnoses

*Opportunity to enhance adequate bowel elimination pattern
*Opportunity to enhance adequate urinary elimination pattern

Risk Diagnoses

*Risk for constipation
*Risk for altered urinary elimination

Actual Diagnoses

Altered Bowel Elimination
- Constipation
- Colonic Constipation
- Perceived Constipation
- Diarrhea
- Bowel Incontinence

Altered Urinary Elimination
- Urinary Retention

Total Incontinence
Functional Incontinence
Reflex Incontinence
Urge incontinence
Stress Incontinence

4. Activity—Exercise Pattern

Wellness Diagnoses

Potential for enhanced
- *Effective cardiac output
- *Effective diversional activity pattern
- *Effective activity-exercise pattern
- *Effective home maintenance management
- *Effective self-care activities
- *Adequate tissue perfusion
- *Effective breathing pattern

Potential for enhanced infant behavior

Risk Diagnoses

Risk for Disorganized Infant Behavior
Risk for Peripheral Neurovascular Dysfunction
*Risk for altered respiratory function

Actual Diagnoses

Impaired Gas Exchange Activity Intolerance
Ineffective Airway Clearance
Ineffective Breathing Pattern
Decreased Cardiac Output
Decreased Adaptive Intracranial Capacity
Disuse Syndrome
Diversional Activity Deficit
Impaired Home Maintenance Management
Impaired Physical Mobility
Dysfunctional Ventilatory Weaning Response
Inability to Sustain Spontaneous Ventilation
Self-Care Deficit: (Feeding, Bathing/Hygiene, Dressing/Grooming, Toileting)
Altered Tissue Perfusion: (Specify type: Cerebral, Cardiopulmonary, Renal, Gastrointestinal, Peripheral)
Disorganized Infant Behavior

5. Sexuality—Reproductive Pattern

Wellness Diagnosis

*Opportunity to enhance sexuality patterns

Risk Diagnosis

*Risk for altered sexuality pattern

Actual Diagnoses

Sexual Dysfunction
Altered Sexuality Patterns

(* Not on current NANDA list)

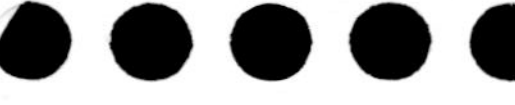

6. Sleep-Rest Pattern

Wellness Diagnosis
*Opportunity to enhance sleep

Risk Diagnosis
***Risk for sleep pattern disturbance**

Actual Diagnosis
Sleep Pattern Disturbance

7. Sensory—Perceptual Pattern

Wellness Diagnosis
*Opportunity to enhance comfort level

Risk Diagnoses
*Risk for pain
Risk for Aspiration

Actual Diagnoses
Pain
Chronic Pain
Dysreflexia
Sensory-Perceptual Alterations: (Specify: visual, auditory, kinesthetic, gustatory, tactile, olfactory)
Unilateral Neglect

8. Cognitive Pattern

Wellness Diagnosis
*Opportunity to enhance cognition

Risk Diagnosis
*Risk for altered thought processes

Actual Diagnoses
Acute Confusion
Chronic Confusion
Decisional Conflict
Impaired Environmental Interpretation Syndrome
Knowledge Deficit (Specify)
Altered Thought Processes
Impaired Memory

9. Role-Relationship pattern

Wellness Diagnoses

Opportunity to enhance:

- *Effective relationships
- *Effective parenting
- *Effective role performance
- *Effective communication
- *Effective social interaction
- *Effective care-giver role
- *Effective grieving

Risk Diagnoses

*Risk for dysfunctional grieving
High risk for Loneliness
Risk for Altered Parent/Infant/Child Attachment

Actual Diagnoses

Impaired Verbal Communication
Altered Family Processes
Altered Family Processes: Alcoholism
Anticipatory Grieving
Dysfunctional Grieving
Altered Parenting
Parental Role Conflict
Altered Role Performance
Impaired Social Interaction
Social Isolation

10. Self-Perception–Self-Concept Pattern

Wellness Diagnoses

*Opportunity to enhance self-perception
*Opportunity to enhance self-concept

Risk Diagnoses

*Risk for hopelessness
*Risk for body image disturbance
*Risk for low self esteem

Actual Diagnoses

Anxiety
Fatigue
Fear
Hopelessness
Powerlessness
Personal Identity Disturbance
Body Image Disturbance
Self-Esteem Disturbance
Chronic Low Self-Esteem
Situational Low Self-Esteem

(* Not on current NANDA list)

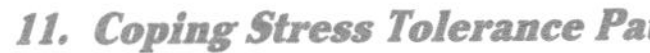

11. Coping Stress Tolerance Pattern

Wellness Diagnoses
- *Opportunity to enhance effective individual coping
- Family Coping: Potential for Growth
- Potential for Enhanced Community Coping

Risk Diagnoses
- *Risk for ineffective coping (individual, family, or community)
- *Risk for self-harm
- *Risk for self-abuse
- Risk for self-mutilation
- *Risk for suicide
- Risk for Violence: Self-directed or directed at others

Actual Diagnoses
- Impaired Adjustment
- Caregiver Role Strain
- Ineffective Individual Coping
- Ineffective Family Coping: Disabling
  - Defensive Coping
  - Ineffective Denial
- Ineffective Family Coping: Compromised
- Ineffective community coping
- Post-trauma Response
- Rape-trauma syndrome
- Relocation Stress Syndrome

12. Value Belief Pattern

Wellness Diagnosis
- Potential for Enhanced Spiritual Well-Being

Risk Diagnosis
- *Risk for spiritual distress

Actual Diagnosis
- Spiritual Distress (distress of the human spirit)

Appendix XV

Collaborative Problems*

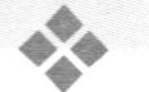

Potential Complication: Cardiac/Vascular

PC: Decreased cardiac output
PC: Dysrhythmias
PC: Pulmonary edema
PC: Cardiogenic shock
PC: Thromboemboli/deep vein thrombosis
PC: Hypovolemia
PC: Peripheral vascular insufficiency
PC: Hypertension
PC: Congenital heart disease
PC: Endocarditis
PC: Pulmonary embolism
PC: Spinal shock
PC: Ischemic ulcers
PC: Angina

Potential Complication: Gastrointestinal-Hepatic-Biliary

PC: Paralytic ileus/small bowel obstruction
PC: Hepatic failure
PC: Hyperbilirubinemia
PC: Evisceration
PC: Hepatosplenomegaly
PC: Curling's ulcer
PC: Ascites
PC: GI bleeding

Potential Complication: Metabolic/Immune/Hematopoietic

PC: Hypoglycemia/hyperglycemia
PC: Negative nitrogen balance
PC: Electrolyte imbalances
PC: Thyroid dysfunction
PC: Hypothermia (severe)
PC: Hyperthermia (severe)
PC: Sepsis
PC: Acidosis (metabolic, respiratory)
PC: Alkalosis (metabolic, respiratory)
PC: Hypo/hyperthryoidism
PC: Allergic reaction
PC: Donor tissue rejection
PC: Adrenal insufficiency
PC: Anemia
PC: Thrombocytopenia
PC: Opportunistic infection
PC: Polycythemia
PC: Sickling crisis
PC: Disseminated intravascular coagulation

Potential Complication: Neurologic/Sensory

PC: Increased intracranial pressure
PC: Stroke
PC: Seizures
PC: Spinal cord compression
PC: Meningitis
PC: Cranial nerve impairment (specify)
PC: Paralysis
PC: Peripheral nerve impairment
PC: Increased intraocular pressure
PC: Corneal ulceration
PC: Neuropathies

Potential Complication: Muscular/Skeletal

PC: Osteoporosis
PC: Joint dislocation
PC: Compartmental syndrome
PC: Pathological fractures

(Carpenito LJ. Nursing Diagnoses: Application to Clinical Practice, 5th ed. Philadelphia, JB Lippincott, 1995.)
*Frequently used collaborative problems are represented on this list. Other situations not listed here could qualify as collaborative problems.

Potential Complication: Renal/Urinary

PC: Acute urinary retention
PC: Renal failure
PC: Bladder perforation
PC: Renal calculi

Potential Complication: Reproductive

PC: Fetal distress
PC: Postpartum hemorrhage
PC: Pregnancy-associated hypertension
PC: Hypermenorrhea
PC: Polymenorrhea
PC: Syphilis
PC: Prenatal bleeding
PC: Preterm labor

Potential Complication: Respiratory

PC: Hypoxemia
PC: Atelectasis/pneumonia
PC: Tracheobronchial constriction
PC: Pleural effusion
PC: Tracheal necrosis
PC: Ventilator dependency
PC: Pneumothorax
PC: Laryngeal edema

Potential Complication: Multisystem

PC: Medication therapy adverse effects
PC: Adrenocorticosteroids therapy adverse effects
PC: Antianxiety therapy adverse effects
PC: Antiarrhythmia therapy adverse effects
PC: Anticoagulant therapy adverse effects
PC: Anticonvulsant therapy adverse effects
PC: Antidepressant therapy adverse effects
PC: Antihypertensive therapy adverse effects
PC: Beta-adrenergic blockers therapy adverse effects
PC: Calcium channel blockers therapy adverse effects

PC: Angiotensin-converting enzyme therapy adverse effects
PC: Antineoplastic therapy adverse effects
PC: Antipsychotic therapy adverse effects

REFERENCES

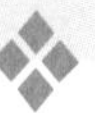

American Academy of Ophthalmology (1992). *Comprehensive adult eye evaluation, preferred practice pattern*. San Francisco.

American Academy of Ophthalmology (1991). *Eye care for the elderly*. San Francisco.

American Academy of Ophthalmology (1990). Policy statement: Frequency of eye examinations. San Francisco.

American Academy of Ophthalmology (1991). Policy statement: Infant & children's vision. San Francisco.

American Cancer Society (1996). *Cancer facts and figures*. Atlanta: American Cancer Society.

American Dental Association (1993). *Caring for your teeth & gums*. Chicago: American Dental Association.

American Dental Association (1990). *Gum disease*. Chicago: American Dental Association.

American Dental Association (1989). *Keeping a healthy mouth: Tips for older adults*. Chicago: American Dental Association.

American Dental Association (1992). *Your child's teeth*. Chicago: American Dental Association.

American Heart Association (1988). Position statement: Dietary guidelines for healthy American adults. Circulation, 77, (3).

American Heart Association (1995). Exercise standards: A statement for health care professionals from the American Heart Association.

American Heart Association (1992). Special Report: Statement on exercise. Dallas, TX: National Center.

Andrews, M., & Boyle, J. (1995). *Transcultural concepts in nursing care* (2d ed). Philadelphia: J. B. Lippincott.

Bates, B. (1995). *A guide to physical examination and history taking* (6th ed). Philadelphia: J. B. Lippincott.

Block, B., & Hunter, M. L. (1981). Teaching physiological assessment of black persons. *Nurse Educator* Jan.–Feb., 24–27.

Briggs, D. C. (1980). *Your child's self-esteem*. Garden City, NY: Doubleday.

Brunner, L. S., & Suddarth, D. S. (1991). *The Lippincott manual of nursing practice* (5th ed). Philadelphia: J. B. Lippincott.

Carpenito, L. J. (1995). *Nursing diagnosis: Application to clinical practice* (6th ed). Philadelphia: J. B. Lippincott.
Caring for your teeth and gums (1993). Chicago: American Dental Association.
Dudek, S. G. (1993). *Nutrition handbook for nursing practice* (2d ed). Philadelphia: J. B. Lippincott.
Erikson, E. (1963). *Childhood and society* (2d ed). New York: W. W. Norton.
Fuller, J., & Schaller-Ayers, J. (1994). *Health assessment: A nursing approach* (2d ed). Philadelphia: J. B. Lippincott.
Gallagher, L. P., & Kreidler, M. C. (1987). *Nursing and health: Maximizing human potential throughout the life cycle.* Norwalk, CT: Appleton & Lange.
Giger, J., & Dairdhizar, R. (1991). *Transcultural nursing: Assessment and intervention.* St. Louis: Mosby Yearbook, Inc.
Gordon, M. (1991). *Manual of nursing diagnosis 1991–1992.* St. Louis: Mosby Yearbook, Inc.
Hill, P. M. & Humphrey, P. (1982). *Human growth and development throughout life: A nursing perspective.* New York: John Wiley & Sons.
Jacobson, N., Gift, A., & Jacox, A. (1990). Advances in physical assessment. *Nursing clinics of North America, 25*(4), 743–833.
Kelley, J., Avant, K. & Frisch, N. (1995). A trifocal model of nursing diagnoses: Wellness reinforced. *Nursing Diagnosis.*
Marshall, W. A. & Tanner, J. M. (1969). Summary of sequence of sexual development: Boys/girls. *Archives of Disease in Childhood, 44,* 291.
Marian, M. E. (1991). *Introductory nutrition and dietary therapy.* Philadelphia: J. B. Lippincott.
Metropolitan Life Insurance Company Build Study (1983). New York: Society of Actuaries and Association of Life Insurance Medical Directors of America.
Murray, R. B., & Zentner, J. P. (1993). *Nursing assessment and health promotion strategies through the life span* (5th ed). Norwalk, CT: Appleton & Lange.
North American Nursing Diagnosis Association. Nursing Diagnoses: Definitions and Classification (1995-1996). Philadelphia: North American Nursing Diagnoses Association.
National Institutes of Health (NIH Publication No. 93-1088) (1994). National high blood pressure education program: The 5th report of the Joint National Committee on Detection, Evaluation and Treatment of High Blood Pressure. Bethesda, MD.
Overfield, T. (1985). *Biological variation in health and illness: Race, age, and sex differences.* Menlo Park, CA: Addison-Wesley.
Physical growth NCHS percentile charts (1982). Columbus, OH: Ross Laboratories (a Division of Abbott Laboratories).
Piaget, J. (1967). *Six psychological studies.* New York, Vintage Books.
Rice, E. M. (1989, May–June). Geriatric assessment. *Advancing Clinical Care,* 8–15.

Ross Laboratories (1986). *Guidelines for anthropometric measurements* (Brochure G623). Columbus, OH: Ross Laboratories.

Task Force on Blood Pressure Control in Children (1987). Report of the second Task Force on Blood Pressure Control in Children-1987. *Pediatrics 79:* 1–25.

U. S. Department of Agriculture, U. S. Department of Health and Human Services (1990). Nutrition and your health: Dietary guidelines for Americans.

Wong, D., & Whaley, L. (1990). *Clinical handbook of pediatric nursing* (2d ed). St. Louis: C. V. Mosby.

Index

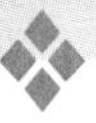

Page numbers followed by *f* indicated figures; page numbers followed by *t* indicate tables.

POWERS and MOORE's

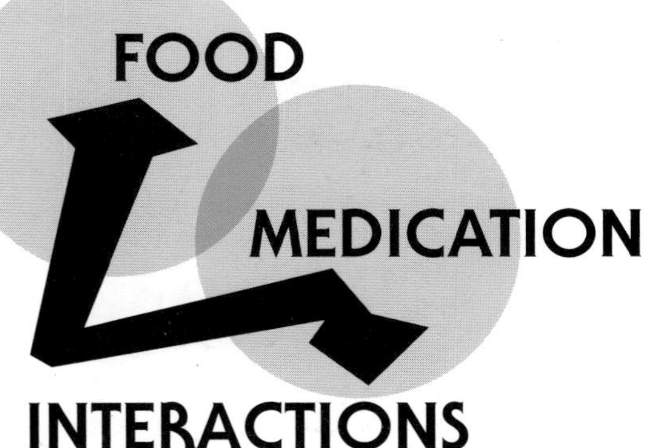

9th Edition

by

ZANETA M. PRONSKY, M.S., R.D.

Published and distributed by: FOOD-MEDICATION INTERACTIONS
PO Box 659
Pottstown, PA 19464 Phone: 610-970-7143

Library of Congress Cataloging-in Publications Number: 95-060960
ISBN: 0-9606164-5-4 Printed in USA

First Edition, December 1978
Second Edition, May, 1979
Third Edition, May 1981
Fourth Edition, October, 1983
Fifth Edition, March, 1986
Sixth Edition, August, 1988
Authors: Dorothy Powers, R.D. & Ann O. Moore, M.S., R.D.

Seventh Edition, January, 1991
Author: Ann Moore Allen, M.S., R.D.

Author: Zaneta M. Pronsky, M.S., R.D.

Contact the author/publishers for orders, information about <u>Computerized Food-Medication Interactions</u> software or specific references at: PO Box 659, Pottstown, PA 19464 or (610) 970-7143.

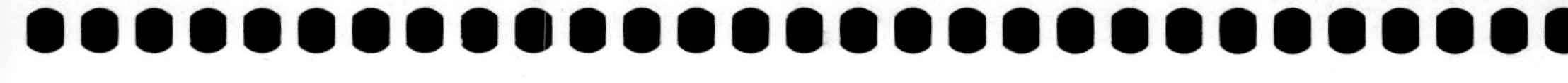

AUTHOR: Zaneta M. Pronsky, M.S., R.D.

SENIOR EDITOR: Sr. Jeanne P. Crowe, Pharm.D., R.Ph., Director of Pharmacy, Camilla Hall Nursing Home; Faculty, Graduate Division; Immaculata College, Immaculata, PA

EDITORS:

Sol Epstein, M.D., F.R.C.P., F.A.C.P., Head of Endocrinology and Metabolism, Albert Einstein Medical Center; Professor of Medicine, Temple University, Philadelphia, PA

Leroy C. Knodel, Pharm. D., Director, Drug Information Service; Associate Professor, Department of Pharmacology, The University of Texas Health Science Center at San Antonio, San Antonio, TX

Christine Hamilton Smith, Ph.D., R.D., Professor, The Marilyn Magaram Center for Food Science, Nutrition & Dietetics, Department of Family Environmental Studies, California State University Northridge Northridge, CA

TABLE RESEARCH EDITOR:

Nancy Feldgus, M.A., R.D., Clinical Dietitian, Holy Redeemer Hospital, Meadowbrook, PA

ACKNOWLEDGMENTS

Special thanks go to Ann Moore Allen and Bob Allen; Margaret Humphreys, reviewer; Marilyn Chapis, Librarian, Pottstown Memorial Medical Center; Nancy Powers-Siler, M.S., R.D., University of Illinois; Joanna Steinman, Polybytes; and John Pinto, PhD., Sloan Kettering Memorial for their help, encouragement and/or contributions.

PREFACE

Any procedure or practice described in this book should be applied by the health-care practitioner under appropriate supervision in accordance with professional standards of care used with regard to the unique circumstances that apply in each practice situation. Care has been taken to confirm the accuracy of information presented and to describe generally accepted practices. However, the authors, editors and publishers cannot accept responsibility for errors or omissions or for any consequences from applications of the information in this book and make no warranty, expressed or implied, with respect to the contents of the book.

Every effort has been made to ensure that the information herein is in accordance with current recommendations and practice. Because of ongoing research, change in government regulations and the constant flow of information on drug interactions, reactions and therapy, the reader is cautioned to check the package insert of each drug for indications, dosages, warnings and precautions, particularly if the drug is new or infrequently used.

For orders, information about **Computerized Food-Medication Interactions** software, requests for specific references, or suggestions for improvements contact the author/publishers at:

Food-Medication Interactions
PO Box 659, Pottstown, PA 19464 (610) 970-7143.
Fax: (610) 970-5470

TABLE OF CONTENTS

INTRODUCTION TO FOOD MEDICATION INTERACTIONS

Medications can affect and be affected by food. Recognition of the interaction of drugs and nutrition plays a vital role in the expanding medical services available for patients. The Joint Commission on Accreditation of Health Care Organizations and other agencies are currently focusing more attention on this topic by mandating that health care professionals document and advise patients about food-medication interactions.

Patients must be assessed individually for the effect of food on medication action and the effect of medication on nutritional status. These two aspects of medication use can be complicated by: special diets, nutritional supplements, non-nutrients in food, alcohol intake, tube feeding, underlying illness, polypharmacy, general physical condition, and other factors.

Please note that food and medication interactions are only possibilities. Inclusion of an effect does not imply that this effect will occur in each patient. An effect is included if the reported incidence is $\geq$ 1% more than that reported with a placebo. If the % incidence is available, the effect is underlined if the incidence is $\geq$ 5%. It is capitalized and underlined if $\geq$ 20%.

Medications in the same therapeutic classifications generally exhibit similar effects. Therefore a drug may be referred to a master drug of that classification with the notation "See listing for ...". For example, many thiazides are referred to hydrochlorothiazide with "See listing for hydrochlorothiazide p 102".

The following information provides a review of various aspects of food-medication interactions to enable the health professional to optimize dietary and drug regimens. Included are guidelines for counseling medicated patients and dietary suggestions to aid in the relief of nutrition-related side effects of drugs. Reference tables are added to provide access to supplemental information which augments the text.

Before using the **Food-Medication Interactions** pocketbook please review this information, the Guide to the Use of the Book inside the front cover, and the Table of Contents, (page 5). Drugs are listed alphabetically by generic and Trade names (capitalized). Every effort has been made to include the most commonly used prescription and nonprescription drugs with the most up to date information available on each drug.

MECHANISMS OF FOOD MEDICATION INTERACTIONS

PHARMACOKINETICS AND NUTRIENT KINETICS: The study of the **absorption**, **distribution**, **metabolism** and **excretion** of drugs/nutrients. **Absorption:** Process by which a drug/nutrient proceeds from the site of administration to the systemic circulation. **Distribution:** Movement of the drug/nutrient from one location to another. **Metabolism:** Process by which the drug/nutrient is changed by the action of enzymes (usually in the liver). The compound may become more, less or equally as active as the parent compound. **Excretion:** Process by which the drug/nutrient or metabolites are removed from the body primarily by the kidneys.

EFFECT OF FOOD/NUTRIENTS ON MEDICATION KINETICS

EFFECT OF FOOD/NUTRIENTS ON MEDICATION ABSORPTION

The presence of food in the stomach may decrease the rate and/or extent of drug absorption.

___The absorption of the antihistamine astemizole (Hismanal) may be decreased by 60% when taken with food.

___A high fiber diet may decrease the absorption of tricyclic antidepressants such as amitriptyline (Elavil).

Chelation occurs between certain drugs and divalent/trivalent cations Ca, Mg, Al, Fe, Zn.

___Ciprofloxacin (Cipro) forms an insoluble complex with calcium in some dairy products; Ca, Fe and Mg in supplements; or Ca, Al and/or Mg antacids preventing absorption.

The presence of food in the stomach may enhance the absorption of some drugs.

___The absorption of cefuroxime axetil (Ceftin) is significantly higher with a meal than in a fasting state.

EFFECT OF FOOD/NUTRIENTS ON MEDICATION DISTRIBUTION

A significant decrease in serum albumin may increase the free fraction of highly protein bound drugs.
Hypoalbuminemia (< 3g/dL) provides fewer binding sites for highly bound drugs such as phenytoin (Dilantin) (90% bound) and warfarin (Coumadin) (99% bound). A higher free fraction of drug increases drug effects.

EFFECT OF FOOD/NUTRIENTS ON MEDICATION METABOLISM

Food may alter the hepatic metabolism of some drugs.

___First-pass metabolism of propranolol (Inderal) may decrease if taken with food, increasing drug blood level.

___High pro, low CHO diet induces cytochrome P450 mixed oxidase system, promoting hepatic metabolism of drugs significantly metabolized by this enzyme system, such as theophylline (Theo-Dur). Drug levels may decrease.

EFFECT OF FOOD/NUTRIENTS ON MEDICATION EXCRETION

Foods and nutrients may alter the renal excretion of some drugs.

___Lithium (Eskalith) and sodium compete for tubular reabsorption in the kidney. High sodium intake causes more lithium to be excreted. Low sodium intake will cause the kidney to retain lithium, raising blood levels.

EFFECTS OF MEDICATIONS ON FOOD/NUTRIENT KINETICS

EFFECT OF MEDICATION ON NUTRIENT ABSORPTION

Drug complexes with nutrients preventing the absorption of drug, nutrient or both.

___ Antibiotics tetracycline and ciprofloxacin (Cipro) chelate with divalent or trivalent cations, Ca, Mg, Fe, Zn.

___ Antihyperlipidemic, bile acid sequestrant cholestyramine (Questran) adsorbs fat soluble vits A, D, E, K.

Drug alters gastric acidity.

___ Prolonged use of antiulcer drugs such as cimetidine (Tagamet) may decrease absorption of vit $B_{12,}$ thi, Fe.

Drug damages mucosal surface.

___ Medication induced mucosal damage by antineoplastic drugs may cause decreased nutrient absorption.

EFFECT OF MEDICATION ON NUTRIENT DISTRIBUTION

Drug increases the metabolism of nutrients resulting in higher requirements and danger of deficiency.

___ Anticonvulsants phenobarbital and phenytoin (Dilantin) increase the metabolism of folic Acid, vits D and K.

Drug causes vitamin antagonism.

___ Antituberculosis drug isoniazid (INH) inhibits the conversion of pyridoxine (vit B_6) to the active form. This may cause vit B_6 deficiency and peripheral neuropathy unless a B_6 supplement is also prescribed.

EFFECT OF MEDICATION ON NUTRIENT EXCRETION

Drug increases the urinary loss of nutrients.

___ Loop diuretics, such as furosemide (Lasix), increase excretion of Na, K, Cl, Mg, Ca.

Drug decreases the urinary excretion of nutrients.

___ Thiazide diuretics increase excretion of most electrolytes but decrease excretion of Ca due to ↑ renal reabsorption.

MODIFICATION OF MEDICATION ACTION

ENHANCEMENT OF MEDICATION ACTION

Foods or additives have effects similar to those of a drug, enhancing the effects or toxicity of the drug.

___ High caffeine intake may increase the adverse effects of theophylline (nervousness, tremor, insomnia).

___ Tyramine, dopamine or other vasoconstrictors in food enhance the toxic effects of MAO inhibitors, such as tranylcypromine sulfate (Parnate). This effect may cause a hypertensive crisis, which can be fatal.

ANTAGONISM OF MEDICATION ACTION

Nutrient or food ingredient may oppose the desired action of the drug.

___ Vit K aids the production of clotting factors in direct opposition to the action of warfarin (Coumadin).

___ Caffeine is a stimulant which counteracts the antianxiety effects of tranquilizers.

Diet counteracts the effect of the drug.

___ High fat diet counteracts the effect of antihyperlipidemic drugs such as lovastatin (Mevacor).

EFFECTS OF MEDICATION ON FOOD INTAKE AND NUTRITIONAL STATUS

ORAL AND TASTE/SMELL EFFECTS

Drug may impair salivary flow causing dry mouth and increased caries, stomatitis, glossitis.

___ Tricyclic antidepressants such as amitriptyline (Elavil) cause dry mouth and sour or metallic taste.

Drug may be secreted into the saliva.

___ The antibiotic clarithromycin (Biaxin) enters the saliva causing a bitter taste.

Drug may suppress natural oral bacteria resulting in oral candidiasis.
___ Antibiotics, such as tetracycline, may result in oral yeast overgrowth i.e. candidiasis.

Drug may cause dysgeusia (taste change)
___ Antihypertensive drug captopril (Capoten) causes taste disorder or loss of taste perception.

Drug may damage rapidly proliferating cells.
___ The cytotoxic effects of antineoplastics such as cisplatin or methotrexate cause stomatitis, glossitis, esophagitis.

GASTROINTESTINAL EFFECTS

Drug may irritate the stomach mucosa causing distress, nausea, vomiting, bleeding, ulceration.
___ Nonsteroidal anti-inflammatory drugs (NSAID) such as acetylsalicylic acid (aspirin), ibuprofen (Advil, Motrin) and naprosyn (Aleve, Anaprox) cause stomach irritation, sometimes leading to sudden, serious gastric bleeding.

Drug may affect intestinal peristalsis.
___ Anticholinergic drugs (antipsychotics, antidepressants, antihistamines) may slow peristalsis causing constipation.

Drug may destroy intestinal bacteria.
___ Antibiotics [(eg ciprofloxacin (Cipro)] cause overgrowth of Clostridium difficile and result in pseudomembranous colitis.

APPETITE CHANGES

Drug may suppress appetite.
___ SSRI antidepressant drugs such as fluoxetine (Prozac) may cause anorexia and weight loss.

Drug may increase appetite
___ Tricyclic antidepressants and most antipsychotic drugs, such as amitriptyline (Elavil) and thioridazine (Mellaril), stimulate appetite and weight gain.

Authors: Zaneta M. Pronsky, RD, MS and Sr. Jeanne Patricia Crowe, Pharm.D., R.Ph.

GUIDELINES FOR COUNSELING MEDICATED PATIENTS

The following guidelines provide information about potential medication/food interactions. Examples illustrate possible diet adjustments. Medication information for the patient should include the following:

1. Pertinent **information** about the medication: The **name, purpose** of the drug, and **duration** of therapy.
   Eg: Ciprofloxacin (Cipro), Antibiotic, 10 days therapy.
2. **When** and **how** to take the drug:
   Eg: Take the drug in the AM; PM; 6 hours before bedtime; on an empty stomach; 1 hour before or 2 hours after meals; with food, meals or specific beverages.
   Eg: Take Ca carbonate with meals as a calcium supplement; 1 - 3 hours after meals as an antacid.
3. **Side effects** and possible dietary suggestions to aid in their relief.
   See next section, Dietary suggestions pages 13 - 16.
4. Potential **nutritional problems** that may arise from medication use, especially when dietary intake is inadequate:
   Eg: Potassium-depleting diuretics may cause hypokalemia. Recommend increased intake of foods known to be good sources of potassium.
5. **Dietary changes** that may alter **drug action** (particularly after drug stabilization):
   Eg: High intake of vitamin K-containing foods may impair warfarin action. Regulate intake of foods high in vitamin K.
6. **Foods and beverages to avoid** while taking the drug:
   Eg: Avoid foods high in pressor amines, especially tyramine, with an MAOI such as phenelzine sulfate (Nardil) to prevent a hypertensive crisis. Provide information on specific foods to avoid or limit.

7. **Alcohol:** Concurrent intake of beer, wine, other alcoholic beverages or alcohol used in cooking with some medications may modify the effects of both or may produce undesirable side effects:
   Eg: A disulfiram-like reaction results from concurrent alcohol & chlorpropamide use. Before any alcohol is served to patients the physician should be consulted.
8. Potential **interactions** between medications and **vitamin, mineral and other food supplements:**
   Eg: Concurrent administration of a calcium supplement and an antibiotic such as tetracycline or ciprofloxacin may impair the absorption of both the calcium and the antibiotic. Take separately by 2-4 hours.
9. **Special diet prescribed** for a medical condition must be followed: Antihyperlipidemic drug therapy is an adjunct to a low cholesterol, low fat diet. Insulin or sulfonylurea therapy is an adjunct to a diabetic diet.
   Drug therapy is <u>not</u> a substitute for dietary regulation.
10. A **personal dietary prescription** pertains to that person only.
    Do not follow dietary suggestions prescribed for others.
    Eg: Dietary restrictions with potassium-depleting diuretics differ from those with potassium-sparing diuretics. Serious adverse effects occur if diet prescriptions are interchanged.
11. Before modifying a drug prescription, the prescribing physician must be consulted .
12. A registered dietitian should be consulted for in-depth nutritional information.

Adapted from: 7th edition guidelines by Christine H. Smith, Editor.

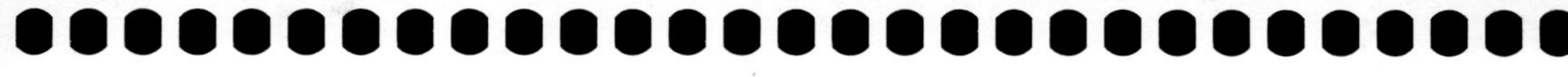

DIETARY SUGGESTIONS TO AID IN THE RELIEF OF NUTRITION-RELATED SIDE EFFECTS OF DRUGS

The following suggestions are intended to reinforce rather than replace information provided by the physician or pharmacist. Some individuals may experience only mild, transient discomforts, while others may be affected by multiple drug side effects. Prior to implementing dietary suggestions consult the physician or pharmacist to determine if the patient's symptom is a possible adverse effect of the drug. The patient may be in need of further medical attention.

Loss of Appetite

1. Question patient regarding factors contributing to appetite loss such as depression.
2. Educate the patient about the importance of an adequate, well balanced diet.
3. Create a pleasant environment for eating. If possible, eliminate distractions and time pressure.
4. If early satiety occurs or meals are not well-tolerated, offer small, frequent, attractive meals or snacks.
5. Provide variety in color, texture, taste and temperature.
6. Enhance flavors by using seasonings. Marinate meats in sauces or fruit juice.
7. Encourage weakened patients to select foods that require minimal eating effort.
8. Consider prescription of calorie-dense nutritional supplements between meals.

Taste/Smell Dysfunction

1. If permissible, mask the taste of a drug with food, pulpy fruits (applesauce, crushed pineapple), fruit juices or milk. Use sugarless gum or candy, water or lemon juice as mouth rinses.
2. Encourage good oral hygiene.

Dry or Sore Mouth

1. Decrease dry or salty foods/snacks. Moisten (dunk) dry foods in beverages or swallow with liquid.
2. Offer moist, soft-textured foods: mashed potatoes, pureed food, custards, puddings or fruit whips.
3. Avoid spicy, rough textured or highly acidic foods.
4. Add milk-flavored sauces, gravies or syrups to food.
5. Lick or suck ice chips. Incorporate cold foods or beverages into meals or snacks: sherbets, ice cream, ice milk, frozen yogurt, melons, fruit ices, popsicles.
6. Suggest sugarless gum/candy. Warm water rinses or saliva substitutes, such as Optimoist, may help.
7. Stress the importance of good oral hygiene. Severe or long-term decreased salivation can cause tooth decay, gum disease, fungal infection, ill-fitting dentures and changes in eating habits. If dry mouth lasts 2 weeks a dental consultation is needed. Do dental care cautiously to minimize trauma to the oral mucosa.

Appetite Stimulation or Weight Gain

1. Assess weight gain as a possible reversal of depression-induced weight loss.
2. Educate the patient that certain drugs may increase appetite and the desire for sweets.
3. Encourage a slow rate of eating (at least 20 minutes to finish first portions of a meal).
4. Encourage intake of low calorie foods, condiments, beverages and snacks.
5. Incorporate high fiber foods or snacks which may contribute to early satiety.
6. Instruct patient or food provider to control access to specific high calorie foods, snacks, or beverages.

Epigastric Distress (stomach discomfort, heartburn or indigestion)

1. After drug administration (particularly medications which cause GI irritation) remain upright for 15-30 minutes.
2. Evaluate dietary habits for specific foods or beverages that may contribute to epigastric distress.
3. Offer small quantities of food at frequent intervals in a relaxed environment. Avoid overeating.
4. Avoid extremely hot or extremely cold foods or liquids (may stimulate acid secretion).

5. Limit alcohol, caffeine, decaffeinated coffee, colas, peppermint, chocolate, pepper, chili powder and spicy foods.
6. Limit citrus juices, tomato products and other highly acidic foods.
7. Avoid greasy, fried or fatty foods (may delay gastric emptying).
8. Evaluate the intake of milk or dairy products (may stimulate acid secretion).
9. Avoid eating at least one hour before bedtime.

Nausea

In order to maintain adequate hydration and nutrient intake:

1. Honor food preferences. Disliked foods may aggravate nausea.
2. Offer small quantities of easily digestible foods at frequent intervals. Eat slowly.
3. Reduce food volume at meals. Serve liquids after meals or limit liquid intake with meals.
4. Suggest intake of toasted or dry enriched white bread, crackers or graham crackers, cooked or dry ready-to-eat cereals. To reduce nausea eat one of these foods early in the morning or before rising.
5. Serve cold, clear, or carbonated liquids (ginger ale) or juices. Avoid lukewarm beverages.
6. Avoid any fried, greasy or fatty foods (may delay gastric emptying).
7. Hot aromas may aggravate nausea. Cold foods may be better tolerated than hot foods.
8. If nausea occurs at consistent times each day reschedule meal and snack times.

Diarrhea

1. Focus on fluid and electrolyte replacement.
2. During the acute phase food may be withheld for 24 hours or longer or limit to clear liquids.
3. Intake of frequent small amounts of bland foods (crackers, plain toast) may be allowed as tolerated.
4. Initially restrict or avoid caffeine, alcohol, highly spiced foods, concentrated sweets, raw fruits & vegetables, uncooked foods, fried foods, bran & whole grain cereals, nuts, beans, relishes.
5. Resume normal diet gradually.

Gastrointestinal Gas (flatulence and/or belching)

1. Evaluate for: rapid rate of eating, chewing gum, and situations associated with swallowing large amounts of air.
2. Encourage patient to avoid flatulogenic foods such as beans, bran, cabbage, cauliflower, broccoli, onions, peppers, radishes, apples, celery, eggplant or to use alpha-D-galactosidase enzyme (Beano).
3. Limit consumption of carbonated beverages.

Constipation

1. Avoid prolonged use or overuse of cathartics, laxatives, or enemas which cause laxative dependence (interfere with normal bowel reflexes).
2. Patient may need education concerning misconceptions about constipation.
3. Evaluate the diet for adequacy of fluid, volume, nutrients and fiber.
4. Increase fiber (vegetables, fruits, whole grain cereals) in the diet. May use bran in moderation.
5. Maintain adequate fluid intake (especially water).
6. Stress the importance of daily exercise, regular meals, defecation reflex recognition (usually active after meals, especially breakfast), and regularity in defecation time.

Adapted from: 7th edition Dietary Suggestions by Christine H. Smith, Editor.

FOOD MEDICATION INTERACTIONS

MEDICATION	CLASSIFICATION & DIETARY/RELATED SIGNIFICANCES	
Accupril	ANTIHYPERTENSIVE, ACE Inhibitor	See **quinapril p 172**
Accutane	ANTI-ACNE	See **isotretinoin p 111**
acetaminophen **Aspirin Free Anacin** **Datril** **Aspirin Free Excedrin** **65 mg caffeine** **Panadol** **Tempra** **Tylenol**	ANALGESIC, ANTIPYRETIC **Drug:** May take s̄ regard to food. **Oral/GI:** No GI bleeding. **S/Cond:** Limit alcohol to < 3 drinks/day.[10] **Other:** Rare hepatotoxicity. **Blood/Serum:** Hemolytic anemia, ↓ WBC, ↑ bil, ↑ LDH, ↑ SGOT, ↑ SGPT, ↑ PT, false ↑ uric acid (dose-related). False ↓ glucose c̄ glucose oxidase/peroxidase. **Urinary:** False ↓ glucose c̄ chemstrips. Check brand for alcohol, aspartame, saccharin, sorbitol, starch or sucrose.	

acetazolamide
Diamox
Parenteral—
47 mg Na/150 mg
Diamox Sequels (SR)

DIURETIC, ANTIGLAUCOMA, ANTICONVULSANT,
Carbonic Anhydrase Inhibitor
K-depleting — Oral or Parenteral (IV)

Drug: Take c̄ food to ↓ GI irritation. **Diet:** Insure adequate fluid intake. ↑ K may be needed. Avoid natural licorice. **Nutr:** Anorexia, ↓ wt.
Oral/GI: <u>Metallic taste</u>, dry mouth, <u>N/V</u>, constipation, <u>diarrhea</u>.
S/Cond: Not c̄ lactation. Caution c̄ diabetes. 90% serum pro bound. Caution c̄ G6PD def— risk of hemolytic anemia. **Other:** Drowsiness, confusion, fatigue, paresthesia.
Blood/Serum: ↓ <u>BICARBONATE</u>, ↓ <u>Na</u>, ↓ <u>K</u>, ↑ <u>Cl</u>, ↑ bil, ↑ uric acid, ↑ glucose (c̄ diabetes). Anemias, including rare fatal aplastic anemia, dyscrasias. **Urinary:** ↑ <u>BICARBONATE</u>, ↑ <u>pH</u> ↑ <u>Na</u>, ↑ <u>K</u>, ↓ <u>Cl</u>, ↓ uric acid, ↑ glucose (c̄ diabetes), false + pro, ↑ Thi, ↑ Pyr, ↑ Mg.[11]
Monitor: CBC & platelets, electrolytes, diabetics for hyperglycemia.

acetylsalicylic acid (ASA)
Aspirin
Ascriptin (buffered)
Tab— Starch
Bufferin (buffered)
Ecotrin– enteric-coated
Tab/Cap- Starch

NSAID, ANALGESIC, ANTIPYRETIC, ANTIARTHRITIC

Drug: Take c̄ 8 oz H_2O or milk, after meals or c̄ food to ↓ GI irritation. Food ↓ rate of abs.[4] Swallow enteric-coated tab whole.
Diet: Insure adequate fluid intake. ↑ foods high in Vit C[13] & Fol[11] c̄ LT high dose. **Nutr:** Anorexia.
Oral/GI: May cause sudden, serious gastric bleeding. <u>N/V</u>, <u>DYSPEPSIA</u>.
S/Cond: Avoid alcohol. Caution c̄ lactation. Caution c̄ diabetes. Not for patient prone to Vit K def. > 90% serum pro bound at low serum conc. Caution c̄ G6PD def– risk of hemolytic anemia. **Other:** May contribute to Fe def anemia. LT use may cause occult fecal blood loss.[14]

Reyes syndrome. **Blood/ Serum:** ↓ T_4, ↓ or ↑ uric acid (dose-related), ↓ K, ↑ SGOT, ↑ SGPT, ↑ alk phos. High dose— ↑ or ↓ glucose, ↓ Fol,[11] possible ↓ Vit C. **Urinary:** ↑ Vit C, ↑ K, false ↑ or ↓ glucose (method related). **Monitor:** HCT & renal func c̄ LT use or high dose.[6]

Achromycin-V — ANTIBIOTIC — See **tetracycline p 194**

ACTH, Acthar — HORMONE, Pituitary — See **corticotropin p 61**

Actifed
triprolidine HCl
pseudoephedrine HCl
Tab— lactose & sucrose
Susp— sorbitol

ANTIHISTAMINE, DECONGESTANT, Sympathomimetic

Drug: Take c̄ food or milk to ↓ GI irritation. **Nutr:** Anorexia.
Oral/GI: Dry mouth, taste changes, epigastric distress.
S/Cond: Avoid alcohol. Not c̄ lactation. **Other:** Drowsiness, dizziness, weakness, blurred vision, excitability (children).

Actinomycin-D — ANTINEOPLASTIC — See **dactinomycin p 65**

Acutrim — APPETITE SUPPRESSANT — See **phenylpropanolamine p 160**

acyclovir
Zovirax
200 mg Cap— lactose
Syrup— sorbitol

ANTIVIRAL (Herpes) — Oral or Parenteral (IV)

Drug: May take c̄ food. **Diet:** Insure adequate fluid intake, unless otherwise directed. **Oral/GI:** Medicine taste, sore throat, N/V, constipation, diarrhea. **S/Cond:** Caution c̄ lactation.
Other: Headache, dizziness, fatigue, confusion, edema, rash, ↓ BP, acute renal failure.
Blood/Serum: Transient c̄ IV ↑ BUN, ↑ crea, ↑ SGOT, ↑ SGPT.

Adalat — ANTI-ANGINA, Ca Channel Blocker — See **nifedipine p 142**

Adriamycin — ANTINEOPLASTIC — See **doxorubicin p 78**

Adrucil — ANTINEOPLASTIC — See **fluorouracil p 92**

Advil — ANTI-INFLAMMATORY — See **ibuprofen p 104**

Agoral Plain — LUBRICANT LAXATIVE — See **mineral oil p 133**

albuterol sulfate
Proventil
Ventolin
Tab— Lactose
Syrup— sorbitol or saccharin

BRONCHODILATOR, Sympathomimetic — Oral, Inhalant or Parenteral (IV)

Drug: Take c̄ food if GI distress. Swallow SR tabs whole. **Diet:** Limit caffeine/xanthine, see p 240. **Nutr:** ↑ appetite, anorexia.
Oral/GI: Peculiar taste, sore throat, N/V, dyspepsia, diarrhea.
S/Cond: Not c̄ lactation. Caution c̄ HTN. Caution c̄ diabetes— ↑ glucose.
Other: Tremor, headache, dizziness, bronchospasm, nervousness, edema, nosebleed. Syrup— hyperactivity in children.
Blood/Serum: Transient c̄ IV ↓ K.

Aldactazide — ANTIHYPERTENSIVE, DIURETIC — See **spironolactone p 186 & hydrochlorothiazide p 102**

Aldactone — DIURETIC — See **spironolactone p 186**

Aldomet — ANTIHYPERTENSIVE — See **methyldopa p 130**

Aleve — NSAID — See **naproxen p 139**

Alka-Seltzer — ANTACID — See **sodium bicarbonate p 184**
Flavored Tab— 506 mg Na
c̄ Aspirin— 567 mg Na
Eff. Tab— 311 mg Na
Extra Strength— 588 mg Na

sodium bicarbonate, citric acid, K bicarbonate
Some formulations contain aspirin. See also **acetylsalicylic acid p 18**

Alkeran — ANTINEOPLASTIC — See **melphalan p 125**

allopurinol
Zyloprim
Tab— lactose

ANTIGOUT, Xanthine Oxidase Inhibitor

Drug: Take after meals c̄ fluids to ↓ GI upset.
Diet: Drink 10-12 glassesfluids/day to produce 2 L urine per 24 hrs.[13] Avoid large doses Vit C.[13]
Nutr: To ↓ risk of xanthine calculi, maintain alkaline urine.
Oral/GI: Metallic taste, N/V, abdominal pain, diarrhea.
S/Cond: Limit alcohol. Caution c̄ lactation.
Other: Drowsiness, headache, rash.
Blood/Serum: ↓ URIC ACID. < 1% dyscrasias, ↑ alk phos, ↑ SGOT, ↑ SGPT, ↑ bil, ↑ BUN, ↑ crea.
Urinary: ↓ URIC ACID.
Monitor: CBC, uric acid, renal & hepatic func.

alprazolam
Xanax
Tab— lactose

ANTIANXIETY, ANTI-PANIC, Benzodiazepine

Drug: May take c̄ food or H_2O to ↓ GI distress.
Nutr: ↑ APPETITE, anorexia, ↑ or ↓ wt.
Oral/GI: ↑ Salivation, dry mouth, N/V, gastritis, cramps, constipation, diarrhea.
S/Cond: Avoid alcohol. Not c̄ lactation. May be habit forming c̄ LT use. Hypoalbuminemia (< 3.0 g/dL) may ↑ drug effects.[13]
Other: DROWSINESS, fatigue, ataxia, blurred vision, headache, confusion, dizziness, tremor.
Blood/Serum: High dose— ↑ SGOT, ↑ bil.
Monitor: Hepatic func, CBC.

Altace

ANTIHYPERTENSIVE, ACE Inhibitor See **ramipril p 174**

aluminum hydroxide
Alu-Cap
AlternaGel— < 2.5 mg Na, .7 g sorbitol/5 mL
Amphojel
Tab—- saccharin
Susp— saccharin, sorbitol
Dialume

ANTACID, Phosphate Binder

Drug: Take 1-3 hr after meals. Chew chewable well. **Diet:** Phosphate-binding therapy — take c̄ meals & 8 oz H_2O or fluids. ↓ phosphate diet. Take Fe, Fol, Thi or Vit A suppl separately by 2 hrs. Take separately from citrus fruit/juice by 3 hrs.[22]
Nutr: Inactivates Thi. ↓ abs of Vit A, Fol, P, Fe.
Oral/GI: Chalky taste, N/V, CONSTIPATION, cramps, diarrhea.
S/Cond: LT use c̄ dialysis may cause encephalopathy, neurotoxicity & osteomalacia. Liquid form thickens some tube feedings.[8]
Blood/Serum: ↓ P, ↑ Al c̄ LT use in ESRD.

aluminum hydroxide & magnesium hydroxide ANTACID, ANTIFLATULENT if c̄ simethicone
Drug: Take 1 hr after meals & HS. Chew tab well. **Diet:** Take Fe, Fol, Thi or Vit A suppl separately by 2 hrs.[13] Take separately from citrus fruit/juice by 3 hrs.[22] **Nutr:** ↓ abs of Vit A, Fol, P, & Fe. Inactivates Thi.
Oral/GI: Chalky taste, rare constipation, diarrhea.
S/Cond: Mylanta Double Strength thickens some tube feedings.[8] Not c̄ ESRD —↑ Mg.
LT use may cause encephalopathy, neurotoxicity.
Blood/Serum: ↓ P, ↓ K, ↑ Mg c̄ LT use, ↑ Al c̄ LT use in ESRD.

Aludrox— (simethicone) Susp— saccharin, sorbitol.
Di-Gel— (simethicone) Tab— mannitol, sucrose. Liquid— saccharin, sorbitol.
Gelusil— (simethicone) Liquid— saccharin, sorbitol, sugar, mannitol. Tab— mannitol, sorbitol, sugar.
Maalox Tab— sugar. Susp— saccharin, sorbitol, tartrazine.
Maalox Plus— (simethicone) Tab— sugar, saccharin, sorbitol, starch. Susp— saccharin, sorbitol.
Mylanta/ Mylanta Double Strength (simethicone) Tab— mannitol, saccharin, sorbitol.
Susp— saccharin, sorbitol.

Alupent BRONCHODILATOR See **metaproterenol p 127**

amantadine HCl ANTIPARKINSON, ANTIVIRAL
Symmetrel
Syrup— 3.2 g sorbitol/5 mL

Nutr: Anorexia. **Oral/GI:** Dry mouth, <u>nausea</u>, constipation.
S/Cond: Avoid alcohol. Caution c̄ lactation. ↑ risk of dental problems.
Other: <u>Dizziness</u>, <u>insomnia</u>, blurred vision, depression, ataxia, confusion, fatigue, headache, leg/ankle edema, hallucinations, anxiety.

Ambien SLEEP AID, Hypnotic See **zolpidem tartrate p 217**

amikacin sulfate
Amikin
sulfites

ANTIBIOTIC, Aminoglycoside — Parenteral only (IM or IV)
Diet: Insure adequate fluid intake. **Nutr:** ↑ thirst.
Oral/GI: ↑ Salivation, N/V. **S/Cond:** Not c̄ lactation.
Other: Dizziness, drowsiness, hearing loss, clumsiness.
Blood/Serum: ↑ BUN, ↑ crea. **Urinary:** Pro, ↓ specific gravity.
Monitor: Renal func.

amiloride HCl & hydrochlorothiazide
Moduretic
Tab— lactose

ANTIHYPERTENSIVE, DIURETIC
Drug: Take c̄ meals or milk to prevent GI upset. **Diet:** ↓ Na, ↓ cal diet may be needed. Caution c̄ Ca suppl.[3] Avoid natural licorice. **Nutr:** Anorexia.
Oral/GI: Dry mouth, N/V, dyspepsia, diarrhea, GI pain.
S/Cond: Avoid alcohol. Not c̄ lactation. Not c̄ serum K > 5.5.[7]
Other: Dizziness, headache, rash, weakness, cough.
Blood/Serum: Anemia, ↓ Na, ↓ Cl, ↑ uric acid, ↑ or ↓ K, ↑ BUN, ↑ Ca, ↓ P, ↓ or ↑ Mg, ↓ bicarbonate, ↑ chol, ↑ TG, ↑ glucose.
Urinary: ↑ Na, ↑ Cl, ↑ uric acid, ↓ Ca, ↑ Mg, ↑ or ↓ K, ↑ bicarbonate.
Monitor: Electrolytes, BUN. Diabetics for possible hyperglycemia.

aminophylline

BRONCHODILATOR — See listing for **theophylline p 194**

amiodarone HCl
Cordarone
Tab— lactose.

ANTIARRHYTHMIC
Nutr: Anorexia. **Oral/GI:** Abnormal taste, smell & salivation, N/V, abdominal pain, constipation. **S/Cond:** Not c̄ lactation. Not c̄ hypokalemia.[13]
Other: ATAXIA, dizziness, tremor, pulmonary toxicity, hepatic toxicity,

fatigue, blurred vision, photosensitivity, cough, insomnia, headache, flushing, edema, CHF.
Blood/Serum: ↑ Alk Phos, ↑ SGOT, ↑ SGPT, ↑ T_4, ↓ T_3, ↑ TSH, ↑ crea, dyscrasias. **Monitor:** Hepatic, pulmonary & thyroid func̄.

amitriptyline HCl
Elavil
Tab— lactose

ANTIDEPRESSANT, Tricyclic
Drug: May take c̄ food to ↓ GI distress.
Diet: ↑ fiber may ↓ drug effect.[3] Limit caffeine, see p 240.
Nutr: ↑ WT, ↑ APPETITE especially for sweets, CHO. ↑ need for Rib.[41]
Oral/GI: DRY MOUTH, taste changes, N/V, CONSTIPATION, diarrhea, flatulence.
S/Cond: Avoid alcohol. Not c̄ lactation. ↑ risk of dental problems, see p 9 & 14. 95% serum pro bound.
Other: SEDATION, DROWSINESS, BLURRED VISION, delirium, dizziness, sweating, fine tremor, headache, weakness, confusion, ↑ or ↓ BP, galactorrhea, edema, rash. Rare SIADH, jaundice & hepatitis.
Blood/Serum: Dyscrasias, ↑ or ↓ glucose. ↑ prolactin. Rare ↑ SGOT, ↑ SGPT, ↑ alk phos. **Urinary:** Retention.

amlodipine
Norvasc

ANTIHYPERTENSIVE, ANTIANGINAL, Ca Channel Blocker
Drug: Take s̄ regard to food. **Diet:** ↓ Na, ↓ cal may be recommended. Avoid natural licorice. **Oral/GI:** Dysphagia, nausea, cramps.
S/Cond: Not c̄ lactation. **Other:** Edema, dizziness, flushing, drowsiness, palpitations, muscle pain, rash.

amoxicillin
Amoxil
Susp— 1.67 g sucrose/5 mL
Chew Tab— mannitol, sucrose, saccharin
Trimox
Wymox
Pwd for oral susp— sucrose

ANTIBIOTIC, Penicillin
Drug: Food does not affect abs. May take c̄ food to ↓ GI distress. Chew tab— crush or chew. **Oral/GI:** N/V, diarrhea. Rare stomatitis, glossitis, oral candidiasis or pseudomembranous colitis.
S/Cond: Caution c̄ lactation.
Other: Rash. **Blood/Serum:** Anemias, dyscrasias, ↑ SGOT, ↑ SGOT.
Monitor: LT use— Renal & hepatic func. CBC c̄ diff.[6]

amoxicillin and potassium clavulanate
Augmentin

ANTIBIOTIC, Penicillin — See **amoxicillin above**
Tab 125— 6 mg K, 250 & 500— 25 mg K
250 pwd— 12 mg K &125 pwd— 6 mg K/ 5 mL suspension
Chew Tab & Pwd for susp— saccharin & mannitol.

Amphojel

ANTACID, Phosphate Binder — See **aluminum hydroxide p 22**

amphotericin B
Fungizone

ANTIFUNGAL, ANTIPROTOZOAL — Parenteral only (IV)
Diet: Insure adequate fluid intake. ↑ K, ↑ Mg. **Nutr:** ANOREXIA, ↓ WT.
Oral/GI: N/V, stomach pain, dyspepsia, diarrhea.
S/Cond: Not c̄ lactation.
Other: FEVER, NEPHROTOXICITY, headache, blurred vision, muscle pain, ↑ or ↓ B/P, peripheral neuropathy.
Blood/Serum: Anemia, ↑ BUN, ↑ crea, ↓ K, ↓ Na, ↓ Mg, ↑ Alk Phos, ↑ bil, ↑ SGOT, ↑ SGPT, ↑ GGT.
Urinary: ↑ K, ↑ uric acid, pro.
Monitor: Electrolytes, Mg, renal & hepatic func, CBC & platelets.

ampicillin
Parenteral—64 mg Na/g to 78 mg Na/g
Some cap— lactose
Pwd— sucrose

ANTIBIOTIC, Penicillin — Oral or Parenteral (IM or IV)

Drug: Take $\bar{c}$ 8 oz H_2O on empty stomach 1 hr before or 2 hrs after meal. Acid stable. **Oral/GI:** Taste changes, glossitis, stomatitis, oral candidiasis $\bar{c}$ LT use, N/V, pseudomembranous colitis, diarrhea.
S/Cond: Caution $\bar{c}$ lactation.
Other: Rash. **Blood/Serum:** Anemia, dyscrasias, ↑ SGOT, ↑ SGPT.
Urinary: False + glucose ($CuSO_4$).
Monitor: LT use— CBC $\bar{c}$ diff, hepatic & renal func.

ampicillin sodium & sulbactam sodium
Unasyn
115 mg Na/ 1.5 g

ANTIBIOTIC, Penicillin — Parenteral only (IM or IV)

Oral/GI: Oral candidiasis $\bar{c}$ LT use, N/V, pseudomembranous colitis, diarrhea. **S/Cond:** Caution $\bar{c}$ lactation.[10] **Other:** Rash.
Blood/Serum: Dyscrasias, anemia, ↑ SGOT, ↑ SGPT, ↑ alk phos, ↑ LDH. ↓ alb, ↓ TP, ↑ BUN, ↑ crea.
Urinary: False + glucose ($CuSO_4$).
Monitor: LT use— CBC $\bar{c}$ diff, hepatic & renal func.

Anacin — ANALGESIC, ANTIPYRETIC — See **acetylsalicylic acid p 18 & caffeine p 38**
Tab— 400 mg aspirin, 32 mg caffeine

Anafranil — ANTIDEPRESSANT, Tricyclic — See **clomipramine HCl p 56**

Anaprox — ANTI-INFLAMMATORY, ANALGESIC — See **naproxen p 139**

Ancef — ANTIBIOTIC, cefazolin sodium — See **cephalosporins p 46**

Ansaid Tab— lactose	NSAID	See listing for **ibuprofen p 104**
Antabuse	ALCOHOL DETERRENT	See **disulfiram p 75**
Antivert	ANTINAUSEANT	See **meclizine HCl p 124**
Apresoline	ANTIHYPERTENSIVE	See **hydralazine HCl p 102**
AquaMephyton	VITAMIN	See **vitamin K p 212**
Aquasol A	VITAMIN	See **vitamin A p 208**
ara-C	ANTINEOPLASTIC	See **cytarabine p 64**
Aredia	Ca REGULATOR, Bisphosphonate	See **pamidronate disodium p 151**
Aristocort	CORTICOSTEROID, Triamcinolone	See **corticosteroids p 60**
Artane	ANTIPARKINSON	See **trihexyphenidyl HCl p 201**
ASA	ANALGESIC	See **acetylsalicylic acid p18**
Asacol	ANTI-INFLAMMATORY	See **mesalamine p 126**
ascorbic acid	VITAMIN	See **vitamin C p 210**

Ascriptin — ANALGESIC (buffered) — See **acetylsalicylic acid p 18**
325 mg aspirin, 50 mg each Mg & AlOH, $CaCo_3$

Aspirin — ANALGESIC — See **acetylsalicylic acid p 18**

Aspirin Free Anacin — ANALGESIC — See **acetaminophen p 17**

astemizole
Hismanal
Tab— lactose

ANTIHISTAMINE
Drug: Food ↓ abs by 60%. Take on empty stomach 1 hr before or 2 hrs after food. **Nutr:** ↑ appetite, ↑ wt.
Oral/GI: Dry mouth, nausea, diarrhea.
S/Cond: Caution c̄ lactation. Not c̄ hypokalemia.[13] **Other:** Fatigue.

Atarax — ANTIHISTAMINE, ANTIANXIETY — See **hydroxyzine p 104**

atenolol
Tenormin

ANTIHYPERTENSIVE, ANTIANGINA
Cardioselective Beta-Blocker — Oral or Parenteral (IV)
Drug: Take s̄ regard to food. **Diet:** ↓ Na, ↓ cal may be recommended. Avoid natural licorice. Take separately from Ca suppl & antacids.
Nutr: Ca salts may ↓ abs.[3, 9b] **Oral/GI:** Nausea, diarrhea.
S/Cond: Caution c̄ lactation. Caution c̄ diabetes— may mask signs of hypoglycemia.[13] May inhibit insulin release in hyperglycemia.
Other: Dizziness, drowsiness, fatigue, depression.
Blood/Serum: ↑ TG, ↓ HDL, ↑ lipoproteins, ↑ K, ↑ uric acid, ↑ BUN.
Monitor: BP.

Ativan ANTIANXIETY See **lorazepam p 120**

atovaquone
Mepron
ANTI-PCP in HIV
Drug: Take with high fat meals (23-46 grams fat) to ↑ abs 3-4 fold.
Nutr: Anorexia. **Oral/GI:** Oral candidiasis, taste changes, N/V, dyspepsia, abdominal pain, DIARRHEA.
S/Cond: Caution with lactation.
Other: RASH, FEVER, headache, insomnia, weakness, dizziness, ↓ BP.
Blood/Serum: ↑ glucose, ↑ SGPT, ↑ SGOT, ↑ amylase, ↑ Alk Phos, ↓ Na, anemia, neutropenia. **Monitor:** CBC, hepatic func.

Atrovent BRONCHODILATOR See **ipratropium bromide p 109**

attapulgite
Donnagel—
Liquid— saccharin, sorbitol, 1.4% alcohol
Chew Tab— saccharin, sorbitol
Kaopectate— sucrose
ANTIDIARRHEAL
Diet: Diarrhea may ↑ fluid & electrolyte needs. **Oral/GI:** Constipation.

Augmentin ANTIBIOTIC See **amoxicillin & potassium clavulanate p 26**

Axid ANTIULCER See **nizatidine p 144**

Azactam ANTIBIOTIC, Monobactam See **aztreonam p 31**

azathioprine
Imuran
Tab— lactose

IMMUNOSUPPRESSANT, ANTIARTHRITIC Oral or Parenteral (IV)
Drug: May take c̄ food to ↓ GI upset. **Nutr:** Anorexia.
Oral/GI: Stomatitis, esophagitis, N/V, diarrhea, steatorrhea.
S/Cond: Not c̄ lactation. Do dental care cautiously, see p 10 & 14.
Other: Bone marrow suppression, rash, ↑ infection.
Blood/Serum: ↓ WBC, anemia, ↑ SGOT, ↑ SGPT, ↑ bil, ↑ alk phos, ↓ uric acid, ↑ amylase, ↓ alb. **Urinary:** ↓ uric acid.
Monitor: CBC weekly X 1 mo, then 2X/mo. Hepatic func.

azithromycin
Zithromax
Cap— lactose

ANTIBIOTIC, Macrolide
Drug: Food ↓ abs 52%. Take 1 hr before or 2 hrs after meals.
Diet: Take Mg suppl separately by 2 hrs. **Oral/GI:** N/V, abdominal pain, diarrhea. **S/Cond:** Caution c̄ lactation.
Blood/Serum: ↑ CPK, ↑ SGOT, ↑ SGPT, ↑ GGT, ↑ K.
< 1% dyscrasias, ↑ BUN, ↑ crea, ↑ P, ↑ LDH, ↑ alk phos, ↑ bil, ↑ glucose.

Azmacort — ANTIASTHMA Inhalant — See **triamcinolone acetonide p 200**

AZT (Azidothymidine) — ANTIVIRAL, ANTI-HIV — See **zidovudine p 215**

aztreonam
Azactam
Pwd— Na free

ANTIBIOTIC, Monobactam Parenteral only (IM or IV)
Oral/GI: N/V, diarrhea, pseudomembranous colitis.
S/Cond: Not c̄ lactation. **Other:** Rash.
Blood/Serum: ↑ SGOT, ↑ SGPT, ↑ alk phos, ↑ crea, ↑ LDH, ↑ PT.

Azulfidine — ANTI-INFLAMMATORY See **sulfasalazine p 189**

baclofen
Lioresal
Tab— starch

MUSCLE RELAXANT, ANTISPASMODIC, Oral & Intrathecal
Oral/GI: Dry mouth, altered taste, N/V, constipation. **S/Cond:** Avoid alcohol. Caution c̄ diabetes—may ↑ glucose. Caution c̄ epilepsy.
Other: DROWSINESS, dizziness, weakness, confusion, headache, depression, insomnia, ↓ BP, edema.
Blood/Serum: ↑ Alk Phos, ↑ SGOT, ↑ SGPT, ↑ glucose.
Urinary: ↑ frequency.

Bactrim — ANTIBIOTIC See **trimethoprim c̄ sulfamethoxazole p 202**

beclomethasone dipropionate
Beconase— Nasal
Vancenase— Nasal
Vanceril— Inhalant

ANTIASTHMA, ADRENOCORTICOID Nasal or Inhalant
Oral/GI: ↓ sense of taste, sore throat, N/V. **S/Cond:** Caution c̄ lactation.
Other: NASOPHARYNGEAL IRRITATION, nose bleed, dizziness, headache.

Beepen VK — ANTIBIOTIC See **penicillin p 155**

Benadryl — ANTIHISTAMINE See **diphenhydramine HCl p 74**

benazepril HCl
Lotensin
Tab— lactose, starch

ANTIHYPERTENSIVE, ACE Inhibitor
Drug: Take s̄ regard to food. **Diet:** Insure adequate fluid intake. ↓ Na, ↓ cal may be recommended. Avoid salt subs. Caution c̄ K suppl. Avoid natural licorice.

S/Cond: Limit alcohol. Caution c̄ lactation. 97% serum pro bound.
Other: COUGH, headache, dizziness, angioedema (rare, can be fatal).
Blood/Serum: ↑ K, ↓ Na. Transient ↑ crea. Rare dyscrasias.
Monitor: Serum K, BP.

Bentyl ANTISPASMODIC See **dicyclomine HCl p 70**

benztropine mesylate
Cogentin
Tab— lactose, starch
Parenteral—
4 mg Na/mL

ANTIPARKINSON, ANTI-EPS, Anticholinergic Oral or Parenteral (IM or IV)
Drug: May take c̄ food to ↓ GI upset. **Oral/GI:** DRY MOUTH, N/V, epigastric distress, constipation. **S/Cond:** Avoid alcohol. May inhibit lactation. ↑ risk of dental problems, see p 9 & 14. Caution in hot weather. May aggravate tardive dyskinesia.[7]
Other: CONFUSION, DEPRESSION, drowsiness, blurred vision, ↓ sweating, dizziness, photosensitivity, weakness, muscle cramps.
Urinary: Retention, pain.

beta carotene PROVITAMIN See **vitamin A p 208**
Nutr: Not toxic c̄ high dose.[47] **Other:** Yellow skin c̄ high dose.

Betapace ANTIARRHYTHMIC, Non-Selective Beta-Blocker See **sotalol HCl p 186**

Betapen VK ANTIBIOTIC See **penicillin p 155**

Betaseron ANTI-MULTIPLE SCLEROSIS See **interferon beta-1b p 109**

bethanechol Cl
Urecholine
Tab— lactose, starch
Duvoid
Myotonachol
Tab— tartrazine

CHOLINERGIC STIMULANT, Anti-GERD   Oral or Parenteral (SC)
Drug: Take 1 hr before or 2 hrs after meals to avoid N/V.
Oral/GI: ↑ salivation, ↑ GASTRIC MOTILITY, belching, N/V, abdominal cramps, borborygmi, diarrhea. **S/Cond:** Not c̄ lactation.
Other: Blurred vision. High dose— dizziness, flushing, ↓ BP, headache, insomnia, seizures. **Blood/Serum:** ↑ lipase, ↑ amylase, ↑ SGOT.
Urinary: STIMULATES EMPTYING OF THE BLADDER. ↑ frequency.

Biaxin ANTIBIOTIC, Macrolide See **clarithromycin p 54**

Bicillin ANTIBIOTIC See **penicillin p 155**

BiCNU ANTINEOPLASTIC See **carmustine p 43**

bisacodyl
Dulcolax
Enteric-Coated
Tab— lactose
sucrose

STIMULANT LAXATIVE
Drug: Take on empty stomach c̄ 8 oz H_2O or juice. Swallow tab whole. Do not crush. Do not take within 1 hr of milk, Ca or Mg suppl.
Diet: High fiber c̄ 1500-2000 mL fluid/day to prevent constipation.
Nutr: ↓ intestinal abs of amino acids, & glucose.[11] ↓ wt.
Oral/GI: Nausea, belching, abdominal cramps, diarrhea. LT use— laxative dependence, malabsorption, steatorrhea.
S/Cond: Caution c̄ lactation. Caution c̄ diabetes.
Blood/Serum: LT use— ↓ K, ↓ Ca.

bismuth subsalicylate **Pepto-Bismol** liquid— saccharin Tab— mannitol saccharin Caplet— saccharin	ANTIDIARRHEAL, ANTINAUSEANT See also **acetylsalicylic acid p 18** **Drug:** Chew tabs. **Oral/GI:** Temporary darkening of tongue & stool. Impaction (debilitated elderly & children). **S/Cond:** Caution c̄ lactation c̄ chronic use. Not c̄ salicylate allergy. **Blood/Serum:** ↑ or ↓ uric acid, ↓ K, ↓ T_4, ↓ T_3. **Urinary:** False + glucose ($CuSO_4$).
bleomycin sulfate **Blenoxane**	ANTINEOPLASTIC, Antibiotic Parenteral only (IM, IV or SC) **Diet:** Insure adequate fluid intake. **Nutr:** ANOREXIA, ↓ wt. **Oral/GI:** STOMATITIS, NAUSEA/VOMITING. **S/Cond:** Not c̄ lactation. **Other:** SKIN TOXICITY, RASH, FEVER, CHILLS, pulmonary toxicity (↑ IN ELDERLY ≥ 70), pulmonary fibrosis (may be fatal), dyspnea. **Monitor:** Hepatic & renal func, pulmonary x-rays.
Brethine	ANTIASTHMA See **terbutaline sulfate p 193**
Bricanyl	ANTIASTHMA See **terbutaline sulfate p 193**

bromocriptine **Parlodel** Cap— sulfites Tab & cap— lactose	ANTIPARKINSON, GROWTH HORMONE SUPPRESSANT **Drug:** Take c̄ food or milk to ↓ GI irritation. **Nutr:** Anorexia. **Oral/GI:** Dry mouth, dyspepsia, NAUSEA/vomiting, abdominal cramps, constipation, diarrhea, GI bleeding. **S/Cond:** Avoid alcohol. Will inhibit lactation. > 90% serum albumin bound. **Other:** Drowsiness, fatigue, headache, dizziness, fainting, ↓ BP, hallucinations, confusion. **Blood/Serum:** ↓ PROLACTIN. Transient ↑ BUN, ↑ SGOT, ↑ SGPT, ↑ alk phos, ↑ CPK, ↑ uric acid. **Monitor:** BP. LT use— Hepatic, renal & cardiovascular func. CBC c̄ diff.
Bromo-Seltzer buffered	ANALGESIC, ANTACID — See **acetaminophen p 17** 761 mg Na/ 325 mg dose. **Drug:** Dissolve in 120 mL cool water.
brompheniramine maleate **Dimetane** **Dimetane Extentabs** (SR)	ANTIHISTAMINE, Alkylamine See listing for **chlorpheniramine maleate p 49** Oral & Parenteral (IV, IM or SC) **S/Cond:** Elixir precipitates tube feeding. Tab— lactose. Extentab— sucrose, wheat flour. Elixir — 3% alcohol, glucose, saccharin.
Bufferin	ANALGESIC, ANTIPYRETIC — See **acetylsalicylic acid p 18** 325 mg aspirin, $CaCO_3$, $MgCO_3$, Mg Oxide
bumetanide **Bumex** Tab— lactose Vial— 1% benzyl alcohol	DIURETIC— Loop (K-depleting) — Oral & Parenteral (IM or IV) **Drug:** May take c̄ food to ↓ GI irritation. **Diet:** Possible ↓ Na, ↑ K, ↑ Mg, ↓ cal. **S/Cond:** Caution c̄ alcohol. Not c̄ lactation. 95% serum protein bound. **Other:** ↓ BP, dizziness, headache. Rare gout.

Blood/Serum: ↓ Na, ↓ Cl, ↓ K, ↓ Mg, ↑ crea, ↑ BUN, ↑ URIC ACID, ↓ Ca, ↑ LDH. <1%— Dyscrasias, ↑ SGOT, ↑ SGPT, ↑ alk phos, ↑ bil, ↑ chol. **Urinary:** ↑ Na, ↑ Cl, ↑ K, ↑ Mg, ↑ Ca , ↑ P, ↓ uric acid.
Monitor: BP, electrolytes, uric acid, renal & hepatic func, CBC c̄ diff, CO_2.

buprenorphine
Buprenex

ANALGESIC, Narcotic, Opioid — Parenteral only (IM or IV)
Oral/GI: Delayed gastric emptying. N/V. **S/Cond:** Avoid alcohol. Caution c̄ lactation. 96% serum protein (globulin) bound.
Other: SEDATION, DROWSINESS, dizziness, headache, ↓ BP, respiratory depression. **Blood/Serum:** ↑ amylase, ↑ lipase.

bupropion HCl
Wellbutrin

ANTIDEPRESSANT
Drug: May take c̄ food to ↓ GI irritation. **Nutr:** Anorexia, ↓ wt. ↑ appetite, ↑ wt. **Oral/GI:** Dry mouth, stomatitis, dyspepsia, N/V, constipation. **S/Cond:** Avoid alcohol. Not c̄ lactation. Not c̄ seizures, anorexia or bulimia. > 80% albumin bound. **Other:** Tremor, dizziness, agitation, sweating, confusion, blurred vision, insomnia, rash, headache, tachycardia, ataxia, edema. **Blood/Serum**: ↓ WBC.[13]

buspirone HCl
BuSpar
Tab— lactose

ANTIANXIETY
Drug: Take s̄ regard to food. **Oral/GI:** Sore throat, nausea, diarrhea. **S/Cond:** Caution c̄ alcohol. Not c̄ lactation. 95% serum pro bound. **Other:** Dizziness, drowsiness, confusion, nervousness, tremor, ataxia, blurred vision, headache, rash. **Blood/Serum**: <1%— ↑ SGOT, ↑ SGPT.

busulfan
Myleran
Tab— NaCl

ANTINEOPLASTIC, Alkylating Agent
Drug: Take s̄ regard to food. May take on empty stomach to ↓ N/V.[7]
Diet: ↑ fluid intake essential to ↑ uric acid excretion.[13]
Nutr: Anorexia, ↓ wt. **Oral/GI:** N/V, stomatitis, diarrhea.
S/Cond: Not c̄ lactation. **Other:** BONE MARROW SUPPRESSION, fatigue, skin darkening, dizziness, pulmonary fibrosis, gout.
Blood/Serum: Anemias, dyscrasias, ↓ WBC, ↑ uric acid. Rare ↑ SGOT, ↑ SGPT, ↑ bil, ↑ alk phos. **Urinary:** ↑ uric acid.
Monitor: Weekly CBC c̄ diff & platelets,[10] uric acid.[13] Hepatic func.

Cafergot

ANTIMIGRAINE — See **ergotamine tartrate & caffeine p 82**

caffeine
Caffedrine
Cap— SR
No Doz
Tab— sucrose
Vivarin
Tab— dextrose

STIMULANT, Methylxanthine
Drug: Swallow SR form whole. **Diet:** Limit dietary caffeine sources, see p 240. Take Ca or Fe suppl separately by 2 hrs.[13] High cruciferous vegetable intake ↑ caffeine metabolism.[35] **Nutr:** May ↓ Ca & Fe abs.
Oral/GI: N/V, GI DISTRESS, dyspepsia, diarrhea. **S/Cond:** Not c̄ lactation.[13] Caution c̄ diabetes— ↑ glucose. Dependence may develop c̄ LT use of dose ≥ 130 mg.[24] **Other:** INSOMNIA, ↑ HEART RATE, tremor, nervousness, irritability. **Blood/Serum:** ↑ glucose, ↓ K. False ↑ uric acid.
Urinary: ↑ VMA, ↑ Na, ↑ H_2O.

Calan

ANTIARRHYTHMIC, ANTIHYPERTENSIVE — See **verapamil p 206**

Calcijex

Ca REGULATOR — See **calcitriol p 39**

calcitonin
Calcimar
Miacalcin

Ca REGULATOR, ANTI PAGET'S DISEASE, Hormone bone resorption inhibitor — Parenteral (IM or SC) & Nasal

Drug: Use HS to ↓ N/V. **Diet:** To ↓ bone loss— Adequate Vit D & Ca intake essential. Take suppl 4 hrs after drug. To ↓ hypercalcemia— May need ↓ Ca, ↓ Vit D diet. Avoid Ca & Vit D suppls. **Nutr:** Anorexia. **Oral/GI:** Metallic or salty taste, epigastric discomfort, NAUSEA/V, diarrhea. **S/Cond:** Not c̄ lactation. **Other:** Flushing, edema of feet, headache, rash. **Blood/Serum:** ↓ ALK PHOS, ↓ Ca, ↓ P. **Urinary:** ↑ frequency, ↑ P, ↑ or ↓ Ca, ↓ HYDROXYPROLINE, ↑ Mg, ↑ K, ↑ Cl. Transient ↑ Na, ↑ H_2O. **Monitor:** Serum alk phos & Ca. Urinary hydroxyproline.

calcitriol
Rocaltrol
cap— sorbitol
Calcijex
Parenteral (IV)

Ca REGULATOR, Active Vit D_3 (1,25 $[OH]_2$—D_3) — Oral or Parenteral (IV)

Diet: Dialysis— Low P diet. Not c̄ Vit D or Mg suppl. Rickets or Osteomalacia—add Ca suppl. **Nutr:** ↑ Ca abs, anorexia, ↓ wt, ↑ thirst. **Oral/GI:** Dry mouth, metallic taste, N/V, constipation, diarrhea. **S/Cond:** Not c̄ lactation. **Other:** Weakness, ataxia, headache, bone pain. **Blood/Serum:**, ↑ Ca, ↑ P, ↓ alk phos , ↑ Mg, ↑ BUN, ↑ crea, ↑ SGOT, ↑ SGPT, ↑ Chol. **Urinary:** ↑ Ca, ↑ P, ↑ alb. **Monitor**: Serum Ca, P, Mg, alk phos, renal func. Urinary Ca & P.

calcium acetate
Phos-Lo

PHOSPHATE BINDER — See also listing for **Ca carbonate p 40**

Drug: Take c̄ meals. **Diet:** Avoid Ca suppl. **Nutr:** ↓ Fe abs, anorexia. Does not promote Al abs. **Oral/GI:** N/V, constipation. **Other:** Kidney stones. **Blood/Serum:** ↑ Ca & ↓ P in ESRD. **Monitor:** Serum Ca, P.

calcium carbonate **Tums** Tab— Na-free, sucrose **OsCal** **Rolaids Calcium Rich/Sodium Free** Tab— mannitol, sucrose Fruit flavored— tartrazine	ANTACID, Ca SUPPLEMENT, PHOSPHATE BINDER **Drug:** Take c̄ meals as suppl and P binder. Take 1-3 hr after meals as antacid. Chew tabs. **Diet:** Insure adequate fluid intake. Take separately from large amounts high fiber, high oxalate or high phytate foods, see p 241 & 242. Take Fe or Fl separately by 1-2 hrs. (may ↓ abs). Vit D— ↑ Ca abs— concurrent & LT use may cause milk-alkali syndrome. **Nutr:** NIH adult recommendation = 1,000 - 1,500 mg.[73] Contains 40% Ca. Anorexia. Infrequent hypercalcemia c̄ alkalosis. **Oral/GI:** Chalky taste, dry mouth. Excessive dose— N/V, abdominal pain, constipation. **S/Cond:** Limit alcohol & caffeine (< 8 cups coffee/day)— large amounts ↓ abs. **Other:** Kidney stones c̄ LT high dose. **Blood/Serum:** ↑ Ca & ↓ P in ESRD. **Urinary:** ↑ Ca. **Monitor:** Serum Ca, P.
calcium citrate **Citracal** Tab— sugar	Ca SUPPLEMENT, PHOSPHATE BINDER See **$CaCO_3$ above** Contains 21% Ca. **Drug:** Take s̄ regard to food. Food does not affect abs.
calcium gluconate	ANTACID, Ca SUPPLEMENT Contains 9% Ca. See **$CaCO_3$ above**
calcium polycarbophil **FiberCon** 100 mg Ca/tab, Na Free	BULK FORMING LAXATIVE, ANTIDIARRHEAL **Drug:** As laxative— take c̄ 8 oz H_2O or other liquid. **Diet:** High fiber c̄ 1500-2000 mL fluid/day to prevent constipation. Take Fe or Fl separately by 1-2 hrs. **Nutr:** Ca is partially absorbed. Provides significant dietary Ca. **Oral/GI:** ↑ PERISTALSIS & BOWEL MOTILITY. Rare bowel obstruction.

captopril
Capoten
Tab— lactose

ANTIHYPERTENSIVE, ANTI-DIABETIC NEPHROPATHY, ACE Inhibitor

Drug: Take on empty stomach 1 hr before meals (food ↓ abs by 30-40%).
Diet: Insure adequate fluid intake. ↓ Na, ↓ cal may be recommended. Avoid salt subs. Caution c̄ K suppl. Take Mg suppl separately by 2 hrs. Avoid natural licorice.
Nutr: Anorexia, ↓ wt.
Oral/GI: Dysgeusia, metallic or salty taste, N/V, peptic ulcer, abdominal pain, constipation, diarrhea.
S/Cond: Limit alcohol. Not c̄ lactation. Caution c̄ diabetes— ↓ glucose.
Other: ↓ BP, COUGH, rash, dizziness, headache, fatigue, insomnia, angioedema (rare, can be fatal).
Blood/Serum: Dyscrasias, ↑ K, ↓ Na, ↑ SGOT, ↑ SGPT,↑ alk phos, ↑ bil, ↑ prolactin, ↑ uric acid, ↓ glucose in diabetics. Transient ↑ BUN, ↑ crea.
Urinary: Pro. False + acetone.
Monitor: BP, electrolytes, renal func, WBC c̄ diff, diabetics for ↓ glucose.

Carafate ANTIULCER See **sucralfate p 188**

carbamazepine
Tegretol
Chewable Tab—
sucrose
Susp—
sucrose, sorbitol

ANTICONVULSANT Also used as antimanic, antipsychotic

Drug: Take c̄ food or milk to ↓ GI distress. **Nutr:** Anorexia.
Oral/GI: Dry mouth, stomatitis, glossitis, N/V, abdominal pain, constipation, diarrhea. **S/Cond:** Avoid alcohol.[13] Not c̄ lactation. ↑ risk of dental problems, see p 9 & 14. **Other:** Dizziness, ataxia, drowsiness, blurred vision, double vision, rash, SIADH, edema, water intoxication.
Blood Serum: ↓ WBC, dyscrasias, ↑ BUN, ↑ SGOT, ↑ SGPT, ↑ alk phos, ↑ bil, ↓ T_3, ↓ T_4, ↓ Na, ↑ chol, ↑ HDL, ↑ TG. Aplastic anemia (rare, can be fatal). **Urinary:** ↑ frequency. Glucose in diabetics, pro.
Monitor: CBC c̄ diff, renal & hepatic func, serum Fe & Na, urinalysis.

carboplatin
Paraplatin
mannitol

ANTINEOPLASTIC, Alkylating Agent — Parenteral only (IV)

Diet: Insure adequate fluid intake to ↑ urinary output. **Nutr:** ANOREXIA.
Oral/GI: Altered taste, STOMATITIS, NAUSEA/VOMITING, GI pain, diarrhea, constipation. **S/Cond:** Not c̄ lactation. Do dental care cautiously, see p 10 & 14.
Other: BONE MARROW SUPPRESSION, WEAKNESS, infections, peripheral neuropathy, ↓ BP, blurred vision.
Blood/Serum: DYSCRASIAS, ANEMIA, ↑ BUN, ↑ crea, ↑ ALK PHOS, ↑ bil, ↑ SGOT, ↓ Ca, ↓ Mg, ↓ K, ↓ Na. **Urinary:** ↓ output.
Monitor: Renal func & CBC c̄ diff before each dose. Electrolytes, Mg.

Cardene — ANTIANGINAL, Ca Channel Blocker — See **nicardipine p 141**

Cardizem — ANTIANGINAL, Ca Channel Blocker — See **diltiazem HCl p 73**

Cardura
ANTIHYPERTENSIVE — See **doxazosin mesylate p 77**

carisoprodol
Soma
Tab— starch
MUSCLE RELAXANT
Drug: May take c̄ food to ↓ GI distress. **Oral/GI:** N/V, epigastric distress, hiccups. **S/Cond:** Avoid alcohol. Not c̄ lactation. **Other:** DROWSINESS, dizziness, tremor, headache, insomnia, flushing, depression.

carmustine
BiCNU
10% alcohol
ANTINEOPLASTIC, Alkylating Agent — Parenteral only (IV)
Diet: Insure adequate fluid intake. **Nutr:** Anorexia. **Oral/GI:** Stomatitis, dysphagia, N/V, diarrhea. **S/Cond:** Not c̄ lactation. Do dental care cautiously, see p 10 & 14. **Other:** Drowsiness, dizziness, ataxia, flushing, bone marrow depression (often delayed), MILD HEPATIC TOXICITY, jaundice, rash, pulmonary toxicity.
Blood/Serum: ↑ SGOT, ↑ SGPT, ↑ bil, DYSCRASIAS, anemia, ↑ BUN.
Monitor: Weekly CBC c̄ diff. Hepatic, renal & pulmonary func.

Catapres
ANTIHYPERTENSIVE — See **clonidine p 57**

Ceclor
ANTIBIOTIC — See **cefaclor below**

cefaclor
Ceclor
Susp— 3 g sucrose/5mL
ANTIBIOTIC, Cephalosporin — Oral only
Drug: Take s̄ regard to food. **Oral/GI:** Oral candidiasis & sore mouth & tongue c̄ LT use, N/V, cramps, diarrhea, pseudomembranous colitis. **S/Cond:** Caution c̄ lactation. **Blood/Serum:** ↑ alk phos, ↑ SGOT, ↑ SGPT. **Urinary:** False + glucose ($CuSO_4$).

cefadroxil
Duricef

ANTIBIOTIC, Cephalosporin
Suspension— 2 g sucrose/5mL

See listing for **cephalexin p 45**
S/Cond: Caution c̄ lactation.

cefixime
Suprax
Susp— sucrose
Tab— starch

ANTIBIOTIC, Cephalosporin — Oral only

Drug: Take s̄ regard to food. May take c̄ food if GI upset.
Oral/GI: Oral candidiasis & sore mouth & tongue c̄ LT use, dry mouth, N/V, dyspepsia, abdominal pain, flatulence, DIARRHEA. Rare pseudomembranous colitis.
S/Cond: Caution c̄ lactation.
Other: Headache, dizziness. rash.
Blood/Serum: ↑ amylase. Transient ↑ SGOT, ↑ SGPT, ↑ alk phos, ↑ BUN, ↑ crea, dyscrasias.
Urinary: False + glucose ($CuSO_4$).

cefmetazole

ANTIBIOTIC — see **cephalosporins p 46**

cefprozil
Cefzil
Susp— aspartame — 28 mg phenylalanine/ 5 mL, Na, sucrose

ANTIBIOTIC, Cephalosporin — Oral only

Drug: Take s̄ regard to food.
Oral/GI: Oral candidiasis & sore mouth and tongue c̄ LT use, N/V, diarrhea, pseudomembranous colitis.
S/Cond: Caution c̄ lactation.
Other: Dizziness, rash.
Blood/Serum: ↑ SGOT, ↑ SGPT, eosinophilia.
Urinary: False + glucose ($CuSO_4$).

cefuroxime axetil **Ceftin**— Tab Susp— sucrose **cefuroxime sodium** **Zinacef**— Parenteral 54 mg Na/g	ANTIBIOTIC, Cephalosporin — Oral or Parenteral (IM or IV) **Drug:** Take c̄ food to enhance abs. (may crush tab & mix c̄ food, milk or juice). **Oral/GI:** Oral candidiasis & sore mouth & tongue c̄ LT use, bitter taste, N/V, diarrhea. Rare pseudomembranous colitis. **S/Cond:** Caution c̄ lactation. **Other:** Dizziness. **Blood/Serum:** (↑ incidence c̄ Parenteral) ↓ Hgb, ↓ HCT, eosinophilia, ↑ SGOT, ↑ SGPT, ↑ LDH, ↑ alk phos. **Urinary:** False + glucose ($CuSO_4$).
Cefzil	ANTIBIOTIC, Cephalosporin — See **cefprozil above**
cephalexin **Keflex** Susp— 3 g sucrose /5 mL	ANTIBIOTIC, Cephalosporin — Oral only **Drug:** May be taken s̄ regard to food. **Oral/GI:** Oral candidiasis & sore mouth/ tongue c̄ LT use. Dyspepsia, gastritis, diarrhea, pseudomembranous colitis. **S/Cond:** Caution c̄ lactation. **Other:** Dizziness, headache, fatigue, rash. **Blood/Serum:** ↑ SGOT, ↑ SGPT. **Urinary:** False + glucose ($CuSO_4$).

cephalosporins ANTIBIOTIC

Parenterals Only (IM or IV)
All contain Na— 35-83 mg/g.

Diet: May need ↑ Vit K or supplement especially c̄ cefamandole, cefmetazole, cefoperazone, or cefotetan. Consider Na content c̄ ↓ Na diet.
Oral/GI: Oral candidiasis & sore mouth & tongue c̄ LT use. N/V, diarrhea, pseudomembranous colitis.
S/Cond: No alcohol— disulfiram-like reaction c̄ cefamandole, cefmetazole, cefoperazone, cefotetan. Caution c̄ lactation. LT use in malnourished— ↓ Vit K synthesis.
Cefazolin, cefonicid, cefoperazone, cefotetan & ceftriaxone are ≥ 85% serum pro bound.
Other: Rash < 1% headache, dizziness.
Blood/Serum: Dyscrasias, eosinophilia, ↓ H/H, Transient ↑ SGOT, ↑ SGPT, ↑ LDH, ↑ alk phos, ↑ GGT, ↑ BUN, ↑ crea (possible false ↑ c̄ Jaffe method except c̄ ceftazidime). Rare ↑ PT.
Urinary: False + glucose ($CuSO_4$), (possible false ↑ crea c̄ Jaffe method except c̄ ceftazidime).
Monitor: PT, CBC c̄ diff if used > 10 days.

cefamandole nafate
Mandol
cefazolin sodium
Ancef
Kefzol
cefmetazole
Zefazone

cefonicid sodium
Monocid
cefoperazone sodium
Cefobid
cefotaxime sodium
Claforan
cefotetan disodium
Cefotan

cefoxitin
Mefoxin
ceftazidime
Ceptaz
Fortaz
Tazicef
Tazidime

ceftizoxime sodium
Cefizox
ceftriaxone sodium
Rocephin

cephradine — ANTIBIOTIC, Cephalosporin — Oral only

Velosef

Susp— 3 g sucrose/ 5 mL

Drug: Take s̄ regard to food. Food delays but does not ↓ abs.
Oral/GI: Oral candidiasis & sore/ tongue c̄ LT use, dyspepsia, diarrhea, pseudomembranous colitis.
S/Cond: Caution c̄ lactation.
Other: Dizziness. **Blood/Serum:** ↑ SGOT, ↑ SGPT, ↑ bil.
Urinary: False + glucose ($CuSO_4$).

Cephulac — ANTIHYPERAMMONEMIC — See **lactulose p 114**

Cerubidine — ANTINEOPLASTIC — See listing for **doxorubicin p 78**

Parenteral only 100 mg mannitol/ vial

Chemet — ANTI-LEAD POISONING, Chelating Agent — See **succimer p 187**

chloral hydrate — SEDATIVE, Hypnotic, Sleep Aid — Oral & suppositories

Supp— tartrazine
Syrup— saccharin, sucrose

Drug: Swallow caps whole c̄ 8 oz H_2O or juice. Dilute syrup in 4 oz H_2O or juice.
Oral/GI: Unpleasant aftertaste, epigastric distress, N/V, flatulence, diarrhea.
S/Cond: Avoid alcohol. Not c̄ lactation.
May be habit forming c̄ use > 2 wks.
Other: DROWSINESS, ataxia, headache, confusion, dizziness, rash.
Urinary: False + glucose ($CuSO_4$).
Blood/Serum: ↓ T_4,[7] ↓ T_3,[7] ↓ WBC, ↑ eosinophils.

chlorambucil
Leukeran
Tab— lactose, sucrose

ANTINEOPLASTIC, Alkylating Agent

Drug: Take c̄ chilled liquid. **Diet:** Insure adequate fluid intake.
Oral/GI: Stomatitis, N/V, GI pain, diarrhea. **S/Cond:** Not c̄ lactation. Do dental care cautiously, see p 10 & 14. 99% serum pro bound.
Other: BONE MARROW SUPPRESSION, confusion, tremor. Rare hepatic or pulmonary toxicity.
Blood/Serum: ↓ WBC, ↓ platelets, ↑ uric acid, ↑ SGOT, ↑ alk phos.
Urinary: ↑ uric acid. **Monitor:** Weekly CBC c̄ diff, hepatic func, uric acid.

chloramphenicol
Chloromycetin
Cap— lactose
Susp— 2 g sucrose/5 mL, alcohol
Pwd— 52 mg Na/1g

ANTIBIOTIC — Oral or Parenteral (IV)

Drug: Take 1 hr before or 2 hrs after meals c̄ 8 oz H_2O. May take c̄ food to ↓ GI distress. **Diet:** Caution c̄ Fe suppl— ↑ risk of Fe overload.
Nutr: Delays response to Fe, Fol or Vit B_{12}.[6] **Oral/GI:** Bad taste, glossitis, stomatitis, N/V, enterocolitis, diarrhea. **S/Cond:** Caution c̄ alcohol—mild disulfiram-like reaction.[1] Not c̄ lactation. Do dental care cautiously, see p 10 & 14. **Other:** Confusion, headache, depression, rash, bone marrow suppression, grey syndrome especially in infants.
Blood/Serum: Dyscrasias, ↑ Fe, aplastic anemia (rare, can be fatal).
Urinary: False + glucose ($CuSO_4$).
Monitor: CBC c̄ diff q 2 days, Fol level.

chlordiazepoxide
Librium
Cap— lactose

ANTIANXIETY, Benzodiazepine — Oral or Parenteral (IM or IV)

Drug: May take c̄ food to ↓ GI distress. **Diet:** Ca or Mg suppl may ↓ rate, but not extent of abs. **Nutr:** ↑ appetite, ↑ wt, ↑ thirst, ↓ wt.
Oral/GI: Dry mouth, ↑ salivation, bitter taste, nausea, GI distress,

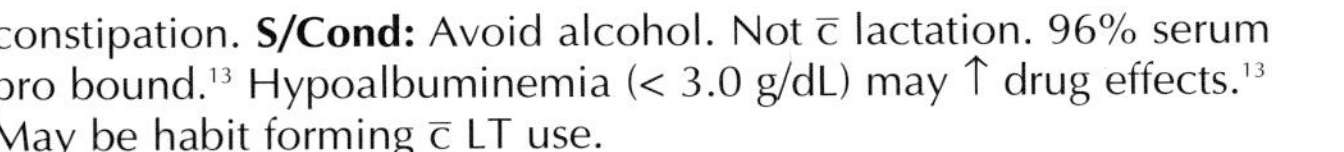

constipation. **S/Cond:** Avoid alcohol. Not $\bar{c}$ lactation. 96% serum pro bound.[13] Hypoalbuminemia (< 3.0 g/dL) may ↑ drug effects.[13] May be habit forming $\bar{c}$ LT use.
Other: Drowsiness, ataxia, dizziness, confusion, blurred vision, edema, rash, EPS. **Blood/Serum:** Dyscrasias, anemia, ↑ alk phos, ↑ bil, ↑ LDH ↑ SGOT, ↑ SGPT, ↑ glucose,↑ CPK $\bar{c}$ IM.
Monitor: CBC $\bar{c}$ diff & hepatic func $\bar{c}$ LT use.[10]

Chloromycetin — ANTIBIOTIC — See **chloramphenicol above**

chlorothiazide
Diuril

ANTIHYPERTENSIVE, DIURETIC (K-depleting) — Oral or Parenteral. (IV)
250 mg Tab— lactose. Susp— saccharin, sucrose, alcohol 0.5%.
See listing for **hydrochlorothiazide p 102**

chlorpheniramine maleate
Chlor-Trimeton
Tab— lactose, sucrose
Syrup— 7% alcohol
Teldrin (SR)
Cap— sucrose, benzyl alcohol

ANTIHISTAMINE, Alkylamine — Oral or Parenteral. (IM, IV or SC)
Drug: Take $\bar{c}$ food to ↓ GI distress. Do not crush SR form— swallow whole.
Nutr: Anorexia. **Oral/GI:** Dry mouth, ↓ salivation, oral candidiasis $\bar{c}$ LT use, N/V, GI distress, constipation.
S/Cond: Avoid alcohol. Not $\bar{c}$ lactation. ↑ risk of dental problems, see p 9 & 14.
Other: Drowsiness, dizziness, excitability in children, headache (IV).
Blood/Serum: Dyscrasias, anemia.

chlorpromazine HCl
Thorazine
Parenteral— sulfites, benzyl alcohol
Tab— lactose
Syrup— sucrose
Conc— saccharin
Spansule (cap)— sucrose, benzyl alcohol

ANTIPSYCHOTIC, ANTIEMETIC, Phenothiazine Oral or Parenteral (IM, IV)

Drug: May take c̄ food or 8 oz milk or H_2O to ↓ GI distress. Swallow spansule whole. Dilute oral conc in 4 oz drink or soft food. **Diet:** Take Mg suppl separately by 2 hrs.[13] **Nutr:** ↑ appetite, ↑ wt. ↑ need for Rib.[41] May ↓ abs of Vit B_{12}. **Oral/GI:** DRY MOUTH, N/V, CONSTIPATION.
S/Cond: Avoid alcohol. Not c̄ lactation. Conc precipitates tube feedings.[8] ↑ risk of dental problems, see p 9 & 14. 90% serum pro bound.
Other: SEDATION, EXTRAPYRAMIDAL SYMPTOMS, BLURRED VISION, restlessness, drowsiness, dizziness, hives, ↓ BP, tachycardia, headache, photosensitivity, edema, jaundice, ocular changes. Tardive dyskinesia c̄ LT use.
Blood/Serum: Dyscrasias, ↓ WBC, ↑ chol, ↑ bil, ↑ or ↓ glucose, ↑ prolactin. **Urinary:** Retention, + glucose, ↑ Rib.
Monitor: Hepatic func. CBC c̄ diff. BP.

chlorpropamide
Diabinese
Tab— starch

ORAL HYPOGLYCEMIC, Sulfonylurea

Drug: Usually given at breakfast. **Diet:** Prescribed diet compliance important. Mg suppl may ↑ rate of abs. **Nutr:** ↑ appetite, ↑ wt, anorexia.
Oral/GI: Dyspepsia, N/V, diarrhea. **S/Cond:** No alcohol— DISULFIRAM-LIKE REACTION. Not c̄ lactation. 90% serum pro bound. Hypoalbuminemia (< 3.0 g/dL) may ↑ drug effects.[44] Exercise & wt control may modify drug dosage. **Other:** Dizziness, drowsiness, SIADH, edema, jaundice, rash.
Blood/Serum: ↓ GLUCOSE, dyscrasias, ↑ alk phos, ↑ SGOT, ↑ LDH, ↑ BUN, ↑ crea, ↓ Na. **Urinary:** ↓ glucose, ↓ Na.
Monitor: Glucose, possibly glycosylated Hgb, Na.

chlorthalidone **Hygroton** Tab— lactose	ANTIHYPERTENSIVE, DIURETIC (K-depleting) See listing for **hydrochlorothiazide p 102** Structurally & pharmacologically similar to thiazides. **Drug:** Take c̄ food in AM. Longer duration of action than thiazides.
Chlor-Trimeton	ANTIHISTAMINE See **chlorpheniramine maleate p 49**
chlorzoxazone **Paraflex** Caplet— lactose **Parafon Forte DSC** Caplet— lactose	MUSCLE RELAXANT **Drug:** May take c̄ food to ↓ GI distress. May be crushed & added to food. **Oral/GI:** Dyspepsia, stomach cramps, N/V, diarrhea, constipation. Rare GI bleeding. **S/Cond:** Avoid alcohol. Caution c̄ lactation. **Other:** Drowsiness, dizziness, headache, rash. **Blood/Serum:** Rare dyscrasias. **Urinary:** Orange or purple-red color.

cholestyramine
Questran
3.8 g sucrose/9 g

Questran Light—
aspartame
16.8 mg phenylalanine,
0.7 g sucrose/5 g

ANTIHYPERLIPIDEMIC, ANTIDIARRHEAL bile acid sequestrant

Drug: Take before meals. Mix pwd in 2-6 ozs H_2O, non-carbonated beverage, fluid soup or pureed fruit. NEVER TAKE POWDER DRY.

Diet: ↓ Fat, ↓ chol, ↑ fluids, ↑ fiber, ↓ cal if needed. Fat soluble vit & Fol suppls recommended.[1] Take suppls 1 hr before or 4 hrs after drug.

Nutr: May ↓ abs of fat, Ca, Fe, Zn, Mg,[1] Vits A, D, E, & K, MCT,[11] Fol. Anorexia, ↑ or ↓ wt. **Oral/GI:** Belching, N/V, dyspepsia, pain, CONSTIPATION, flatulence, diarrhea. Rare GI bleeding, steatorrhea.

S/Cond: ↓ abs of vits may ↓ vit content of breast milk.

Other: Drowsiness, dizziness, headache, osteomalacia/osteoporosis c̄ LT use, ↑ thyroid hormone degradation.

Blood/Serum: ↓ CHOL, ↓ LDL, ↑ HDL, ↓ Ca, ↓ T_4, ↓ K, ↓ Na, ↑ P, ↑ Cl, ↓ Fol, ↑ PT. Transient ↑ TG, ↑ alk phos, ↑ SGOT, ↑ SGPT.

Urinary: ↑ Ca, ↑ Mg. **Monitor:** Chol, TG, PT, Ca, electrolytes.

Chronulac

LAXATIVE

See **lactulose p 114**

cimetidine
Tagamet—
Tab— starch
cimetidine HCl
Tagamet
Liquid,
2.8% alcohol,

ANTISECRETORY, ANTIULCER, ANTIGERD

Histamine H_2 antagonist — Oral or Parenteral (IM or IV)

Drug: Take s̄ regard to meals. **Diet:** May need bland diet. Take Fe suppl 1 hr before drug.[3] Take Ca or Mg suppl separately by 1 hr. Limit caffeine/ xanthine, see p 240. **Nutr:** ↓ abs of Vit B_{12}.[74] **Oral/GI:** ↓ GASTRIC ACID SECRETIONS, ↑ GASTRIC pH, N/V, diarrhea. **S/Cond:** Caution c̄ alcohol. Not c̄ lactation. Avoid or limit smoking. Liquid precipitates tube feeding.[8]

sorbitol,
saccharin

Other: Drowsiness, dizziness, headache, confusion, hallucinations. **Blood/Serum:** ↑ SGOT, ↑ SGPT, ↑ alk phos, ↑ crea, ↓ Vit B_{12}, ↓ PTH, ↑ prolactin.

ciprofloxacin
Cipro
Cipro I.V.

ANTIBIOTIC, Fluoroquinolone — Oral or Parenteral (IV)

Drug: Take s̄ regard to food. Avoid milk & yogurt.[3] **Diet:** Insure adequate fluid intake. Limit caffeine/xanthine— drug causes ↑ caffeine effect, see p 240. Take antacids, Mg, Ca, Fe or Zn suppl or MVI + minerals separately by 2-4 hrs.
Nutr: Milk or yogurt ↓ abs & bioavailability.[3]
Oral/GI: N/V, abdominal pain, diarrhea. Rare oral candiasis, pseudomembranous colitis. **S/Cond:** Not c̄ lactation.
Other: Headache, dizziness, restlessness, rash, photosensitivity.
Blood/Serum: ↑ SGOT, ↑ SGPT, ↑ BUN, ↑ crea, ↑ CPK, ↑ TG. < 1% dyscrasias, ↑ alk phos, ↑ LDH, ↑ GGT, ↑ bil, ↑ uric acid.
Monitor: Renal & hepatic func, CBC c̄ diff.[6]

cisapride
Propulsid
Tab - lactose

ANTIGERD, GI Stimulant

Drug: Take with beverage 15 to 30 minutes before meals & HS.
Oral/GI: ↑ RATE OF GASTRIC EMPTYING, dyspepsia, N/V, abdominal pain, diarrhea, constipation.
S/Cond: Limit alcohol. Caution with lactation. 98% serum pro bound. **Other:** Headache, abnormal vision.

cisplatin
Platinol

ANTINEOPLASTIC, resembles Alkylating Agent Parenteral only. (IV)

Diet: Insure adequate fluid intake. May need mineral suppls.
Nutr: Anorexia, ↓ wt. **Oral/GI:** Altered taste, stomatitis, SEVERE N/V, diarrhea. **S/Cond:** Not c̄ lactation. Do dental care cautiously, see p 10 & 14. 90% serum pro bound.
Other: RENAL TOXICITY, WEAKNESS, OTOTOXICITY, PERIPHERAL NEUROPATHY, INFECTIONS, BONE MARROW SUPPRESSION.
Blood/Serum: ↓ WBC, ↓ PLATELETS, ANEMIA, ↑ BUN, ↑ CREA, ↑ URIC ACID, ↑ ALK PHOS, ↑ SGOT, ↑ bil, ↓ Mg, ↓ K, ↓ Na, ↓ Zn, ↓ Ca, ↓ P.
Urinary: ↑ Mg, ↑ Ca, ↑ K, ↑ Zn, ↑ Cu, ↑ amino acids.
Monitor: Weekly CBC c̄ diff. Renal & hepatic func, Ca, P, Mg, K, uric acid.

Citracal — Ca SUPPLEMENT — See **calcium citrate p 40**

Citrucel — LAXATIVE, Bulk Forming — See **methylcellulose p 129**

Claforan — ANTIBIOTIC, cefotaxime sodium — See **cephalosporins p 46**

clarithromycin
Biaxin
Susp— sucrose
Tab— starch

ANTIBIOTIC

Drug: Take s̄ regard to meals. **Oral/GI:** Abnormal taste, dyspepsia, N/V, abdominal pain, diarrhea. **S/Cond:** Caution c̄ alcohol— ↑ sedative effect. Caution c̄ lactation. **Other:** Headache.
Blood/Serum: ↑ BUN, ↑ PT. < 1% ↑SGOT, ↑ SGPT, ↑ LDH, ↑ alk phos, ↑ bil, ↑ GGT, ↑ crea, ↓ WBC.

Claritin — ANTIHISTAMINE — See **loratadine p 120**

clemastine fumarate — ANTIHISTAMINE
Tavist
Tab— lactose
Syrup— 5.5% alcohol, saccharin, sorbitol

Drug: Take c̄ food to ↓ GI distress. **Nutr:** Anorexia. **Oral/GI:** Dry mouth, epigastric distress, N/V, diarrhea, constipation. **S/Cond:** Avoid alcohol. Not c̄ lactation. **Other:** SEDATION, drowsiness, ataxia, dizziness, confusion, blurred vision, headache, insomnia. **Blood/Serum:** Dyscrasias.

clindamycin — ANTIBIOTIC — Oral or Parenteral (IV)
Cleocin
Cap— lactose
75 & 150 mg— tartrazine
Soln— sucrose
Parenteral— benzyl alcohol 9.45 mg/mL

Drug: May take c̄ food or 8 oz H_2O to ↓ esophageal irritation.
Nutr: Anorexia, ↓ wt, ↑ thirst. **Oral/GI:** Metallic taste, esophagitis, N/V, cramps, severe pseudomembranous colitis, flatulence, bloating, DIARRHEA. **S/Cond:** Not c̄ lactation. 93% serum pro bound.
Other: RASH. **Blood/Serum:** Transient dyscrasias, ↑ SGPT, ↑ SGOT, ↑ alk phos. **Monitor:** Renal & hepatic func & CBC c̄ LT use.

Clinoril — NSAID — See **sulindac p 189**

clofazimine — ANTIBIOTIC, ANTILEPROSY
Lamprene

Drug: Take c̄ meals or milk. **Nutr:** Anorexia, ↓ wt.
Oral/GI: INTOLERANCE, PAIN, N/V, DIARRHEA. **S/Cond:** Not c̄ lactation.
Other: SKIN & FLUID DISCOLORATION, rash.
Blood/Serum: ↑ glucose. < 1% ↑ SGOT, ↑ SGPT, ↑ alk phos, ↑ alb,[13] ↑ bil, ↓ K, eosinophilia.
Urinary: DISCOLORATION.

clomipramine HCl
Anafranil
Cap— starch

ANTI-OCD, ANTIDEPRESSANT, Tricyclic
Drug: May take c̄ food to ↓ GI distress. **Diet:** Limit caffeine, see p 240. ↑ fiber may ↓ drug effect.[3]
Nutr: ↑ WT ↑ APPETITE especially for sweets. Anorexia, ↓ wt.
Oral/GI: Sour/metallic taste, DRY MOUTH, gingivitis, dysphagia, dyspepsia, NAUSEA/V, abdominal pain, CONSTIPATION, diarrhea, flatulence.
S/Cond: Avoid alcohol. Not c̄ lactation. ↑ risk of dental problems, see p 9 & 14. 97% serum pro bound.
Other: SEDATION, DROWSINESS, DIZZINESS, FATIGUE, TREMOR, headache, blurred vision, ↓ BP, nervousness, seizures, confusion, rash. Rare SIADH.
Blood/Serum: Dyscrasias, ↑ SGOT, ↑ SGPT.
<1% ↑ or ↓ glucose ↑ chol, ↑ uric acid, ↓ K, ↓ Na.
Urinary: Retention.
Monitor: Renal & hepatic func & CBC c̄ LT use.

clonazepam
Klonopin
Tab— lactose

ANTICONVULSANT, Benzodiazepine (also used as an anti-panic agent)
Drug: May take c̄ food to ↓ GI distress. **Nutr:** Anorexia, ↑ or ↓ wt, ↑ thirst **Oral/GI:** ↑ salivation, dry/sore mouth, coated tongue, nausea, diarrhea, constipation. **S/Cond:** Avoid alcohol. Not c̄ lactation. May be habit forming c̄ LT use. **Other:** DROWSINESS, ATAXIA, BEHAVIORAL DISTURBANCES, HYPERACTIVITY IN CHILDREN, dizziness, sedation, headache, blurred vision, confusion, congestion, EPS, edema, rash.
Blood/Serum: Dyscrasias. Transient ↑ SGOT, ↑ SGPT, ↑ alk phos.
Monitor: CBC c̄ diff c̄ LT use.

clonidine
Catapres
Tab— lactose
Catapres TTS

ANTIHYPERTENSIVE — Oral & Transdermal patch.

Diet: ↓ Na & ↓ cal may be recommended. Avoid natural licorice.
Nutr: ↑ wt due to edema, anorexia.
Oral/GI: DRY MOUTH, N/V, constipation.
S/Cond: Avoid alcohol. Not $\bar{c}$ lactation. ↑ risk of dental problems, see p 9 & 14.
Other: DROWSINESS, dizziness, sedation, weakness, headache, edema, rash. **Blood/Serum:** Mild transient ↑ SGOT, ↑ SGPT. **Urinary:** ↓ Na, ↓ H_2O
Monitor: BP.

clorazepate dipotassium
Tranxene
Tab— lactose

ANTIANXIETY, Benzodiazepine — See listing for **chlordiazepoxide p 48**

Drug:. Oral form only.

clotrimazole
Mycelex
Oral lozenge— dextrose

ANTIFUNGAL (Anti Oral Candidiasis)

Drug: Dissolve slowly in mouth over 15-30 minutes, swallow saliva. Do not chew. **Oral/GI:** N/V, cramps, diarrhea.
Blood/Serum: ↑ SGOT.
Monitor: Hepatic func.

clozapine
Clozaril
Tab— lactose, starch

ANTIPSYCHOTIC

Drug: Take s regard to food. **Nutr:** ↑ WT. **Oral/GI:** Dry mouth ↑ SALIVATION, N/V, dyspepsia, SEVERE CONSTIPATION, impaction, diarrhea. **S/Cond:** Avoid alcohol. Not c̄ lactation. 95% serum pro bound. Hypoalbuminemia (< 3 g/dL) may ↑ drug effects. **Other:** DROWSINESS, TACHYCARDIA, dizziness, sedation, tremor, fever, visual changes, ↓ BP, EPS,[25] ↑ BP, ataxia, agitation, confusion, headache, seizures, rash. **Blood/Serum:** Agranulocytosis, ↓ WBC (rare, can be fatal), eosinophilia. Mild ↑ SGOT, ↑ SGPT.
Monitor: Baseline WBC c̄ diff, weekly WBC c̄ diff.

codeine
Parenteral— sulfites

ANTITUSSIVE, ANALGESIC, NARCOTIC   Oral or Parenteral (IM, or SC)

Drug: Take c̄ food or milk to ↓ GI distress.
Nutr: Anorexia. Delays digestion.
Oral/GI: Dry mouth, N/V, CONSTIPATION.
S/Cond: Avoid alcohol. Caution c̄ lactation. ↑ risk of dental problems, see p 9 & 14. May be habit forming c̄ LT use.
Other: Drowsiness, sedation, dizziness, confusion, headache, blurred vision, respiratory depression.

Cogentin ANTIPARKINSON See **benztropine mesylate p 33**

Cognex ANTI-ALZHEIMER'S See **tacrine p 190**

Colace STOOL SOFTENER See **docusate sodium p 76**

colchicine ANTIGOUT Oral or Parenteral (IV)
Colchicine
Tab— sucrose

Diet: ↓ purine diet during acute attack[14]. ↓ cal if wt loss needed.
Nutr: May ↓ abs of Vits A & B_{12}, Fe, Ca, K, Na, fat, N. Anorexia, ↓ wt. **Oral/GI:** Sore throat, NAUSEA/VOMITING, STOMACH PAIN, DIARRHEA.
S/Cond: Avoid alcohol. Caution $\bar{c}$ lactation.
Other: Peripheral neuritis, ↑ BP, weakness, rash, bone marrow depression $\bar{c}$ LT use.
Blood/Serum: Dyscrasias, ↓ B_{12}, ↑ alk phos, ↑ SGOT, ↑ CPK, ↓ chol.
Urinary: False + RBC or Hgb.
Monitor: CBC $\bar{c}$ diff $\bar{c}$ LT use.

Combipres ANTIHYPERTENSIVE, DIURETIC See **chlorthalidone p 51 & clonidine p 57**

Compazine ANTIEMETIC, ANTIPSYCHOTIC See **prochlorperazine p 167**

Cordarone ANTIARRHYTHMIC See **amiodarone p 24**

Corgard ANTIHYPERTENSIVE, ANTIANGINAL, Beta-Blocker See **nadolol p 138**

Correctol LAXATIVE, STOOL SOFTENER See **phenolphthalein p 160 & docusate sodium p 76**
8 mg Na/Tab
sugar, wheat flour

corticosteroids ANTI-INFLAMMATORY, IMMUNOSUPPRESSANT, hormone
Oral or Parenteral (IM, IV, SC, intralesional, intra-articular)

Drug: Take c̄ food to ↓ GI effects. **Diet:** ↓ Na, ↑ pro.[7] May need ↑ K, ↑ Vits A, C, D, ↑ Ca, ↑ P, ↑ Pyr, ↑ Fol (or suppl).[1] **Oral/GI:** Esophagitis, N/V, dyspepsia, peptic ulcer, bloating, GI bleeding/perforation.
Nutr: ↑ APPETITE, ↑ WT, except c̄ triamcinolone— ANOREXIA.[13] Negative N balance & myopathy due to pro catabolism. Ca wasting—osteoporosis/necrosis c̄ LT use. ↑ Fol requirement.[13] **S/Cond:** Avoid alcohol. Not c̄ lactation. Caution c̄ diabetes — ↑ glucose. Highly pro bound. Hypoalbuminemia (< 3 g/dL) may ↑ drug effects.[6] **Other:** EDEMA, ↑ BP, insomnia, bruising, slow healing, weakness, dizziness, headache, masking of infection, convulsions, psychological disturbances, acne, rash. LT use— Cataracts, pancreatitis, Cushing's syndrome, osteoporosis, ↓ growth in children. **Blood/Serum:** ↑ Na, ↓ K, ↓ Ca, ↑ glucose, ↓ Zn,[12] ↓ uric acid, ↓ Vit C,[6] ↓ Vit A,[6] ↑ TG, ↑ chol, ↓ T_3, ↓T_4, ↓ TSH, ↑ Hgb,[4] ↑ RBC,[4] dyscrasias.
Urinary: ↓ Na, ↑ K, ↑ Ca, ↑ uric acid, ↑ glucose, ↑ N, ↑ Zn, ↑ Vit C.
Monitor: LT use— Electrolytes, glucose, BP, wt, children's growth.

cortisone
dexamethasone — Low mineralocorticoid effects — less Na retention, edema, K loss, or HTN.
  Decadron Tab— lactose, starch. Parenteral— Acetate— 9 mg benzyl alcohol & 1 mg Na bisulfite/mL. Phosphate— 1 mg Na bisulfite/mL. Elixir— 5% alcohol, saccharin.
  Hexadrol Elixir— 5% alcohol, sorbitol. Tab— lactose. Parenteral— Na sulfite.
hydrocortisone (cortisol)—Cortef Tab— lactose, sucrose; Susp— sucrose.
  Solu-Cortef Parenteral— benzyl alcohol.
methylprednisolone— Low mineralocorticoid effects— less Na retention, edema, K loss, or HTN.
  Depo-Medrol Parenteral— benzyl alcohol. **Medrol** Tab— lactose, sucrose, 24 mg Tab— tartrazine.
  Solu-Medrol Parenteral— benzyl alcohol.
prednisolone **prednisone— Deltasone** Tab— lactose, sucrose.
triamcinolone– Aristocort Tab– lactose. Parenteral– benzyl alcohol. **Kenalog**– Parenteral— benzyl alcohol.

corticotropin (ACTH) **Acthar**	HORMONE, ADRENOCORTICOTROPIC Parenteral only (IV, IM or SC) See listing for **corticosteroids above** Pituitary hormone which stimulates adrenal secretion of corticosteroids. Effects are those of corticosteroids.
cortisol	CORTICOSTEROID, Hydrocortisone See **corticosteroids above**
Cosmegen	ANTINEOPLASTIC See **dactinomycin p 65**
Cotrim	ANTIBIOTIC See **trimethoprim $\bar{c}$ sulfamethoxazole p 202**
Coumadin	ANTICOAGULANT See **warfarin sodium p 213**
Cozaar	ANTIHYPERTENSIVE, Angiotensin Receptor Antagonist See **losartan p 120**
cromolyn sodium **Gastrocrom** Oral cap **Intal** Aerosol spray Pwd for inhalation—lactose **Nasalcrom**	ANTIASTHMA, ANTIMASTOCYTOSIS (Oral form) Oral, Aerosol or Nebulizer **Drug:** Oral— Take 1/2 hr before meals— open caps & dissolve pwd in 4 oz hot H_2O. Add 4 oz cold H_2O. Not $\bar{c}$ juice, milk or food. **Oral/GI:** Unpleasant taste. Aerosol/nebulizer— Dry mouth/throat, sore throat. Oral cap— Nausea, abdominal pain, diarrhea. **S/Cond:** Caution $\bar{c}$ lactation. **Other:** Headache, joint pain, rash, insomnia. Aerosol/nebulizer—bronchospasm, ↓ pulmonary func, cough, nasal congestion, drowsiness.
Crystodigin	CARDIOTONIC See **digitoxin p 72**

Cuprimine — METAL CHELATING AGENT — See **penicillamine p 154**

cyanocobalamin — VITAMIN — See **vitamin B_{12} p 210**

cyclobenzaprine HCl
Flexeril
Tab— lactose, starch

MUSCLE RELAXANT

Oral/GI: DRY MOUTH, unpleasant taste, dyspepsia, nausea, constipation.
S/Cond: Avoid alcohol. Caution c̄ lactation. 93% serum pro bound. ↑ risk of dental problems, see p 9 & 14.
Other: DROWSINESS, dizziness, fatigue, blurred vision, headache, confusion, nervousness.

cyclophosphamide
Cytoxan
Tab— lactose, starch
Parenteral— mannitol

ANTINEOPLASTIC, Alkylating Agent — Oral or Parenteral (IV)

Drug: Take c̄ food only if GI distress.
Diet: ↑ fluid intake essential to cause frequent voiding.
Nutr: Anorexia, ↓ wt.
Oral/GI: Dry mouth, stomatitis, N/V, abdominal pain, diarrhea.
S/Cond: Not c̄ lactation. Do dental care cautiously, see p 10 & 14.
Other: BONE MARROW SUPPRESSION, delayed wound healing, weakness, headache, SIADH. Acute hemorrhagic cystitis (rare, can be fatal).
Blood/Serum: ↓ WBC, dyscrasias, anemia, ↑ uric acid, ↑ SGOT, ↑ SGPT, ↑ bil, ↑ LDH, ↑ BUN, ↑ crea.
Monitor: Hepatic & renal func, CBC c̄ diff, uric acid. Urine for RBC.

cyclosporine **Sandimmune** Oral Soln— 12.5 % alcohol, olive oil Cap— 12.7% alcohol, sorbitol	IMMUNOSUPPRESSANT — Oral or Parenteral (IV) **Drug:** Soln— mix c̄ 1 glass milk, chocolate milk or orange juice at room temp. Drink immediately. **Diet:** No K suppl or salt sub. Avoid grapefruit juice.[3] **Nutr:** Anorexia. **Oral/GI:** Gum hyperplasia, N/V, diarrhea. **S/Cond:** Not c̄ lactation. 90% serum pro bound. Do dental care cautiously. Caution c̄ diabetes— ↑ glucose. **Other:** NEPHROTOXICITY, TREMOR, HYPERTENSION, headache, confusion, flushing, sinusitis, edema, convulsions, infections. **Blood/Serum:** ↑ BUN, ↑ CREA, ↑ CHOL, ↑ SGPT, ↑ SGOT, ↑ alk phos, ↑ bil, ↑ GGT, ↑ K, ↓ Mg, ↓ bicarb, ↑ uric acid, ↑ glucose, anemia, ↓ WBC, ↑ amylase. **Monitor:** Renal & hepatic func, BP, CBC, Mg, K.
Cycrin	HORMONE, Progestin — See **medroxyprogesterone acetate p 124**
Cylert	STIMULANT, ANTI-ADHD — See **pemoline p 153**
cyproheptadine HCl **Periactin** Syrup — 5% alcohol, saccharin, sucrose Tab— lactose, starch	ANTIHISTAMINE, ANTIPRURITIC (also used as an appetite stimulant) **Drug:** Take c̄ food or milk. **Nutr:** ↑ APPETITE, ↑ WT. **Oral/GI:** Dry mouth, N/V, constipation, diarrhea. **S/Cond:** Avoid alcohol. Not c̄ lactation. ↑ risk of dental problems, see p 9 & 14. **Other:** DROWSINESS, SEDATION, dizziness, blurred vision, confusion, tremor, edema, ↓ BP, headache, rash.

cytarabine (ara-C)
Cytosar-U
benzyl alcohol

ANTINEOPLASTIC — Parenteral only (IV or SC)

Diet: ↑ fluid intake essential. **Nutr:** ANOREXIA, ↓ wt.
Oral/GI: STOMATITIS, esophagitis, NAUSEA/VOMITING, diarrhea, anal inflammation or ulceration. **S/Cond:** Not c̄ lactation. Do dental care cautiously, see p 10 & 14.
Other: BONE MARROW DEPRESSION, INFECTION, fatigue, dizziness, headache, fever, rash, renal toxicity.
Blood/Serum: DYSCRASIAS, ↓ WBC, anemia, ↑ uric acid, ↑ alk phos, ↑ SGOT, ↑ SGPT, ↑ bil, ↓ K, ↓ Ca. **Urinary:** ↑ uric acid.
Monitor: Daily leukocytes, platelets during induction. Bone aspiration q 2 wks. Renal & hepatic func, uric acid.

Cytotec — ANTIULCER — See **misoprostol p 134**

Cytovene — ANTIVIRAL — See **ganciclovir p 97**

Cytoxan — ANTINEOPLASTIC — See **cyclophosphamide p 62**

dacarbazine
DTIC-Dome
mannitol
citric acid

ANTINEOPLASTIC, Alkylating agent — Parenteral Only (IV)

Drug: Avoid food 4-6 hrs prior to IV to ↓ N/V. **Nutr:** ANOREXIA.
Oral/GI: Stomatitis, SEVERE NAUSEA/VOMITING, diarrhea.
S/Cond: Not c̄ lactation. **Other:** BONE MARROW SUPPRESSION, flu-like syndrome, facial numbness, photosensitivity.
Blood/Serum: Anemia. Rare ↑ alk phos, ↑ SGOT, ↑ SGPT, ↑ BUN.
Monitor: CBC, platelets.

dactinomycin
(actinomycin-D)
Cosmegen
20 mg mannitol/ vial

ANTINEOPLASTIC, Antibiotic — Parenteral Only (IV)

Diet: Insure adequate fluid intake. ↑ need for Vit B_{12} & high calorie snacks. **Nutr:** ↓ abs of Ca, Fe, fat.[11] ↓ effects of Vit K.[13] Anorexia, ↓ wt.
Oral/GI: Dry mouth, STOMATITIS, taste changes, glossitis, SEVERE ESOPHAGITIS, dysphagia, SEVERE NAUSEA/VOMITING, dyspepsia, pain, diarrhea.
S/Cond: Not c̄ lactation. Do dental care cautiously, see p 9 & 14.
Other: FATIGUE, BONE MARROW DEPRESSION, rash, ascites.
Blood/Serum: ↓ WHITE BLOOD CELLS, ↓ PLATELETS, ANEMIA, ↑ uric acid, ↓ Ca. Rare ↑ SGOT,↑ SGPT, ↑ LDH, ↑ bil. **Urinary:** ↑ uric acid.
Monitor: CBC c̄ diff, platelets, hepatic & renal func, uric acid.

Dalmane

HYPNOTIC, Benzodiazepine — See **flurazepam HCl p 93**

danazol
Danocrine
Cap— lactose, benzyl alcohol, starch

HORMONE, Androgen

Nutr: ↑ appetite, ↑ wt.
S/Cond: Not c̄ lactation. Caution c̄ diabetes— may ↑ glucose.
Other: EDEMA, MENSTRUAL DISTURBANCES, headache, ↑ BP, dizziness, fatigue, acne, visual changes, hepatic toxicity c̄ high dose > 2 mos.[4]
Blood/Serum: ↓ HDL, ↑ LDL, ↑ SGOT, ↑ SGPT, ↑ bil, ↑ CPK, ↑ glucose, ↑ HCT, ↓ T_3, ↓ T_4. (No effect on total chol or TG.)
Monitor: Hepatic func.

dapsone (DDS)
Dapsone

ANTIBACTERIAL, ANTILEPROTIC

Nutr: Anorexia. **Oral/GI:** N/V, abdominal pain. **S/Cond:** Not c̄ lactation. Caution c̄ G6PD deficiency — risk of hemolytic anemia. > 90% serum pro bound. Hypoalbuminemia (< 3.0 g/dL) may ↑ drug effects.
Other: Dizziness, blurred vision, headache, tachycardia, insomnia.
Blood/Serum: Dyscrasias, hemolytic anemia, ↓ Hgb, ↓ alb, methemoglobinemia, ↑ SGOT, ↑ SGPT, ↑ bil, ↑ glucose. Rare ↑ BUN, ↑ crea. **Urinary:** Alb, Pro.
Monitor: CBC q wk x 1 mo; q mo x 6 mos, then 2 x/ yr. Hepatic func.

Darvocet-N — ANALGESIC — See **propoxyphene HCl p 168 & acetaminophen p 17**

Darvon/ Darvon-N — ANALGESIC — See **propoxyphene HCl p 168**

Datril — ANALGESIC, ANTIPYRETIC — See **acetaminophen p 17**

daunorubicin HCl
Cerubidine

ANTINEOPLASTIC, ANTI-LEUKEMIA, Antibiotic Parenteral Only (IV)
100 mg mannitol/ vial — See listing for **doxorubicin p 78**

Daypro — NSAID — See **oxaprozin p149**

DDAVP — ANTIDIURETIC, ANTIHEMORRHAGIC — See **desmopressin acetate p 68**

DDC — ANTIVIRAL, ANTI-HIV — See **zalcitabine p 214**

ddI — ANTIVIRAL, ANTI-HIV — See **didanosine p 71**

Decadron CORTICOSTEROID, dexamethasone See **corticosteroids p 60**

Deltasone CORTICOSTEROID, prednisone See **corticosteroids p 60**

Demerol ANALGESIC, NARCOTIC See **meperidine HCl p 125**

Demulen CONTRACEPTIVE, oral See **estrogen p 83**
The last 7 days of the 28 day pack are placebos which contain sucrose.

Depakene/ Depakote ANTICONVULSANT See **valproic acid p 204**

Depen HEAVY METAL ANTAGONIST See **penicillamine p 154**

Depo-Medrol CORTICOSTEROID, methylprednisolone See **corticosteroids p 60**

Depo-Provera HORMONE, ANTINEOPLASTIC See **medroxyprogesterone acetate p 124**

desipramine HCl ANTIDEPRESSANT, Tricyclic See listing for **imipramine p 106**
Norpramin
Tab— sucrose, mannitol
The active metabolite of **imipramine**, **desipramine** is less sedating and has lower anticholinergic effects.

DES HORMONE See **diethylstilbestrol p 71**

desmopressin acetate
DDAVP

ANTIDIURETIC, Hormone, ANTIHEMORRHAGIC, ANTI-ENURESIS
Parenteral (IV or SC) or Nasal Spray

Diet: Drink only enough H_2O to satisfy thirst. **Oral/GI:** Nausea, GI distress, cramps. **S/Cond:** Caution c̄ alcohol— may ↓ antidiuretic effect. Caution c̄ lactation. **Other:** <u>Headache</u>, flushing, dizziness, chills, weakness, ↓ or ↑ BP, H_2O intoxication.
Blood/Serum: ↓ <u>Na</u>. **Monitor**: Electrolytes c̄ use > 7 days.

Desogen
Tab - lactose

ORAL CONTRACEPTIVE — See **estrogen p 83**

Desyrel

ANTIDEPRESSANT — See **trazodone HCl p 199**

dexamethasone

CORTICOSTEROID — See **corticosteroids p 60**

Dexatrim

APPETITE SUPPRESSANT — See **phenylpropanolamine p 160**

dextroamphetamine sulfate
Dexedrine
Tab— lactose, sucrose, tartrazine
Spansule — sucrose, starch, benzyl alcohol, tartrazine

STIMULANT, Amphetamine (Anti-narcolepsy, Anti-ADHD, Anorectic)

Drug: Take at least 6 hrs before bedtime. Swallow SR cap whole. As anorectic take 1/2-1 hr before meals. **Diet:** Limit caffeine. Vit C or acidic juice may ↓ abs of drug. Ca or Mg suppl may ↑ drug levels. **Nutr:** <u>Anorexia</u>, ↓ <u>wt</u>. **Oral/GI:** Dry mouth, metallic taste, N/V, GI distress, diarrhea, constipation. **S/Cond:** Avoid alcohol. Not c̄ lactation. May be habit forming c̄ LT use. **Other:** <u>Dizziness</u>, <u>tremor</u>, <u>headache</u>, <u>nervousness</u>, <u>confusion</u>, <u>insomnia</u>, ↑ <u>or</u> ↓ <u>BP</u>, <u>tachycardia</u>, ↓ growth in children. **Monitor**: Children's growth.

d4T ANTIVIRAL, ANTI-HIV See **stavudine p 187**

DiaBeta ORAL HYPOGLYCEMIC See **glyburide p 99**

Diabinese ORAL HYPOGLYCEMIC See **chlorpropamide p 50**

Dialose STOOL SOFTENER, LAXATIVE See **docusate sodium p 76**

Dialume ANTACID, PHOSPHATE BINDER See **aluminum hydroxide p 22**

Diamox DIURETIC, ANTIGLAUCOMA See **acetazolamide p 18**

diazepam
Valium
Intensol— 19% alcohol
Parenteral—
ethyl & benzyl alcohols

ANTIANXIETY, MUSCLE RELAXANT, Benzodiazepine — Oral or Parenteral (IM or IV)

Drug: May take c̄ food. Swallow SR cap whole. Mix conc c̄ H20, juice, carbonated beverage or semi-solid food. **Diet:** Limit caffeine to < 500 mg/day, see p 240. **Oral GI:** Dry mouth, ↑ salivation, nausea, constipation. **S/Cond:** Avoid alcohol. Not c̄ lactation. May be habit forming c̄ LT use > 4 wks.[7] 98% serum pro bound. Hypoalbuminemia (< 3 g/dL) may ↑ drug effects.

Other: Drowsiness, ataxia, fatigue, dizziness, tremor,blurred vision. Rare rash, jaundice, EPS.

Blood/Serum: ↓ T_4,[7] ↑ SGOT, ↑ SGPT, ↑ LDH, ↑ bil. Rare dyscrasias.

Monitor: CBC c̄ diff & hepatic func c̄ use > 4 wks.

diclofenac sodium **Voltaren** Tab— lactose Enteric-coated for delayed release	NSAID, ANALGESIC, ANTIARTHRITIC **Drug:** Take c̄ food, milk or 8 oz H_2O to ↓ GI irritation. Food delays rate, but not extent of abs. Swallow whole. Do not crush or chew. **Diet:** Caution c̄ GI irritants eg K suppl (↑ risk of GI irritation). **Oral/GI:** Nausea, dyspepsia, GI ulcers & bleeding (may be sudden & serious), abdominal pain, constipation, diarrhea, flatulence. **S/Cond:** Avoid alcohol. Not c̄ lactation. 99% serum pro bound. **Other:** Headache, edema, dizziness, rash, arrhythmia. Rare jaundice, hepatitis. **Blood/Serum:** ↑ SGOT, ↑ SGPT. Rare↑ BUN, ↑ crea. **Monitor:** Hepatic & renal func c̄ LT use.
dicloxacillin sodium 12 mg Na/ 250 mg **Dynapen**	ANTIBIOTIC, penicillin **Drug:** Take c̄ 8 oz H_2O 1 hr before or 2 hrs after food. **Oral/GI:** N/V, diarrhea, flatulence, Rare pseudomembranous colitis. **S/Cond:** Caution c̄ lactation. 98% serum pro bound. **Other:** Rash, fever. **Blood/Serum:** EOSINOPHILIA, ↑ alk phos, ↑ SGOT, ↑ SGPT. Rare dyscrasias. **Monitor:** CBC c̄ diff. Hepatic func.
dicyclomine HCl **Bentyl** Cap, Tab— lactose Syrup— glucose, saccharin	ANTISPASMODIC, ANTICHOLINERGIC Oral or Parenteral (IM) **Drug:** Take 30 min to 1 hr before food. **Oral/GI:** DRY MOUTH/THROAT, ↓ taste acuity, nausea, constipation. **S/Cond:** Limit alcohol. Not c̄ lactation. ↑ risk of dental problems, see p 9 & 14. Syrup precipitates tube feeding.[8] **Other:** DIZZINESS, BLURRED VISION, drowsiness, weakness, headache, nervousness, tachycardia, ↑ heat sensitivity. **Urinary:** Retention.

didanosine (ddI)
Videx
Tab— sugar, aspartame = 23-34 mg phenylalanine/ tab, 264.5 mg Na/ tab
Pwd— 1380 mg Na /pkt, sucrose

ANTIVIRAL, ANTI-HIV

Drug: Take on empty stomach (food ↓ abs by 50%). Do not swallow tab whole. Chew or crush & mix c̄ > 1 oz H_2O. Do not mix c̄ acidic liquid.
Diet: Caution c̄ ↓ Na diet. **Nutr:** ANOREXIA, ↓ wt. **Oral/GI:** Dry mouth, stomatitis, ↓ taste acuity, dyspepsia, NAUSEA/VOMITING, PAIN, DIARRHEA, constipation, flatulence. **S/Cond:** Avoid alcohol. Not c̄ lactation.
Other: Pancreatitis (may be fatal), PERIPHERAL NEUROPATHY, HEADACHE, WEAKNESS, INSOMNIA, RASH, arthritis, pain, dizziness, congestion, chills/ fever, blurred vision, cough, confusion, anxiety, edema, ↑ BP, seizures.
Blood/Serum: DYSCRASIAS, anemia, ↑ SGOT, ↑ SGPT, ↑ alk phos, ↑ bil, ↑ uric acid, ↑ amylase, ↑ lipase, ↓ K,[13] ↑ TG, ↑ CPK.
Monitor: Amylase, lipase, uric acid, K, TG.

Didronel

Ca REGULATOR, ANTIBONE RESORPTION See **etidronate disodium p 85**

diethylstilbestrol (DES)
Diethylstilbestrol
Tab— lactose
diethylstilbestrol diphosphate
Stilphostrol
Tab— lactose

ANTINEOPLASTIC, Hormone, Estrogen

Oral or Parenteral (IV— diphosphate)

Drug: Take c̄ food to ↓ nausea. Enseals— do not break, crush or chew.
Diet: Encourage ↓ Na. Caution c̄ Ca suppl. **Nutr:** Anorexia, ↑ or ↓ wt, ↑ Ca abs. **Oral/GI:** N/V, abdominal cramps, bloating, diarrhea.
S/Cond: Not c̄ lactation. Caution c̄ diabetes— ↓ CHO tolerance.
Other: Edema, dizziness, depression, headache.
Blood/Serum: ↑ Ca (may be severe), ↑ glucose, ↓ Fol, ↑ TG, ↑ Na, ↑ PT.

Diflucan

ANTIFUNGAL See **fluconazole p 91**

diflunisal **Dolobid** Tab— starch	NSAID, ANALGESIC, ANTIARTHRITIC **Drug:** Take c̄ food or milk to ↓ GI irritation. Swallow tab whole. Do not crush or chew. **Diet:** Caution c̄ GI irritants eg K suppl (↑ risk of GI irritation).[13] **Oral/GI:** Dry or sore mouth, <u>N</u>/V, GI ulcers & bleeding (may be sudden & serious), <u>GI pain</u>, <u>diarrhea</u>, constipation, flatulence **S/Cond:** Avoid alcohol. Not c̄ lactation. 98% serum pro bound. **Other:** <u>Headache</u>, <u>rash</u>, fatigue, insomnia, dizziness. Rare jaundice, hepatitis, renal toxicity. **Blood/Serum:** ↑ <u>SGOT</u>, ↑ <u>SGPT</u>, ↓ <u>uric acid</u>, ↑ K. <1% dyscrasias. **Urinary:** ↑ <u>uric acid</u>, pro. **Monitor:** Hepatic & renal func c̄ LT use.
Di-Gel	ANTACID See **aluminum hydroxide** & **magnesium hydroxide p 23**
digitalis **digitoxin** **Crystodigin** Tab— lactose **Digitoxin** **digoxin** **Digoxin** **Lanoxin** Tab— lactose Elixir— sucrose, 10% alcohol IV— 10% alcohol	CARDIOTONIC, ANTIARRHYTHMIC Inotropic agent Oral or Parenteral (IV) **Drug:** Take separately from high bran fiber or high pectin foods.[10] **Diet:** Maintain diet ↑ K, ↓ Na & adequate Mg & Ca. Avoid natural licorice.[14] Mg suppl may ↓ abs of drug.[3] Caution c̄ Ca &/or Vit D suppl. **Nutr:** <u>Anorexia</u>, ↓ <u>wt</u>. Ca & Vit D induced hypercalcemia may ↑ drug effects. **Oral/GI:** <u>N/V</u>, <u>diarrhea</u>. **S/Cond:** Caution c̄ lactation. Caution c̄ some herbal products, see p 244. Caution- Hypokalemia, hypomagnesemia & hypercalcemia ↑ drug toxicity. Hypocalcemia ↓ drug effects. Digitoxin is 97% serum pro bound. Hypoalbuminemia (<3.0 g/dL) may ↑ digitoxin effects **Other:** Drowsiness, blurred (yellow) vision, confusion, depression,weakness,headache. **Blood/Serum:** ↑ or ↓ K, ↓ Zn, ↓ Mg.[11b] Rare eosinophilia. **Urinary:** ↑ Zn.[11b] **Monitor:** Electrolytes especially K, Ca, Mg. Renal func.

dihydrotachysterol
Hytakerol
VITAMIN D — See listing for **calcitriol p 39**
S/Cond: Caution c̄ lactation.[10]

Dilacor XR
ANTIANGINAL, ANTIHYPERTENSIVE — See **diltiazem below**

Dilantin
ANTICONVULSANT — See **phenytoin p 161**

Dilaudid
ANALGESIC — See **hydromorphone HCl p 103**

diltiazem HCl
Cardizem
Tab— lactose
Cardizem SR & CD
Cap— sucrose
Dilacor XR (SR)

ANTIANGINA, ANTIHYPERTENSIVE, Ca Channel Blocker
Drug: Take tab or XR form before meals. Swallow SR, CD or XR cap whole— do not crush, break or chew. **Diet:** ↓ Na, ↓ cal may be needed. Avoid natural licorice. **Nutr:** Anorexia. **Oral/GI:** Dry mouth, dyspepsia, N/V, constipation, diarrhea. **S/Cond:** Not c̄ lactation.
Other: ↓ BP, edema, dizziness, headache, drowsiness, weakness, flushing, insomnia, rash. **Blood/Serum:** < 1% ↑ alk phos, ↑ SGOT, ↑ SGPT, ↑ LDH, ↑ CPK. **Monitor:** BP.

dimenhydrinate
Dramamine
Liquid — sucrose
Chewable Tab—
aspartame—
(1.5 mg phenylalanine)
tartrazine, sorbitol
Parenteral— benzyl alcohol

ANTIVERTIGO, ANTIEMETIC — Oral or Parenteral (IM or IV)
Drug: Take c̄ food or H_2O.
Oral/GI: Dry mouth, nausea, epigastric distress.
S/Cond: Avoid alcohol. Not c̄ lactation.
Other: DROWSINESS, dizziness, ataxia, confusion (especially in elderly), blurred vision, headache, palpitations, ↓ BP.
Urinary: Retention.

Dimetane — ANTIHISTAMINE — See **brompheniramine maleate p 36**

Dimetapp — ANTIHISTAMINE, DECONGESTANT — See **brompheniramine maleate p 36 & phenylpropanolamine p 160**
Cap— Mannitol, sorbitol
Elixir— saccharin, sorbitol
Elixir precipitates tube feedings.[8]

Dipentum
olsalazine sodium — ANTI-INFLAMMATORY — See listing for **mesalamine p 126**

diphenhydramine HCl — ANTIHISTAMINE, SLEEP AID — Oral or Parenteral (IM or IV)
Benadryl
Elixir— 5% alcohol, sucrose
Cap— lactose
Nytol

Drug: May take c̄ food to ↓ GI distress. **Nutr:** Anorexia.
Oral/GI: Dry mouth/throat, N/V, epigastric distress, constipation.
S/Cond: Avoid alcohol. Not c̄ lactation. 98% serum pro bound.[13]
Other: DROWSINESS, SEDATION, dizziness, blurred vision, excitability in children, ataxia, confusion, tachycardia.
Blood/Serum: Hemolytic anemia, dyscrasias **Urinary:** Retention.

dipyridamole — PLATELET AGGREGATION INHIBITOR — Oral or Parenteral (IV)
Persantine
Tab— lactose, sucrose

Drug: Take c̄ 8 oz H_2O on empty stomach for faster abs. May take c̄ food or milk to ↓ GI distress. **Oral/GI:** GI distress, N/V, cramps, diarrhea.
S/Cond: Caution c̄ lactation. > 90% serum pro bound.
Other: Dizziness, headache, weakness, flushing, rash.

Disalcid — NSAID — See **salsalate p 179**

disopyramide phosphate
Norpace
Cap— lactose
Norpace-CR
Cap— sucrose

ANTIARRHYTHMIC

Drug: Swallow CR cap whole. **Nutr:** Anorexia. **Oral/GI:** DRY MOUTH/THROAT, oral candidiasis, N/V, GI pain, flatulence, constipation, diarrhea. **S/Cond:** Avoid alcohol. Not c̄ lactation. ↑ risk of dental problems, see p 9 & 14. Hypokalemia— ↓ drug effects. Hyperkalemia— ↑ toxicity.[10] Caution c̄ diabetes— ↓ glucose (rare).
Other: Blurred vision, headache, dizziness, weakness, fatigue, edema, rash, ↓ BP, ↑ heat sensitivity.
Blood/Serum: ↑ chol, ↑ TG, ↓ K, ↓ glucose.
< 1% ↑ SGOT, ↑ SGPT, ↑ BUN, ↑ crea, anemia, dyscrasias.
Urinary: Retention. **Monitor:** K, glucose, hepatic & renal func.

disulfiram
Antabuse
Tab— starch

ALCOHOL ABUSE DETERRENT

Drug: Tab may be crushed & mixed c̄ beverages. **Diet:** Limit caffeine— drug may ↑ caffeine effects, see p 240. No alcohol-containing products— sauces, vinegars, juice or cider, extracts, soups or baked goods c̄ alcohol.
Oral/GI: Transient garlic or metallic taste, dyspepsia.
S/Cond: AVOID ALL ALCOHOL, cough syrups, elixirs. Caution c̄ diabetes.
Other: Peripheral neuropathy. Transient drowsiness, headache, fatigue. Rare hepatitis, rash, psychotic reaction.
Blood/Serum: ↑ chol[13] (dose-related). Rare ↑ SGOT, ↑ SGPT, dyscrasias.
Monitor: SGOT & SGPT, again in 10-14 days. CBC & SMA-12 q 6 mos.

Ditropan

PARASYMPATHOLYTIC See **oxybutynin chloride p 150**

Diuril ANTIHYPERTENSIVE See **chlorothiazide p 49**

DNase ANTI-CYSTIC FIBROSIS See **dornase alfa p 77**

docusate calcium STOOL SOFTENER, LAXATIVE See listing for **docusate sodium below**
Surfak
Sorbitol, 3% alcohol, corn oil, Na free

docusate sodium STOOL SOFTENER, LAXATIVE
Colace
Syrup — 3 g sucrose /5 mL,[29] alcohol (< 1%)
Cap— 2.5 mg Na/50 mg
Dialose Tab— starch

Drug: Mix liquid c̄ milk or juice to mask bitter taste. Take c̄ full glass liquid.
Diet: High fiber c̄ 1500-2000 mL fluid/day to prevent constipation.
Nutr: Alters intestinal abs of H_2O & electrolytes. **Oral/GI:** BITTER TASTE, throat irritation & nausea (liquid forms), cramps, diarrhea.
Blood/Serum: ↑ glucose, ↓ K (LT use).

Dolobid NSAID See **diflunisal p 72**

Dolophine NARCOTIC, ANALGESIC See **methadone HCl p 127**

Donnagel ANTIDIARRHEAL See **attapulgite p 30**

Dopar ANTIPARKINSON See **levodopa p 116**

Doral SLEEP AID, Benzodiazepine See **quazepam p 172**

dornase alfa (DNase) **Pulmozyme** preservative free	ANTI-CYSTIC FIBROSIS, respiratory inhalant **Oral/GI:** Sore throat, laryngitis. **S/Cond**: Caution with lactation. **Other:** Chest pain, mild & transient rash.
doxazosin mesylate **Cardura** Tab— lactose	ANTIHYPERTENSIVE, $Alpha_1$-Adrenergic Blocker **Diet:** ↓ Na, ↓ cal may be recommended. Avoid natural licorice. **Nutr:** ↑ wt. **S/Cond:** Caution c̄ alcohol. Caution c̄ lactation. 98% serum pro bound. **Other:** DROWSINESS, dizziness, fatigue, ↓ BP, edema, arrhythmias, ataxia. **Blood/Serum:** Slightly— ↓ chol, ↓ LDL, ↓ TG, ↑ HDL, ↓ WBC. **Monitor:** BP.
doxepin HCl **Sinequan** Cap— starch Conc— peppermint oil **Zonalan Cream** (topical)	ANTIDEPRESSANT, ANTIANXIETY, Cream— ANTIPRURITIC, Tricyclic **Drug:** May take c̄ food to ↓ GI distress. Oral conc— Dilute in 4 oz H_2O, milk or juice. Incompatible c̄ carbonated beverages or grape juice.[13] **Diet:** Limit caffeine, see p 240. ↑ fiber may ↓ drug effect.[3] **Nutr:** ↑ APPETITE for sweets, ↑ WT, ↑ thirst. **Oral/GI:** DRY MOUTH, metallic/sour taste, nausea, epigastric distress, constipation. **S/Cond:** Avoid alcohol. Not c̄ lactation. ↑ risk of dental problems, see p 9 & 14. **Other:** DROWSINESS, DIZZINESS, blurred vision, fine tremor, fatigue, confusion, headache. Rare SIADH. **Blood/Serum:** ↑ or ↓ glucose, ↑ SGOT, ↑ SGPT, ↑ alk phos. Rare dyscrasias. **Urinary**: Retention. **Monitor:** BP, CBC, hepatic func.

doxorubicin
Adriamycin

ANTINEOPLASTIC, Antibiotic — Parenteral only (IV)

Diet: Insure adequate fluid intake. **Nutr:** Anorexia, ↓ wt.
Oral/GI: Dry mouth, stomatitis, ESOPHAGITIS, ACUTE NAUSEA/VOMITING, GI ulceration, diarrhea. **S/Cond:** Not c̄ lactation.
Do dental care cautiously, see p 9, 10 & 14.
Other: BONE MARROW DEPRESSION, cardiotoxicity, fever.
Blood/Serum: ↓ WBC, ↓ platelets, anemia, ↑ uric acid, ↑ alk phos, ↑ SGOT, ↑ SGPT, ↑ bil. **Urinary:** ↑ uric acid, red color.
Monitor: CBC c̄ diff, hepatic, renal & cardiac func, uric acid.

doxycycline
Vibramycin
Syrup- 7 g sorbitol/dose
Na metabisulfite

ANTIBIOTIC, Tetracycline — Oral or Parenteral (IV)

Drug: Take c̄ food or 8 oz milk 1 hr before bed to ↓ esophageal & GI irritation. Swallow enteric-coated tab whole. **Diet:** Take Ca, Fe, Mg, Zn or MVI + minerals suppls separately by 2-4 hrs (may chelate c̄ drug & ↓ abs of both drug & mineral). **Nutr:** Possible ↓ Vit K due to ↓ bacterial synthesis in intestine.[11] **Oral/GI:** Glossitis, oral candidiasis, dysphagia, N/V, GI distress, diarrhea. Rare pseudomembranous colitis.
S/Cond: Avoid alcohol c̄ IV.[26] Not c̄ lactation. 93% serum pro bound.
Other: PHOTOSENSITIVITY, dizziness, rash. **Blood/Serum:** Dyscrasias, hemolytic anemia c̄ LT use, ↑ PT, ↑ bil, ↑ SGOT, ↑ SGPT, ↑ alk phos.

Dramamine

ANTIVERTIGO, ANTIEMETIC — See **dimenhydrinate p 73**

dronabinol
Marinol
Cap— sesame oil

ANTIEMETIC, APPETITE STIMULANT, marijuana derivative

Drug: Take BID before lunch & dinner. **Nutr:** ↑ APPETITE, ↑ WT.
Oral/GI: Dry mouth, N/V, diarrhea. **S/Cond:** Avoid alcohol.

Not $\bar{c}$ lactation. 97% serum pro bound. May be habit forming $\bar{c}$ LT use. **Other:** EUPHORIA, drowsiness, dizziness, tachycardia, ataxia, headache, hallucinations, mood changes, confusion.

DTIC-Dome — ANTINEOPLASTIC, Alkylating Agent — See **dacarbazine p 64**

Dulcolax — LAXATIVE — See **bisacodyl p 34**

Duragesic patch — ANALGESIC — See **fentanyl patch p 88**

Duricef — ANTIBIOTIC — See **cefadroxil p 44**

Duvoid — CHOLINERGIC STIMULANT — See **bethanechol p 34**

Dyazide — DIURETIC — See **triamterene p 200 & hydrochlorothiazide p 102**

DynaCirc — ANTIHYPERTENSIVE, Ca Channel Blocker — See **isradipine p 111**

Dynapen — ANTIBIOTIC — See **dicloxacillin sodium p 70**

Ecotrin enteric-coated aspirin — ANALGESIC, ANTIARTHRITIC — See **acetylsalicylic acid p 18**
Drug: Swallow whole. Drug has very low sodium content.

Edecrin — DIURETIC, loop — See listing for **furosemide p 96**
Tab- lactose, starch
IV- 63 mg mannitol/vial

EES — ANTIBIOTIC — See **erythromycin p 82**

Effexor — ANTIDEPRESSANT — See **venlafaxine p 205**

Elavil — ANTIDEPRESSANT, Tricyclic — See **amitriptyline HCl p 25**

Eldepryl — ANTIPARKINSON — See **selegiline p 180**

Elixophyllin — BRONCHODILATOR — See **theophylline p 194**

E-Mycin — ANTIBIOTIC — See **erythromycin p 82**

enalapril maleate
Vasotec
Tab— lactose, starch
IV— 9 mg/mL benzyl alcohol

ANTIHYPERTENSIVE, ACE Inhibitor — Oral or Parenteral (IV)

Drug: Take s̄ regard to food. **Diet:** ↓ Na, ↓ cal may be recommended. Avoid salt subs. Caution c̄ K suppl. Avoid natural licorice.
Oral/GI: Stomatitis, N/V, abdominal pain, diarrhea.
S/Cond: Limit alcohol. Caution c̄ lactation. Caution c̄ diabetes— ↓ glucose.[9b] Caution c̄ G6PD def— risk of hemolytic anemia.
Other: <u>COUGH</u>, <u>dizziness</u>, headache, weakness, rash.
Blood/Serum: ↑ K, ↓ Na, ↓ Hgb, ↓ HCT. Transient ↑ <u>BUN</u>, ↑ <u>crea</u>. Rare dyscrasias. **Monitor:** BP, K, renal func.

Entex LA
phenylpropanolamine HCl & guaifenesin

DECONGESTANT, EXPECTORANT

Drug: Drink 8 oz H_2O after each dose. Swallow LA form whole.
Diet: Avoid caffeine.[9b] **Nutr:** Anorexia. **Oral/GI:** Dry mouth, GI distress,

Entex, cap/ liquid
phenylpropanolamine HCl
phenylephrine HCl
guaifenesin

nausea. **S/Cond:** Caution c̄ lactation. Caution c̄ diabetes— possible ↑ glucose. Precipitates tube feedings.[8]
Other: ↑ BP, headache, nervousness, insomnia, dizziness.
Urinary: False + VMA.[1]
Liquid— 5 % alcohol, saccharin, sorbitol, sucrose. Tab— sugar.

epoetin alfa
Epogen

RECOMBINANT HUMAN ERYTHROPOIETIN, ANTIANEMIC

Parenteral only (IV or SC)

Diet: May need Fe, Vit B_{12} or Fol suppl. ESRD— Diet compliance mandatory.
S/Cond: Caution c̄ lactation.
Oral/GI: N/V, diarrhea.
Other: ↑ BLOOD PRESSURE, bone or muscle pain, fever, headache, cough.
Blood/Serum: ↑ RBC, ↑ HEMOGLOBIN, ↑ HEMATOCRIT, ↑ Ca, ↓ Fe, ↓ ferritin.
Monitor: Prior to use— Fe studies, B_{12}, Fol. Adequate levels essential c̄ use— BP, CBC c̄ diff, platelets, Fe studies, renal func, uric acid, K.

ergocalciferol VITAMIN See **vitamin D p 211**

Equanil ANTIANXIETY See **meprobamate p 125**

ergotamine tartrate & caffeine ANTIMIGRAINE Oral or Rectal (suppositories)

Cafergot
Tab— lactose, starch, sorbitol, sucrose
100 mg caffeine/tab

Diet: Limit caffeine, see p 240. **Nutr**: Excessive thirst.
Oral/GI: N/V, dyspepsia, abdominal pain, diarrhea.
S/Cond: Avoid alcohol. Not c̄ lactation. Limit smoking. Caution c̄ diabetes— ↑ glucose. Ergotamine is > 93% serum pro bound.
Other: Dizziness, weakness, localized edema, ↑ or ↓ BP, insomnia, muscle pain, cyanosis, numbness of extremities.

erythromycin ANTIBIOTIC, Macrolide Oral or Parenteral (IV)

Drug: Optimal— Take with full glass H_2O on empty stomach 2 hrs before or after meal. May take c̄ food to ↓ GI distress. Food ↓ abs of base & stearate forms. Swallow enteric-coated tab whole. Chew chewable tab well.
Nutr: Anorexia. **Oral/GI:** Oral candidiasis,[13] epigastric distress, N/V, ABDOMINAL CRAMPS, diarrhea. Rare pseudomembranous colitis. **S/Cond:** Caution c̄ lactation. Estolate form is 96% serum pro bound.
Other: Cholestatic hepatitis (↑ c̄ estolate form), rash. **Blood/Serum:** ↑ alk phos, ↑ bil, ↑ SGOT, ↑ SGPT, eosinophilia. **Monitor:** Hepatic func c̄ high dose, LT use or estolate form.

EES— (ethylsuccinate)— sucrose
E-Mycin— (base)— lactose, sucrose
ERYC— (base)— lactose
Ery-Tab (base)
Erythrocin Stearate (stearate)
Ilosone (estolate) Susp— sucrose
Ilotycin (gluceptate)— IV only
PCE (base)— lactose (333 mg Tab)

Eskalith ANTIMANIC See **lithium carbonate p 118**

Estrace HORMONE See **estrogen next page**

estrogen preparations HORMONE, ORAL CONTRACEPTIVE (OC)

Oral, Parenteral, Skin patch, Cream

Drug: Take c̄ food at same time each day. **Diet:** ↑ food high in Fol, Pyr & Vit B_{12} (OC). Vit C suppl > 1 g/day ↑ estrogen serum levels & possible ↑ toxicity.[9] Limit caffeine (OC), see p 240.
Nutr: ↑ or ↓ wt, appetite changes. ↓ Ca bone loss. ↑ Ca abs. **Oral/GI:** N/V, bloating, cramps, diarrhea.
S/Cond: Limit alcohol (OC).[9b] Not c̄ lactation. Caution c̄ diabetes (OC).
Other: Edema, ↑ BP (OC), dizziness, weakness, headache, rash, jaundice, double vision, gallbladder disease, thromboembolism.
Blood/Serum: ↑ glucose, ↑ TG, ↑ Vit A, ↑ Vit E, ↓ Vit C, ↑ transferrin, ↑ TIBC, ↑ Fe, ↑ ceruloplasmin, ↑ Cu, ↓ Mg, ↓ Zn, ↑ Ca, ↑ T_4, ↑ T_3, ↑ alk phos, ↑ bil, ↑ GGT.
Hormone —- ↓ chol, ↑ HDL, ↓ LDL, ↓ VLDL, ↑ TG.
OC—- ↓ Fol, ↓ Pyr, ↓ B_{12}, altered lipids (OC effect on lipids depends on relative doses of estrogen vs. progestin.)[1]

(Side effects vary depending upon dose, but are common to all estrogen preparations.)

Hormone Replacements
Estrace— lactose, tartrazine in 2 mg Tab
Ogen— lactose
Premarin— lactose, sucrose
Estraderm— transdermal patch
Prempro— lactose
Premphase— lactose

Oral Contraceptives (OC) (estrogen—progestin combinations)
Demulen— sucrose
Desogen— lactose
Loestrin— lactose, sugar, starch
Lo/Ovral— lactose
Nordette— lactose
Norinyl—- lactose, starch
Ortho-Cept— lactose
Ortho-Cyclen— lactose
Ortho-Novum— lactose, starch
Tri-Levlen— lactose
Tri-Norinyl— lactose, starch
Triphasil— lactose

ethacrynic acid
Edecrin

DIURETIC, Loop   Oral or Parenteral (IV)   See listing for **furosemide p 96**
Tab— lactose, starch   IV— mannitol 63 mg/ vial

ethambutol HCl
Myambutol
Tab— sucrose, sorbitol

ANTITUBERCULOSIS
Drug: Take c̄ food to ↓ GI distress. **Nutr:** Anorexia.
Oral/GI: Abdominal pain, N/V, GI distress. **S/Cond:** Caution c̄ lactation.
Other: Optic neuritis, ↓ visual acuity, blurred vision, headache, dizziness, confusion. Rare gout.
Blood/Serum: ↑ URIC ACID.
Urinary: ↓ uric acid.
Monitor: Uric acid, ophthalmologic exams.

ethionamide
Trecator-SC
Tab— lactose, sugar, sucrose

ANTITUBERCULOSIS
Drug: May take c̄ meals to ↓ GI distress. **Diet:** Pyr suppl required, 50-100 mg daily to prevent peripheral neuritis. **Nutr:** ANOREXIA, ↓ wt. **Oral/GI:** Metallic taste, stomatitis, drooling (↑ saliva), NAUSEA/VOMITING, stomach pain, diarrhea. **S/Cond:** Caution c̄ diabetes—management more difficult, ↓ glucose. **Other:** Dizziness, drowsiness, weakness, depression, confusion, hepatitis, jaundice, blurred vision.
Blood/Serum: ↑ SGOT, ↑ SGPT, ↑ bil, ↓ platelets, ↓ T_4.
Urinary: ↑ pyr.[1] **Monitor:** Hepatic func.

ethosuximide
Zarontin
Cap— sorbitol
Syrup — sucrose, saccharin

ANTICONVULSANT

Drug: Take c̄ milk or food. **Nutr:** Anorexia, ↓ wt.
Oral/GI: Gum hypertrophy, swollen tongue, hiccups, N/V, epigastric pain, cramps, diarrhea.
S/Cond: Avoid alcohol.
Other: Drowsiness, dizziness, headache, fatigue, ataxia, lupus, aggressiveness, depression.
Blood/Serum: Dyscrasias, rare aplastic anemia.
Monitor: CBC c̄ diff & platelets. Hepatic & renal func c̄ LT use.[13]

etidronate disodium
Didronel
Tab— starch

Ca REGULATOR, ANTIHYPERCALCEMIC, ANTIBONE RESORPTION, Bisphosphonate — Oral or Parenteral (IV)

Drug: Take c̄ H_2O or fruit juice 2 hrs before or after food. Maintain well balanced diet c̄ adequate intake of Ca & Vit D. Avoid foods high in Ca or suppls c̄ Ca, Fe or Mg within 2 hrs of drug (↓ abs of drug).
Oral/GI: Metallic or altered taste, stomatitis, nausea, diarrhea.
Other: ↓ BONE RESORPTION & FORMATION, bone/joint pain (Pagets), fever, fluid overload, osteomalacia.
S/Cond: Caution c̄ lactation.
Blood/Serum: ↓ CALCIUM, ↓ or ↑ PHOSPHATE, ↓ K, ↓ Mg, ↓ alk phos, ↑ crea, ↑ BUN. **Urinary:** ↓ hydroxyproline.
Monitor: Ca, renal func.

See "Guide to the Use of This Book" inside front cover.

etodolac
Lodine
Cap— lactose
Tab— lactose

NSAID, ANALGESIC, ANTIARTHRITIC

Drug: Take c̄ food or milk to ↓ GI irritation. **Diet:** Caution c̄ GI irritants eg K suppl (↑ risk of GI irritation). **Oral/GI:** Dyspepsia, N/V, GI ulcer & bleeding (may be sudden & serious), abdominal pain, diarrhea, flatulence, constipation. **S/Cond:** Avoid alcohol. Caution c̄ lactation. 99% serum pro bound.

Other: Dizziness, weakness, blurred vision, headache, rash. Rare jaundice, hepatitis. **Blood/Serum:** Anemia, ↑ SGOT, ↑ SGPT, ↓ uric acid, ↑ crea. Rare dyscrasias. **Urinary:** False + bil, false + ketones (dipstick). **Monitor:** Hepatic & renal func c̄ LT use.

etoposide
VePesid (VP-16)
Cap— sorbitol
IV— 30 mg benzyl alcohol/mL, 30.5% alcohol

ANTINEOPLASTIC — Oral or Parenteral (IV)

Nutr: Anorexia. **Oral/GI:** Stomatitis, dysphagia, NAUSEA/VOMITING, abdominal pain, diarrhea. **S/Cond:** Not c̄ lactation. Do dental care cautiously, see p 10 & 14. 94% serum pro bound. **Other:** BONE MARROW SUPPRESSION, drowsiness, fatigue, peripheral neuropathy, ↑ infection.

Blood/Serum: ↓ PLATELETS, ↓ WHITE BLOOD CELLS, anemia. Transient ↑ bil, ↑ SGOT, ↑ alk phos.[6] **Monitor:** CBC c̄ diff, platelets 2x/ week.[6]

Ex-lax — LAXATIVE — See **phenolphthalein p 160**

famciclovir
Famvir
Tab— lactose

ANTIVIRAL (Herpes Zoster/ Shingles)
Drug: Take s̄ regard to food. **Oral/GI:** N/V, diarrhea.
Other: Headache, paresthesia, fatigue.

Famotidine
Pepcid
Tab—- starch
Susp— sucrose
Pepcid IV—
20 mg mannitol/ mL

ANTISECRETORY, ANTIULCER, ANTIGERD, Histamine H_2 Antagonist
Oral or Parenteral (IV)
Drug: Take s̄ regard to meals, HS if once a day. **Diet:** May need bland diet. Limit caffeine/xanthine, see p 240. **Oral/GI:** ↓ GASTRIC ACID SECRETION, ↑ GASTRIC pH, diarrhea, constipation. **S/Cond:** Avoid alcohol. Not c̄ lactation. Avoid or limit smoking. **Other:** Headache, dizziness. **Blood/Serum:** <1% dyscrasias, ↑ BUN, ↑ crea, ↑ SGOT, ↑ SGPT, ↑ bil, ↑ alk phos.

Famvir ANTIVIRAL See **famciclovir above**

Fastin APPETITE SUPPRESSANT See **phentermine HCl p 160**

Feldene NSAID See **piroxicam p 163**

felodipine
Plendil (SR)
Tab— lactose

ANTIHYPERTENSIVE, Ca Channel Blocker
Drug: Take s̄ regard to food. Swallow whole. Do not crush or chew.
Diet: ↓ Na, ↓ cal may be recommended. Not c̄ grapefruit juice.[50] Avoid natural licorice. **Oral/GI:** Mild gingival hyperplasia.
S/Cond: Not c̄ lactation. 99% serum pro bound. **Other:** ↓ BP, PERIPHERAL EDEMA, headache, flushing, cough, dizziness, weakness, tachycardia.
Monitor: BP.

fenfluramine HCl
Pondimin

APPETITE SUPPRESSANT, ANTI-OBESITY

Drug: Take 1/2-1 hr before meals. **Diet:** Low calorie.
Oral/GI: Dry mouth, N/V, pain abdominal, diarrhea (↑ in first week), constipation. **S/Cond:** Avoid alcohol. Caution c̄ lactation. Caution c̄ diabetes— ↑ muscle uptake of glucose.
Other: DROWSINESS, dizziness, ataxia, headache, ↑ or ↓ BP, confusion, palpitations, depression. **Blood/Serum:** ↓ glucose.

fentanyl patch
Duragesic patch
alcohol—
0.1 mL/ dose

ANALGESIC, Narcotic

Nutr: Anorexia. **Oral/GI:** Dry mouth, dyspepsia, N/V, hiccups, abdominal pain, constipation, flatulence, diarrhea. **S/Cond:** Avoid alcohol. Not c̄ lactation. May be habit forming c̄ LT use.
Other: Sedation, respiratory depression, drowsiness, confusion, weakness, anxiety, depression, amnesia, ↑ or ↓ BP, ataxia, edema, rash.
Blood/Serum: ↑ amylase, ↑ lipase. **Urinary:** Retention.

ferrous salts

HEMATINIC, ANTIANEMIC, Mineral Supplement, Iron

Drug: Take c̄ 8 oz H_2O or juice on empty stomach. May take c̄ food to ↓ GI distress, but food ↓ abs 50%.[6] Drink liquid form c̄ straw to ↓ dental stains. Do not take c̄ bran, high phytate foods, see p 242, fiber suppl, tea, coffee, dairy products or egg. **Diet:** 200 mg Vit C/ 30 mg Fe will ↑ abs.[6] Meat ↑ abs. Take Ca , Zn or Cu suppl separately. **Nutr:** Anorexia. RDA— Men & women 51+ = 10 mg; Women = 15; Children = 10; Pregnancy = 30; Lactation = 15. **Oral/GI:** DENTAL STAINS c̄ liquid forms, NAUSEA/V, DYSPEPSIA, bloating, CONSTIPATION, diarrhea, DARK STOOLS. **S/Cond:** Limit alcohol. 90% serum pro bound. Feosol Elixir precipitates tube feedings. Not c̄ hemochromatosis, hemolytic anemia or thalassemia. **Other:** Fatal poisoning can occur c̄ ≥ 200 mg Fe in children or 200-250 mg/kg in adult in one dose. Iron overload (hemosiderosis) & toxicity may result from LT use of high dose.

Blood/Serum: ↑ Hgb, ↑ HCT, ↑ ferritin, ↑ Fe, ↑ % transferrin saturation. False ↓ Ca.[13]
Urinary: Dark color. **Monitor:** Hgb/HCT, ferritin, Fe.

ferrous fumarate	ferrous gluconate	ferrous sulfate
33% elemental Fe	12% elemental Fe	20% elemental Fe
Ferro-Sequels (SR)	**Fergon**	**Feosol**
(+ 100 mg docusate Na)	Tab— starch, sucrose	Tab— starch. Cap— benzyl alcohol, starch, sucrose.
Tab— lactose, starch		Elixir— 5% alcohol, glucose, saccharin, sucrose.

Fiberall powder LAXATIVE, bulk forming See **psyllium p 171**

FiberCon LAXATIVE, bulk forming See **calcium polycarbophil p 40**

filgrastim
Neupogen
mannitol
50 mg/mL

COLONY STIMULATING FACTOR (↑ production & activity of WBC)
Parenteral only (IV or SC)
Other: BONE PAIN, splenomegaly, fever. Transient ↓ BP.
Blood/Serum: ↑ NEUTROPHILS, ↑ WBC. Transient ↑ uric acid, ↑ LDH, ↑ alk phos, ↓ platelets. **Urinary:** Blood, pro.
Monitor: CBC c̄ diff & platelets 2-3x/week.

finasteride
Proscar
Tab— lactose, starch

ANTI-PROSTATE HYPERPLASIA, Androgen Hormone Inhibitor
Drug: Take s̄ regard to meals. **S/Cond:** 90% serum pro bound.
Not for women or children. No nutritionally-related effects reported.

Fioricet
50 mg butalbital
40 mg caffeine &
325 mg acetaminophen

ANALGESIC, SEDATIVE, Barbiturate — See also **acetaminophen p 17**

Drug: Take s̄ regard to food. **Oral/GI:** Dyspepsia, N/V, flatulence.
S/Cond: Avoid alcohol. Caution c̄ lactation.
May be habit forming c̄ LT use.
Other: Drowsiness, dizziness.

Fiorinal
Tab— lactose
50 mg butalbital
40 mg caffeine &
325 mg aspirin

ANALGESIC, SEDATIVE, Barbiturate — See also **acetylsalicylic acid p 18**

Drug: Take c̄ food. **Oral/GI:** Dyspepsia, N/V, flatulence.
S/Cond: Avoid alcohol. Caution c̄ lactation.
May be habit forming c̄ LT use.
Other: Drowsiness, dizziness.
Blood/Serum: ↑ or ↓ uric acid (dose-related), ↓ T_4, ↓ K.

5-ASA — ANTI-INFLAMMATORY — See **mesalamine p 126**

5-FU — ANTINEOPLASTIC — See **fluorouracil p 92**

Flagyl — ANTIBIOTIC — See **metronidazole p 132**

Fleet Phospho-soda — LAXATIVE — See **sodium phosphate p 184**

Flexeril — MUSCLE RELAXANT — See **cyclobenzaprine HCl p 62**

Floxin — ANTIBIOTIC, Fluoroquinolone — See **ofloxacin p 146**

fluconazole
Diflucan
Susp— sucrose, natural orange flavor

ANTIFUNGAL, ANTI-CANDIDIASIS — Oral or Parenteral (IV)

Drug: Take s̄ regard to food. **Oral/GI:** Taste changes, dry mouth, N/V, abdominal pain, diarrhea. **S/Cond:** Not c̄ lactation.
Caution c̄ diabetics on sulfonylurea— hypoglycemia.
Other: Headache, rash, tremor, ↑ sweating, hepatotoxicity.
Blood/Serum: ↑ SGOT, ↑ SGPT, ↑ alk phos, ↑ bil, ↑ GGT.

Flumadine

ANTIVIRAL, ANTI-INFLUENZA — See **rimantadine HCl p 177**

fluoride (F)
Sodium Fluoride
Luride
Pediaflor
Drops - sorbitol, < 0.5% alcohol

MINERAL SUPPLEMENT

Drug: Take separately from dairy products, Ca, Fe or Mg suppl.[7]
Tab- dissolve in mouth, chew or swallow whole or add to water or juice.
Drops - Take undiluted or mix with fluids or food.
Nutr: Estimated safe & adequate adult intake = 1.5 to 4.0 mg/day F.[47] Ca, Fe or Mg ions ↓ abs. High conc of dietary Ca forms insoluble complexes c̄ F.[73] Caution—- swallowed F toothpaste provides significant fluoride. **Oral/GI:** Gastric distress.
S/Cond: Do not use in areas c̄ > 0.7 ppm F in water.[10]
Other: In children— 0.1 mg/kg body wt daily causes dental fluorosis. Acute dose of 10-20 mg NaF causes ↑ salivation & GI upset, ≥ 500 mg can be fatal.[10] In adults— 20 to 80 mg F/day lead to chronic toxicity after years of use.[47] Lethal dose is 70 to 140 mg/kg.

fluorouracil
(5-FU)
Adrucil
Fluorouracil

ANTINEOPLASTIC Parenteral only (IV)

Diet: Bland diet may ↓ GI distress. Pyr 100-150 mg may treat hand-foot syndrome. **Nutr:** ANOREXIA, ↓ wt. May ↑ Thi requirement.
Oral/GI: Bitter/sour taste, STOMATITIS, esophagitis, dyspepsia, severe NAUSEA/VOMITING, enteritis, GI ulceration & bleeding, DIARRHEA.
S/Cond: Not c̄ lactation. Do dental care cautiously, see p 10 & 14. Contraindicated c̄ poor nutritional status.
Other: BONE MARROW SUPPRESSION, WEAKNESS, RASH, fatigue, ataxia, photosensitivity, hand-foot syndrome.
Blood/Serum: ↓ WHITE BLOOD CELLS, ↓ platelets, anemia, ↓ alb, ↑ alk phos, ↑ SGOT, ↑ SGPT, ↑ bil, ↑ LDH, ↓ T_3, ↓ T_4.
Monitor: WBC c̄ diff & platelets before each dose, CBC, hepatic func.

fluoxetine
Prozac
Cap— starch
liquid—
0.23% alcohol

ANTIDEPRESSANT, ANTI-OCD, SSRI

Drug: Take in AM s̄ regard to meals. **Diet:** No tryptophan suppl— will ↑ side effects.[13] **Nutr:** Anorexia, ↓ wt.
Oral/GI: Dry mouth, taste changes, dyspepsia, N/V, diarrhea, constipation.
S/Cond: Avoid alcohol. Not c̄ lactation. Caution c̄ diabetes-hypoglycemia. Caution c̄ elderly— ↑ incidence of ANOREXIA.[21] 94% serum pro bound.
Other: Tremor, headache, drowsiness, dizziness, insomnia, weakness, visual disturbances, photosensitivity, rash.
Blood/Serum: ↑ or ↓ glucose, ↓ Na.
Urinary: ↑ frequency.

fluoxymesterone
Halotestin
Tab— tartrazine
lactose, sucrose

ANTINEOPLASTIC, Androgen Hormone

Drug: Take c̄ food to ↓ GI distress. **Diet:** Adequate cal & pro important. May need ↓ Na. **Nutr:** ↑ appetite, ↑ wt. **Oral/GI:** N/V, diarrhea.
S/Cond: Not c̄ lactation. Caution c̄ diabetes— ↓ glucose. Caution c̄ children— ↑ bone maturation s̄ ↑ growth. **Other:** Edema, headache, anxiety, depression, insomnia, hepatitis, jaundice, paresthesia.
Blood/Serum: ↑ Na, ↑ Cl, ↑ K, ↑ P, ↑ Ca, ↑ RBC, ↑ Hgb, ↑ HCT, ↓ FSH, ↓ LD, ↑ alk phos, ↑ SGOT, ↑ bil, ↑ crea, ↑ chol, ↑ LDL, ↓ HDL, ↑ or ↓ glucose, ↓ total T_4.
Urinary: ↓ Ca. **Monitor:** CBC, hepatic func, serum & urinary Ca- women.

fluphenazine HCl
Prolixin
Oral or Parenteral (IM)

ANTIPSYCHOTIC, Phenothiazine See listing for **perphenazine p 158**
Elixir & Conc— 14% alcohol Parenteral— benzyl alcohol
Elixir— 3 g sucrose/5 mL Tab— lactose, sucrose
2.5, 5 & 10 mg— tartrazine

flurazepam HCl
Dalmane
Cap— lactose

SEDATIVE, HYPNOTIC, SLEEP AID, Benzodiazepine

Drug: Take HS. **Nutr:** ↑ or ↓ appetite, ↑ or ↓ wt. **Oral/GI:** N/V, dyspepsia, GI pain, diarrhea, constipation. **S/Cond:** Avoid alcohol. Not c̄ lactation. May be habit forming c̄ LT use. **Other:** DROWSINESS, ataxia, dizziness, weakness, headache, confusion, blurred vision.
Blood/Serum: Rare ↑ SGOT, ↑ SGPT, ↑ alk phos, ↑ bil.

flurbiprofen
Ansaid

NSAID, ANTIARTHRITIC See listing for **ibuprofen p 104**
Tab— lactose

fluvastatin
Lescol
Cap— starch, benzyl alcohol

ANTIHYPERLIPIDEMIC, HMG-CoA Reductase Inhibitor
Drug: Take single dose HS s̄ regard to food. **Diet:** ↓ fat, ↓ cholesterol (↓ cal if needed).
Oral/GI: Dyspepsia, abdominal cramps. **S/Cond:** Not c̄ lactation.
Other: Muscle pain.
Blood/Serum: ↓ CHOL, ↓ LDL, ↑ HDL, ↓ TG, ↑ SGOT, ↑ SGPT.
Monitor: Chol, lipid profile, hepatic func.

fluvoxamine
Luvox

ANTI-OCD, selective serotonin reuptake inhibitor (SSRI)
Drug: Take single dose HS s̄ regard to food. **Diet:** No tryptophan suppl.
Nutr: Anorexia. **Oral/GI:** Dry mouth, taste changes, NAUSEA/V, dyspepsia, diarrhea, constipation. **S/Cond:** Caution c̄ lactation. Smoking ↑ drug metabolism 25%. **Other:** Headache, weakness, drowsiness, insomnia, nervousness, dizziness, tremor.
Blood/Serum: < 1% dyscrasias, ↑ Chol. **Urinary:** ↑ frequency.

folic acid
(folate)
Parenteral— benzyl alcohol

B COMPLEX VITAMIN, ANTIANEMIC Oral or Parenteral (IM, IV or SC)
Drug: Usual therapeutic dose— 1 mg daily for megaloblastic/macrocytic anemia. **Diet:** Well balanced diet. Take Zn suppl separately by 2 hr.
Nutr: RDA— Men = 200 mcg; Women = 180; Pregnancy = 400; Lactation = 280. **S/Cond:** ↑ need in alcoholism, celiac disease, chronic diarrhea, sprue. Fol inhibited by def of Pyr, Vits B_{12}, C &/or E. HIV— ↓ abs of Fol. **Blood/Serum:** ↓ B_{12} c̄ LT high dose. ↑ RBC, ↑ WBC, ↑ Hgb, ↑ HCT, ↓ MCH, ↓ MCV when used to treat anemia.
Monitor: CBC. B_{12} c̄ LT high dose.

Fortaz — ANTIBIOTIC, ceftazidime — See **cephalosporins p 46**

foscarnet sodium
Foscavir

ANTIVIRAL (ANTI CMV Retinitis in HIV) Parenteral only (IV)

Diet: Insure adequate fluid intake. **Nutr:** Anorexia, ↓ wt, ↑ thirst.
Oral/GI: Dry mouth, taste changes, stomatitis, dysphagia, NAUSEA/VOMITING, abdominal pain, DIARRHEA, constipation.
S/Cond: Caution c̄ lactation. Do dental care cautiously, see p 9 & 14.
Other: FEVER, HEADACHE, bone marrow suppression, seizures, paresthesia, weakness, confusion, cough, dizziness, anxiety, rash, visual changes, tremor, ataxia, edema, drowsiness, insomnia.
Blood/Serum: ↑ CREA, ANEMIA, ↑ BUN, dyscrasias, ↓ WBC, ↓ Ca, ↓ Mg, ↑ or ↓ P, ↓ K, ↓ Na, ↑ alk phos, ↑ LDH, ↑ SGOT, ↑ SGPT.
Urinary: Pro. **Monitor:** Renal func closely, electrolytes, Ca, P, Mg.

fosinopril sodium
Monopril
Tab— lactose

ANTIHYPERTENSIVE, ACE Inhibitor

Diet: ↓ cal, ↓ Na may be recommended. Avoid salt subs. Caution c̄ K suppl. Insure adequate fluid intake. Take Ca or Mg suppl separately by 2 hrs. Avoid natural licorice. **S/Cond:** Limit alcohol. Not c̄ lactation. 97% serum pro bound. **Other:** ↓ BP, COUGH, dizziness, fatigue.
Blood/Serum: ↑ K, ↓ Na, ↑ alk phos, ↑ bil, ↑ SGOT, ↑ SGPT. Transient ↑ BUN, ↑ crea. **Monitor:** BP, electrolytes.

Fulvicin — ANTIFUNGAL — See **griseofulvin p 100**

Fungizone — ANTIBIOTIC — See **amphotericin B p 26**

furosemide
Lasix
Tab— lactose
Liquid — 11.5% alcohol, sorbitol
Parenteral— benzyl alcohol

DIURETIC (Loop K-depleting), ANTIHYPERTENSIVE
Oral or Parenteral (IM or IV)

Drug: May take c̄ food or milk to ↓ GI distress. IV— pH must be > 5.5.
Diet: ↑ K, ↑ Mg (or K, Mg suppl), ↓ cal, ↓ Na may be recommended. Avoid natural licorice. **Nutr:** Anorexia, ↑ thirst.
Oral/GI: Stomach cramps, Sorbitol in soln may cause diarrhea c̄ high dose.
S/Cond: Limit alcohol. Caution c̄ lactation. Caution c̄ diabetes— ↑ glucose.
Other: Dizziness, blurred vision, headache, rash, weakness, photosensitivity. Rare gout.
Blood/Serum: ↓ K, ↓ Mg, ↓ Na, ↓ Cl, ↓ Ca, ↑ glucose, ↓ Zn,[11b] ↑ BUN, ↑ uric acid, dyscrasias, anemia. ↑ Chol, ↑ LDL, ↑ VLDL, ↑ TG.[6]
Urinary: ↑ K, ↑ Na, ↑ CL, ↑ Mg, ↑ Ca, ↑ glucose.
Monitor: Electrolytes, Mg, Ca, glucose, uric acid, CO_2, renal func.

gabapentin
Neurontin
Cap - lactose

ANTICONVULSANT

Drug: Take s̄ regard to food. Take Mg suppl separately by 2 hrs.
Nutr: ↑ WT, ↑ APPETITE.
Oral/GI: Dry mouth or throat, dyspepsia.
S/Cond: Caution c̄ alcohol. Not c̄ lactation.
Other: Drowsiness, dizziness, fatigue, ataxia, tremor, edema, visual changes, amnesia.
Blood/Serum: <1%— ↓ WBC, dyscrasias.
Urinary: False + pro c̄ dipstick.

ganciclovir sodium
Cytovene

ANTIVIRAL, (ANTI-CMV retinitis in HIV) Oral & Parenteral (IV)
Drug: Take $\bar{c}$ food. **Diet:** Insure adequate fluid intake. **Nutr:** Anorexia. **Oral/GI:** NAUSEA/V, abdominal pain, GI hemorrhage, flatulence, DIARRHEA. **S/Cond:** Not $\bar{c}$ lactation. **Other:** Headache, FEVER, rash, neuropathy, paresthesia, weakness. **Blood/Serum:** ↓ WHITE BLOOD CELLS, ANEMIA, ↓ platelets, ↑ crea, ↑ BUN, ↑ SGOT, ↑ SGPT, ↑ alk phos, ↑ bil. < 1% ↓ glucose, ↓ K. **Monitor:** CBC $\bar{c}$ diff, platelets, renal & hepatic func.

Gantanol
ANTIBIOTIC See **sulfamethoxazole p 188**

Gantrisin
Tab— lactose
ANTIBIOTIC See listing for **sulfamethoxazole p 188**
Pediatric susp— 0.3% alcohol, invert sugar, sucrose
Syrup— 0.9% alcohol, sucrose

Garamycin
ANTIBIOTIC See **gentamicin sulfate p 98**

Gastrocrom
ANTIMASTOCYTOSIS See **cromolyn sodium p 61**

Gaviscon
aluminum hydroxide
ANTACID See **aluminum hydroxide p 22**
Various forms contain magnesium carbonate or trisilicate.
S/Cond: Thickens some tube feedings.[8]

Gelusil
Sodium Free
ANTACID, ANTIFLATULENT
contains simethicone
See **aluminum hydroxide & magnesium hydroxide p 23**

gemfibrozil
Lopid
Tab— starch

ANTIHYPERLIPIDEMIC (Types IIb, IV & V hyperlipidemia)
Drug: Take 1/2 hr before breakfast & supper. **Diet:** ↓ fat, low sucrose, cal controlled. **Oral/GI:** Taste changes, dyspepsia, abdominal pain, N/V, diarrhea, constipation, flatulence. **S/Cond:** Not c̄ lactation. Caution c̄ diabetes— possible ↑ glucose.[6] 95% serum pro bound.
Other: Headache, dizziness, blurred vision, fatigue, rash, gallstones, paresthesia, muscle pain.
Blood/Serum: ↓ TG, ↑ HDL, ↓ LDL, ↓ CHOL, ↑ SGOT, ↑ alk phos, ↑ SGPT, ↑ bil, ↑ LDH, ↑ CPK. Slightly ↑ glucose, ↓ K, ↓ Hgb/HCT, ↓ WBC.
Monitor: CBC, hepatic func, TG, chol.

gentamicin sulfate
Garamycin
3.2 mg
Na bisulfite/mL

ANTIBIOTIC, Aminoglycoside — Parenteral only (IM or IV)
Diet: Insure adequate fluid intake. **Nutr:** Anorexia, ↓ wt.
Oral/GI: Stomatitis, ↑ salivation, N/V. **S/Cond:** Not c̄ lactation.
Other: Nephrotoxicity, hearing loss, dizziness, ataxia, headache, confusion, depression, peripheral neuropathy, ↑ or ↓ BP, rash, convulsions.
Blood/Serum: ↑ BUN, ↑ crea, ↑ N, ↑ SGOT, ↑ SGPT, ↑ LDH, ↑ bil, ↑ alk phos, ↓ Mg, ↓ K, ↓ Na, ↓ Ca.
Urinary: Pro.
Monitor: Renal func, electrolytes, Ca, Mg, urinalysis.

glipizide
Glucotrol
Tab— lactose

ORAL HYPOGLYCEMIC, Sulfonylurea– 2nd generation
Drug: Take on empty stomach 30 minutes before breakfast (food delays abs).
Diet: Prescribed ADA diet. Caution c̄ high dose nicotinic acid— ↑ glucose.

Nutr: ↑ or ↓ appetite, ↑ wt. **Oral/GI:** Dyspepsia, nausea, diarrhea, constipation. **S/Cond:** Limit alcohol. Not c̄ lactation. ≥ 98% serum pro bound. Hypoalbuminemia (< 3 g/dL) may ↑ drug effects.
Other: Dizziness, headache, drowsiness Rare SIADH.
Blood/Serum: ↓ GLUCOSE, ↑ SGOT, ↑ LDH, ↑ alk phos, ↑ BUN, ↑ crea, ↓ Na. Rare dyscrasias.
Urinary: ↓ GLUCOSE. **Monitor:** Glucose, possibly glycosylated Hgb.

Glucophage — ORAL HYPOGLYCEMIC, Biguanide — See **metformin p 127**

glyburide
DiaBeta
Glynase PresTab
Tab— lactose
Micronase

ORAL HYPOGLYCEMIC, Sulfonylurea– 2nd generation
Drug: Take with breakfast. **Diet:** Prescribed ADA diet. Caution c̄ high dose nicotinic acid— ↑ glucose. **Nutr:** ↑ or ↓ appetite, ↑ wt.
Oral/GI: Dyspepsia, nausea, diarrhea, constipation.
S/Cond: Limit alcohol. Not c̄ lactation. ≥ 97% serum pro bound. Hypoalbuminemia (< 3 g/dL) may ↑ drug effects.
Other: Blurred vision, rash. Rare SIADH, jaundice.
Blood/Serum: ↓ GLUCOSE, ↑ SGOT, ↑ SGPT, ↓ Na. Rare dyscrasias.
Urinary: ↓ GLUCOSE. **Monitor:** Glucose, possibly glycosylated Hgb.

granisetron HCl
Kytril
Tab— lactose

ANTINAUSEANT, ANTIEMETIC — Oral or Parenteral (IV)
Oral/GI: Taste disorder, abdominal pain, constipation, diarrhea.
Other: Headache, weakness, transient ↓ or ↑ BP, fever.
Blood/Serum: Transient ↑ SGOT, ↑ SGPT.

griseofulvin
Fulvicin P/G
Tab— lactose
Grifulvin V Tab— starch
Susp— .2% alcohol, saccharin, sucrose
Grisactin Tab— starch
Cap— lactose

ANTIFUNGAL

Drug: Take microsize forms c̄ or after high fat meal or whole milk to ↑ abs.
Nutr: ↑ thirst. **Oral/GI:** Taste loss, oral candidiasis, dry mouth, stomach pain, N/V, diarrhea. **S/Cond:** Avoid alcohol.
Other: Headache, confusion, dizziness, fatigue, insomnia, photosensitivity, peripheral neuritis. Rare hepatotoxicity, nephrosis.
Blood/Serum: Rare ↓ WBC. **Urinary:** Pro.
Monitor: c̄ LT use— CBC, hepatic & renal func

guaifenesin
Robitussin syrup
corn syrup, glucose, saccharin
Humibid LA (SR tab)
Humibid Sprinkle (SR cap)

EXPECTORANT

Drug: Take c̄ 8 oz H_2O. Swallow SR tab whole. Swallow Sprinkle cap whole or open & put on small amount soft food.
Oral/GI: N/V, GI distress, diarrhea. **S/Cond:** Precipitates tube feedings.[8]
Other: Headache, drowsiness, dizziness, rash.
Urinary: False + VMA.

guanfacine HCl
Tenex
Tab— lactose

ANTIHYPERTENSIVE

Drug: Take HS. **Diet:** ↓ Na, ↓ cal may be recommended. Avoid natural licorice. **Oral/GI:** DRY MOUTH, nausea, constipation. **S/Cond:** Caution c̄ alcohol. Caution c̄ lactation. ↑ risk of dental problems, see p 9 & 14.
Other: Sedation, drowsiness, fatigue, dizziness, headache, insomnia. weakness. **Monitor:** BP.

Habitrol — SMOKING DETERRENT — See **nicotine transdermal patch p 142**

Halotestin — ANTINEOPLASTIC, Androgen Hormone — See **fluoxymesterone p 93**

haloperidol
Haldol

ANTIPSYCHOTIC, Butyrophenone — Oral or Parenteral (IM)

Drug: Take c̄ food or milk to ↓ GI distress. Do not mix conc c̄ coffee, tea or fruit juice— drug may precipitate.[13] **Nutr:** ↑ appetite, ↑ wt, anorexia.
Oral/GI: DRY MOUTH, ↑ salivation, dyspepsia, N/V, constipation, diarrhea.
S/Cond: Avoid alcohol. Not c̄ lactation. ↑ risk of dental problems, see p 9 & 14. 92% serum pro bound. **Other:** EXTRAPYRAMIDAL SYMPTOMS (EPS), DROWSINESS, restlessness, blurred vision, ↑ or ↓ BP, lactation, dizziness, headache, photosensitivity. Tardive dyskinesia c̄ LT use.
Blood/Serum: ↑ prolactin, ↓ WBC, anemia, ↑ or ↓ glucose, ↓ Na.
Urinary: Retention, hesitancy.

heparin sodium
Heparin sodium
< 10 mg benzyl alcohol/mL
7 mg Na/2 mL vial

ANTICOAGULANT — Parenteral only (IV or SC)

Oral/GI: N/V, abdominal pain, GI bleeding, constipation, black tarry stools.
S/Cond: Limit alcohol.[9b] Caution c̄ diabetes & ESRD— hyperkalemia.[7] Do dental care cautiously— ↑ bleeding.
Other: BLEEDING, hemorrhage, dizziness, headache, osteoporosis, bone & muscle pain c̄ LT use (> 3 mos).
Blood/Serum: ↓ PLATELETS, ↑ SGOT, ↑ SGPT, ↑ PT, ↓ TG, ↑ FFA, ↓ chol, ↓ T_4. **Monitor:** APTT, platelet count, HCT, occult blood.

Hexadrol — CORTICOSTEROID — See **dexamethasone p 68**

Hismanal — ANTIHISTAMINE — See **astemizole p 29**

Hivid — ANTIVIRAL, ANTI-HIV — See **zalcitabine p 214**

Humibid LA or Sprinkle — EXPECTORANT — See **guaifenesin p 100**

Humulin — ANTIDIABETIC, HYPOGLYCEMIC — See **insulin p 108**

hydralazine HCl
Apresoline
Tab— tartrazine, lactose, starch, mannitol

ANTIHYPERTENSIVE, Vasodilator — Oral or Parenteral (IM or IV)

Drug: Take c̄ meals. **Diet:** ↓ cal, ↓ Na may be recommended. Avoid natural licorice. Pyr suppl (100-200 mg) may correct drug-induced peripheral neuropathy.[13] **Nutr:** Anorexia, ↓ or ↑ wt, ↑ thirst.
Oral/GI: Dry mouth,[26] unpleasant taste,[26] N/V, GI distress, diarrhea, constipation. **S/Cond:** Limit alcohol. Caution c̄ lactation. May cause lupus-like syndrome. 90% serum pro bound.[26] **Other:** ↓ BP, edema, headache, tachycardia, dizziness, tremor, rash. Rare hepatotoxicity, peripheral neuropathy. **Blood/Serum:** Dyscrasias, + ANA.
Urinary: ↑ Mn,[12] ↑ Pyr, difficult urination. **Monitor:** BP, ANA.

hydrochlorothiazide (HCTZ)
Esidrix
Tab— lactose, sucrose, starch
HydroDIURIL
Tab— lactose, starch
Oretic
Tab— lactose

ANTIHYPERTENSIVE, DIURETIC, Thiazide (K-depleting)

Drug: Take in AM c̄ food or milk.
Diet: May need ↓ Na, ↓ cal, ↑ K, ↑ Mg (or K or Mg suppl).
Avoid natural licorice. Caution c̄ Ca &/or Vit D suppl.[3]
Nutr: Anorexia, ↑ thirst.
Oral/GI: Dry mouth, N/V, GI irritation, diarrhea, constipation.
S/Cond: Limit alcohol. Not c̄ lactation. Caution c̄ diabetes— ↑ glucose.
Other: ↓ BLOOD PRESSURE, dizziness, weakness, photosensitivity.
Rare gout, pancreatitis, jaundice.

Blood/Serum: ↑ GLUCOSE,[18] ↓ NA, ↓ Cl, ↓ K, ↓ Mg, ↑ Ca, dyscrasias, ↑ uric acid, ↑ bil, ↑ chol, ↑ LDL, ↑ TG, ↑ BUN, ↑ crea.
Urinary: ↑ NA, ↑ Cl, ↑ K, ↑ Mg, ↓ Ca, ↑ glucose, ↓ uric acid, ↑ Zn, ↑ bicarb.
Monitor: Electrolytes, Mg, BUN, uric acid, BP, glucose.

hydrocortisone — CORTICOSTEROID — See **corticosteroids p 46**

HydroDIURIL — ANTIHYPERTENSIVE, DIURETIC — See **hydrochlorothiazide above**

hydromorphone HCl — ANALGESIC, ANTITUSSIVE, Narcotic — See listing for **morphine p 136**
Dilaudid
Tab & liquid— Na bisulfite
Tab— lactose, Liquid— sucrose — Oral, Parenteral or Suppository
Cough Syrup— 5% alcohol, 2.5 mg sucrose/ 5 mL, tartrazine

hydroxychloroquine sulfate
Plaquenil
Tab— starch

ANTIMALARIAL, ANTIARTHRITIC (rheumatoid), ANTI-LUPUS
Drug: Take c̄ meals or milk to ↓ GI distress. May crush & mix c̄ 1 t jam, jelly or jello. **Nutr:** Anorexia, ↓ wt.
Oral/GI: Blue black mouth, N/V, abdominal cramps, diarrhea.
S/Cond: Caution c̄ lactation. Caution c̄ G6PD def— risk of hemolytic anemia. Not for LT use in children.
Other: Headache, itching (↑ BLACK PATIENTS), dizziness, visual changes, fatigue, muscle weakness, emotional changes, rash, blue-black skin, nails.
Blood/Serum: Dyscrasias.
Monitor: CBC, ophthalmologic exams.

hydroxyzine
Atarax
Tab— lactose, sucrose, starch
Syrup— 0.5% alcohol, sucrose
Vistaril
Cap— sucrose, starch
Oral Susp— sorbitol

ANTIHISTAMINE, ANTIANXIETY, ANTINAUSEANT (IM)
Oral or Parenteral (IM)

Oral/GI: Dry mouth, bitter taste, nausea.
S/Cond: Not c̄ lactation. ↑ risk of dental problems, see p 9 & 14.
Other: DROWSINESS, ataxia, dizziness, headache, weakness, wheezing. Rare tremor, seizures.

Hygroton — ANTIHYPERTENSIVE, DIURETIC — See **chlorthalidone p 51**

Hytakerol
dihydrotachysterol — VITAMIN D ANALOG — See listing for **calcitriol p 39**

Hytrin — ANTIHYPERTENSIVE — See **terazosin HCl p 192**

ibuprofen
Advil— sucrose
Ibu-
Tab 400 & 600- starch
800— lactose
Midol IB

NSAID, ANTIARTHRITIC, ANALGESIC
Drug: Take c̄ food or milk to ↓ GI effects.
Diet: Caution c̄ GI irritants eg K suppl (↑ risk of GI irritation).[13]
Nutr: ↓ appetite.
Oral/GI: N/V, dyspepsia, abdominal pain, constipation, diarrhea, flatulence, GI ulcers & bleeding (may be sudden & serious).
S/Cond: Avoid alcohol. Not c̄ lactation. 99% serum pro bound.

Motrin
Tab— starch

Other: Dizziness, rash, edema, depression. **Blood/Serum:** ↑ SGOT, ↑ SGPT, ↑ alk phos, ↓ Hgb (> 20% c̄ LT high dose), ↓ HCT, ↑ K, ↑ BUN, ↑ crea, ↓ glucose. Rare dyscrasias, ↑ PT.
Monitor: Hepatic & renal func c̄ LT use.

ifosfamide
Ifex

ANTINEOPLASTIC, Alkylating Agent — Parenteral only (IV)
Diet: Insure adequate fluid (minimum 2 L/day).[26]
Other: BONE MARROW SUPPRESSION, UROTOXICITY, encephalopathy, drowsiness, confusion, dizziness, fatigue, fever, nephrotoxicity (↑ INCIDENCE IN CHILDREN[1]).
Blood/Serum: ↓ WHITE BLOOD CELLS, ↓ PLATELETS, ↑ BUN, ↑ crea, ↑ SGOT, ↑ SGPT, ↑ LDH, ↑ bil.
Urinary: HEMATURIA.
Monitor: Urine for RBC, CBC c̄ diff & platelets before each dose. Renal & hepatic func.

Iletin — ANTIDIABETIC, HYPOGLYCEMIC — See **insulin p 108**

Ilosone — ANTIBIOTIC — See **erythromycin p 82**

Ilotycin — ANTIBIOTIC — See **erythromycin p 82**

Imitrex — ANTIMIGRAINE — See **sumatriptan succinate p 190**

imipenem & cilastatin — ANTIBIOTIC — Parenteral only (IM or IV)

Primaxin
IV— 250— 19 mg Na
IV— 500— 38 mg Na

Oral/GI: IV— N/V, cramps, diarrhea. Rare pseudomembranous colitis. **S/Cond:** Caution c̄ lactation. **Other:** Seizures. **Blood/Serum:** ↑ alk phos, ↑ SGOT, ↑ SGPT, ↑ BUN, ↑ crea, ↑ K, ↑ Cl, ↓ Na, eosinophilia. Rare dyscrasias, ↓ Hgb, ↓ HCT, ↑ bil, ↑ LDH.
Urinary: Pro, RBC. **Monitor:** CBC c̄ diff, hepatic & renal func.

imipramine HCl — ANTIDEPRESSANT, Tricyclic — Oral or Parenteral (IM)

Tofranil
Tab— sucrose
IM- 1 mg Na bisulfite & 1 mg Na sulfite/2 mL
Tofranil PM
Cap— starch

Drug: May take c̄ food to ↓ GI distress. **Diet:** Limit caffeine, see p 240. ↑ fiber may ↓ drug effect.[3] **Nutr:** ↑ need for Rib.[41] ↑ APPETITE especially for sweets, ↑ WT. **Oral/GI:** DRY MOUTH, unpleasant taste, N/V, epigastric distress, diarrhea, constipation.
S/Cond: Avoid alcohol. Not c̄ lactation. ↑ risk of dental problems, see p 9 & 14. ≥ 89% serum pro bound.
Other: DROWSINESS, blurred vision, weakness, ↓ BP, fine tremor, sweating, headache, dizziness, ataxia, fatigue, confusion. Rare SIADH, jaundice.
Blood/Serum: ↑ SGOT, ↑ SGPT, ↑ alk phos, ↑ or ↓ glucose. eosinophilia. Rare dyscrasias.
Urinary: Retention, ↑ Rib.
Monitor: CBC c̄ diff & hepatic func c̄ LT use.

Imodium — ANTIDIARRHEAL — See **loperamide HCl p 119**

Imuran — IMMUNOSUPPRESSANT — See **azathioprine p 31**

indapamide
Lozol
Tab— lactose, starch

ANTIHYPERTENSIVE, DIURETIC, Sulfonamide (K-depleting)

Drug: May take c̄ food to ↓ GI distress. **Diet:** May need ↓ Na, ↓ cal, ↑ K, ↑ Mg (or K or Mg suppl). Avoid natural licorice. **Nutr:** Anorexia, ↓ wt.
Oral/GI: Dry mouth, N/V, GI irritation, constipation, diarrhea.
S/Cond: Limit alcohol. Not c̄ lactation. Caution c̄ diabetes— ↑ glucose.
Other: Headache, dizziness, muscle cramps, fatigue, agitation, peripheral neuritis, insomnia, drowsiness, blurred vision, rash. Rare gout.
Blood/Serum: ↓ POTASSIUM, ↓ Na, ↓ Cl, ↓ Mg, ↑ glucose, ↑ uric acid, ↑ BUN, ↑ crea. Slight ↑ Ca, ↓ P .
Urinary: ↑ Na, ↑ POTASSIUM, ↑ Cl, ↑ Mg, ↓ Ca, ↓ uric acid, ↑ glucose.
Monitor: BP, electrolytes, Mg, uric acid, BUN, glucose.

Inderal

ANTIHYPERTENSIVE, Beta-Blocker See **propranolol HCl p 168**

Indomethacin
Indocin
Cap— lactose
Susp— 1% alcohol, sorbitol
Indocin SR
Cap— sugar, starch

NSAID, ANTIARTHRITIC

Drug: Take c̄ food to ↓ GI distress. Swallow SR Cap whole.
Diet: Caution c̄ GI irritants eg K suppl (↑ risk of GI irritation).
Oral/GI: N/V, dyspepsia, abdominal pain, diarrhea, constipation, GI ulcers & bleeding (may be sudden & serious). **S/Cond:** Avoid alcohol. Not c̄ lactation. Caution c̄ diabetes— ↑ glucose. 99% serum pro bound.
Other: Severe HEADACHE, dizziness, edema, drowsiness, depression.
Blood/Serum: ↑ SGOT, ↑ SGPT. <1% dyscrasias, ↑ K, ↑ BUN, ↑ glucose. **Urinary:** < 1% ↑ glucose, pro.
Monitor: Hepatic & renal func c̄ LT use.

INH ANTITUBERCULOSIS See **isoniazid p 110**

Insulin
Humulin
Iletin
Lente, NPH
Novolin
Regular

ANTIDIABETIC, HYPOGLYCEMIC Parenteral only (IM)

Diet: Diabetic meal plan to balance food c̄ insulin. **S/Cond:** Limit alcohol (↑ hypoglycemic effect). Caution c̄ lactation. Exercise, illness or pregnancy ↑ insulin needs. **Other:** HYPOGLYCEMIA. Transient edema, vision changes. **Blood/Serum:** ↓ GLUCOSE, ↓ K, ↓ Mg, ↓ P,[13] ↑ T_4.[7] **Urinary:** ↓ GLUCOSE.

Monitor: Glucose, possibly glycosylated Hgb.

Intal ANTIASTHMA See **cromolyn sodium p 61**

interferon
alfa 2a
Roferon-A

alfa 2b
Intron-A

ANTINEOPLASTIC Parenteral only

Diet: Insure adequate fluid intake. **Nutr:** ANOREXIA, ↓ WEIGHT, ↑ thirst.

Oral/GI: DRY MOUTH, TASTE CHANGES, stomatitis, NAUSEA/V, abdominal pain, DIARRHEA, flatulence, constipation. **S/Cond:** Avoid alcohol. Not c̄ lactation. ↑ risk of dental problems, see p 9, 10 & 14. Caution c̄ diabetes. **Other:** FLU-LIKE SYMPTOMS, BONE MARROW SUPPRESSION, DIZZINESS, COUGH, headache, fatigue, rash, confusion, blurred vision, peripheral neuropathy, ↑ or ↓ BP.

Blood/Serum: ↓ WHITE BLOOD CELLS, ↓ PLATELETS, ↑ SGOT, ↑ SGPT, ↑ alk phos, ↑ LDH, ↑ bil, ↓ Hgb, ↓ HCT, ↑ BUN, ↑ crea, ↑ fasting glucose, ↑ P, ↓ Ca, ↑ uric acid, ↑ or ↓ TSH.

Urinary: Pro. **Monitor:** CBC c̄ diff, hepatic func, TSH, BP.

interferon beta-1b
Betaseron
pwd— dextrose,

ANTI-MULTIPLE SCLEROSIS — Parenteral only (SC)

Nutr: ↑ or ↓ wt.
Oral/GI: Vomiting, GI upset, abdominal pain, diarrhea, constipation.
S/Cond: Not c̄ lactation.
Other: FLU-LIKE SYMPTOMS, chills, muscle ache, fever, headache, weakness, ↑ sweating, ↑ BP, palpitations, photosensitivity, edema.
Blood./Serum: ↓ WBC, ↑ SGOT, ↑ SGPT, ↑ bil, ↑ or ↓ glucose, dyscrasias.
Monitor: CBC c̄ diff, hepatic func.

Ionamin

APPETITE SUPPRESSANT — See **phentermine resin p 160**

ipratropium bromide
Atrovent
soya lecithin

BRONCHODILATOR, Anticholingeric — Oral Inhalant

Oral/GI: Dry mouth/throat, metallic/bitter taste, nausea, dyspepsia.
S/Cond: Caution c̄ lactation.
Other: COUGH, headache, dizziness, blurred vision, palpitations, nervousness.

iron

MINERAL SUPPLEMENT — See **ferrous salts p 88**

ISMO

ANTIANGINAL — See **isosorbide mononitrate p 110**

isoniazid **INH** **Nydrazid** (Parenteral)	ANTITUBERCULOSIS Oral or Parenteral (IM) **Drug:** Food ↓ abs. Take 1 hr before or 2 hrs after meals. May take c̄ food to ↓ GI distress. **Diet:** Pyr suppl (25-50 mg daily) often prescribed to prevent peripheral neuropathy. MAOI-like activity. Avoid high tyramine or histamine foods, see p 243. **Nutr:** May cause osteoporosis, pellagra— ↑ need Vit D,[11a] Pyr. **Oral/GI:** Dry mouth, N/V, epigastric distress, constipation, diarrhea. **S/Cond:** Avoid alcohol. Caution c̄ lactation. **Other:** Peripheral neuropathy, hepatitis, fatigue, weakness, fever. **Blood/Serum:** ↑ SGOT, ↑ SGPT, ↑ bil, ↑ glucose, ↓ Ca, ↓ P, dyscrasias. **Urinary:** False + glucose ($CUSO_4$), ↑ Pyr, ↑ bil.
Isoptin	ANTIARRHYTHMIC, Ca Channel Blocker See **verapamil HCl p 206**
isosorbide dinitrate **Isordil** **Sorbitrate** Tab— lactose, starch Chewable- mannitol, sugar **isosorbide mononitrate** **ISMO**— Tab— lactose	ANTIANGINAL **Drug:** Take on empty stomach c̄ 8 oz H_2O.[13] Swallow SR tab whole. **S/Cond:** Caution c̄ alcohol. Caution c̄ lactation. **Other:** HEADACHE, ↓ BP, flushing, dizziness, weakness, tachycardia. **Monitor:** BP, heart rate.

isotretinoin
Accutane
Cap— soybean oil

ANTI-ACNE, retinoid

Drug: Take c̄ meals or milk. Do not crush or chew.
Diet: Do not take suppl c̄ Vit A or beta carotene. Do not take MVI.
Nutr: Anorexia, ↑ thirst.
Oral/GI: DRY MOUTH, CHEILITIS (LIP INFLAMMATION), N/V, abdominal pain.
S/Cond: Limit alcohol. Not c̄ lactation. Do dental care cautiously, see p 9 & 14. Caution c̄ diabetes. Not c̄ pregnancy. 99.9% serum pro bound.
Other: CONJUNCTIVITIS, HEADACHE, muscle pain, photosensitivity, rash, fatigue.
Blood/Serum: ↑ TRIGLYCERIDES, ↑ chol, ↓ HDL, ↑ LDL, ↑ VLDL, ↑ LDH, ↑ SGOT, ↑ GGT, ↑ SGPT, ↑ alk phos, ↓ H/H, ↓ WBC, ↑ platelets, ↑ CPK, ↑ glucose, ↑ uric acid.
Monitor: CBC, lipids, hepatic func, diabetes.

israpidine
Dynacirc
Cap— lactose, starch, benzyl alcohol

ANTIHYPERTENSIVE, Ca Channel Blocker

Drug: Take s̄ regard to food. **Diet:** ↓ Na, ↓ cal may be recommended. Avoid natural licorice. **Oral/GI:** N/V, abdominal pain, diarrhea.
S/Cond: Not c̄ lactation. 95% serum pro bound.
Other: ↓ BP, peripheral edema, headache, dizziness, palpitations, fatigue, flushing, rash.
Monitor: BP.

itraconazole
Sporanox
Cap— sucrose, starch

ANTIFUNGAL, ANTI-CANDIDIASIS
Drug: Take c̄ food to ↑ abs. **Diet:** Take Ca or Mg suppl separately by 2 hrs. **Nutr:** Anorexia. **Oral/GI:** N/V, diarrhea. **S/Cond:** Not c̄ lactation. Caution c̄ diabetes— ↑ effect of oral hypoglycemics.[9a] 99% serum pro bound. Caution c̄ achlorhydria (must take in acidic liquid).[13]
Other: Rash, edema, fatigue, fever, headache, dizziness, ↑ BP.
Blood/Serum: ↑ SGOT, ↑ SGPT, ↓ K.
Urinary: Pro. **Monitor:** Hepatic func, K.

Kaopectate — ANTIDIARRHEAL — See **attapulgite p30**

Kayexalate — ANTIHYPERKALEMIA — See **sodium polystyrene sulfonate p 184**

KCl - K-Dur — ELECTROLYTE, potassium supplement — See **potassium chloride p 164**

Keflex — ANTIBIOTIC, Cephalosporin — See **cephalexin p 45**

Kefzol — ANTIBIOTIC, cefazolin sodium — See **cephalosporins p 46**

Kenalog — CORTICOSTEROID, triamcinolone — See **corticosteroids p 60**

ketoconazole
Nizoral
Tab— lactose

ANTIFUNGAL, ANTI-CANDIDIASIS
Drug: Take c̄ food to ↑ abs. Acidic pH < 5.0 needed to dissolve.
Diet: Take Ca or Mg suppl separately by 2 hrs. **Oral/GI:** N/V, abdominal pain. **S/Cond:** Avoid alcohol— possible disulfiram-like

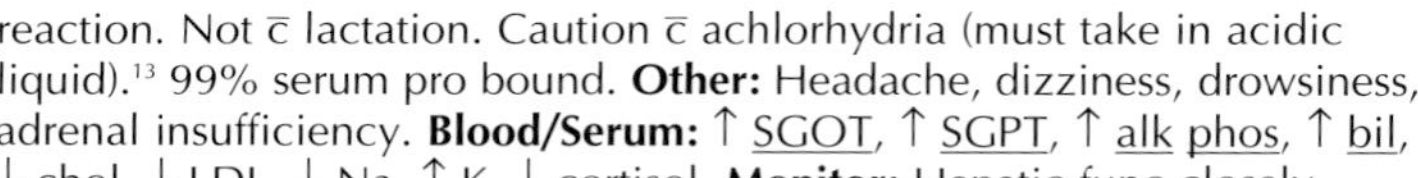

reaction. Not $\bar{c}$ lactation. Caution $\bar{c}$ achlorhydria (must take in acidic liquid).[13] 99% serum pro bound. **Other:** Headache, dizziness, drowsiness, adrenal insufficiency. **Blood/Serum:** ↑ SGOT, ↑ SGPT, ↑ alk phos, ↑ bil, ↓ chol, ↓ LDL, ↓ Na, ↑ K, ↓ cortisol. **Monitor:** Hepatic func closely.

ketorolac tromethamine
Toradol
Parenteral— 10% alcohol
Tab— lactose

NSAID, ANALGESIC (short-term use only)   Oral or Parenteral (IM)

Drug: May take $\bar{c}$ food or milk to ↓ GI distress. **Diet:** Caution $\bar{c}$ GI irritants eg K suppl (↑ risk of GI irritation).[13] **Nutr:** ↑ thirst.
Oral/GI: Dry mouth, stomatitis, taste loss, N/V, dyspepsia, GI pain, diarrhea, flatulence, constipation, GI ulcers & bleeding (may be sudden & serious). **S/Cond:** Avoid alcohol. Caution $\bar{c}$ lactation.
99% serum pro bound.
Other: Edema, drowsiness, headache, dizziness, rash, sweating.
Blood/Serum: ↑ SGOT, ↑ SGPT, ↑ BUN, ↑ crea, ↑ K.

Klonopin — ANTICONVULSANT, Benzodiazepine — See **clonazepam p 56**

K-Lor   Klor-Con   Klotrix   Klorvess   K-Lyte/Cl — ELECTROLYTE, potassium supplement — See **potassium chloride p 164**

K-Phos Neutral
K-Phos Original — ACIDIFIER, PHOSPHOROUS SUPPLEMENT — See **phosphate p 162**

K-Tab — ELECTROLYTE, Potassium Supplement — See **potassium chloride p 164**

Kytril — ANTIEMETIC — See **granisetron HCl p 99**

labetalol HCl
Normodyne
Tab— lactose, starch

ANTIHYPERTENSIVE, $Alpha_1$ & Beta-Blocker — Oral or Parenteral (IV)

Drug: Oral— Take c̄ food. **Diet:** ↓ Na, ↓ cal diet may be recommended. Avoid natural licorice. **Oral/GI:** Dry mouth, taste changes, <u>N</u>/V, dyspepsia. **S/Cond:** Limit alcohol. Caution c̄ lactation. Caution c̄ diabetes— may mask symptoms of & prolong hypoglycemia. May inhibit insulin response to hyperglycemia. **Other:** <u>Dizziness</u>, <u>fatigue</u>, headache, visual changes, rash, ↓ BP. Rare jaundice. **Blood/Serum:** ↓ WBC, ↑ BUN, ↑ crea, ↑ SGOT, ↑ SGPT, ↑ glucose, + ANA, ↑ prolactin (IV).
Monitor: BP, hepatic & renal func.

lactulose
Cephulac
Chronulac
2.2 g galactose, 1.2 g lactose, 1.2 g other sugar/15 mL

ANTIHYPERAMMONEMIC, LAXATIVE

Drug: Take c̄ juice, milk, H_2O or mix c̄ sweet food. Follow c̄ 8 oz H_2O. **Diet:** High fiber c̄ 1500-2000 mL fluid/day to ↓ need for drug. Not c̄ lactose or galactose restricted diet. **Oral/GI:** N/V, <u>belching</u>, <u>cramps</u>, <u>borborygmi</u>, diarrhea, <u>flatulence</u>. **S/Cond:** Caution c̄ lactation. Caution c̄ diabetes. Dilute before use in tube feeding.[6] **Blood/Serum:** ↓ <u>NH_3</u>.
Monitor: Electrolytes in elderly or debilitated c̄ LT use (> 6 mos).[6]

lamotrigine
Lamictal

ANTICONVULSANT

Drug: Take s̄ regard to food. **Oral/GI:** <u>N/V</u>, dyspepsia, abdominal pain, diarrhea. **S/Cond:** Not c̄ lactation. **Other:** <u>Double vision</u>, <u>ataxia</u>, <u>dizziness</u>, <u>headache</u>, <u>blurred vision</u>, <u>rash</u>, drowsiness, insomnia, tremor, hot flashes, fever, depression. **Blood/Serum:** <1%— dyscrasias.

Lamprene ANTIBIOTIC, ANTILEPROTIC See **clofazimine p 55**

Lanoxin CARDIOTONIC See **digoxin p 72**

lansoprazole
Prevacid
Cap (delayed release)
sucrose

ANTIULCER, ANTISECRETORY, Proton Pump Inhibitor
Drug: Take before a meal. Swallow whole. Do not open, chew or crush.
Diet: May ↓ abs of Fe. ↓ abs of Vit B_{12}.
Oral/GI: ↓ GASTRIC ACID SECRETION, ↑ GASTRIC pH, nausea, abdominal pain, diarrhea.
S/Cond: Not c̄ lactation. 97% serum pro bound.
Blood/Serum: Possible ↓ Vit B_{12}.
<1% ↑ SGOT, ↑ SGPT, ↑ alk phos, ↑ crea, dyscrasias.

Larodopa ANTIPARKINSON See **levodopa p 116**

Lasix DIURETIC See **furosemide p 96**

Ledercillin ANTIBIOTIC See **penicillin p 155**

Lente Insulin ANTIDIABETIC, HYPOGLYCEMIC See **insulin p 108**

Lescol ANTIHYPERLIPIDEMIC See **fluvastatin p 94**

Leukeran ANTINEOPLASTIC See **chlorambucil p 48**

leuprolide acetate
Lupron
Soln— benzyl alcohol
Pwd— mannitol

ANTINEOPLASTIC, ANTIENDOMETRIOSIS, Hormone

Parenteral only (IM or SC)

Nutr: Anorexia, ↓ or ↑ wt, ↑ thirst. **Oral/GI:** Dry mouth, sour taste, dysphagia, N/V, GI bleeding, constipation, diarrhea.
S/Cond: Not c̄ lactation. **Other:** HOT FLASHES, ↓ BONE DENSITY, peripheral edema, headache, dizziness, bone pain, weakness.
Blood/Serum: Anemia, ↓ WBC, ↑ SGOT, ↑ LDH, ↑ alk phos, ↑ Ca, ↑ TG, ↑ chol, ↑ LDL, ↓ HDL. **Urinary:** Dysuria, blood, ↑ frequency.

levodopa
Dopar
Cap— tartrazine, lactose
Larodopa

ANTIPARKINSON

Drug: May take c̄ low pro food or juice to ↓ GI distress. Not c̄ high pro food. Protein re-distribution diet of 7:1 CHO to pro may stabilize drug effects.[35,36]
Diet: Limit Pyr to < 5 mg/day (may ↓ drug effect).[1]
Not c̄ amino acids or protein hydrolysates. Take Fe suppl separately (↓ abs of drug).[9b]
Nutr: ANOREXIA, ↓ wt. **Oral/GI:** Dry mouth, TASTE LOSS, ↑ salivation, bitter taste, dysphagia, N/V (80%), epigastric distress, constipation, flatulence. Rare GI ulcers & bleeding. **S/Cond:** Not c̄ lactation.
Other: DYSKINESIA c̄ LT use, FLUSHING, dizziness, ataxia, headache, weakness, insomnia, fatigue, psychological changes, rash, blurred vision.
Blood/Serum: Infrequent— ↓ Hgb, ↓ HCT. Transient ↑ BUN, ↑ SGOT, ↑ SGPT, ↑ alk phos, ↑ LDH, ↑ bil, ↓ K, ↓ WBC.
Urinary: Dark color, false ↓ or ↑ glucose. Retention.
Monitor: CBC, hepatic, renal & cardiovascular func.

levodopa & carbidopa
Sinemet
Tab— starch
Sinemet-CR
sustained release

ANTIPARKINSON — See **levodopa above**

Carbidopa c̄ levodopa ↑ availability of levodopa to the brain by ↓ decarboxylation of levodopa to dopamine. Lower doses of levodopa are needed. Lower dose ↓ incidence of N/V (15%), anorexia, & constipation. Carbiopa prevents negative Pyr effect.
Drug: May break CR tab in 1/2, do not crush or chew.
Diet: No need to limit Pyr.

Levothroid
levothyroxine sodium
Levoxyl

THYROID HORMONE (T_4) — See **thyroid p 196**

Librium

ANTIANXIETY, Benzodiazepine — See **chlordiazepoxide p 48**

Lioresal

ANTISPASMODIC — See **baclofen p 32**

lisinopril
Prinivil
Tab— mannitol
Zestril
Tab— mannitol

ANTIHYPERTENSIVE, ACE Inhibitor

Drug: Take s̄ regard to food. **Diet:** ↓ Na, ↓ cal diet may be recommended. Avoid salt subs. Caution c̄ K suppl. Avoid natural licorice.
Oral/GI: N/V, dyspepsia, diarrhea.
S/Cond: Limit alcohol. Caution c̄ lactation. **Other:** COUGH, dizziness, headache, ↓ BP, chest pain, weakness, rash, edema, paresthesia, gout, angioedema (rare, can be fatal). **Blood/Serum:** ↑ K, ↓ Na, slightly ↓ Hgb/HCT, ↑ BUN, ↑ crea, ↑ uric acid. Rare dyscrasias, ↑ SGOT, ↑ SGPT, ↑ bil. **Monitor:** BP, renal func.

lithium carbonate
Eskalith
Cap, Tab— lactose
Cap— benzyl alcohol
Lithane
Tab— tartrazine
Lithonate
Lithotabs

ANTIMANIC

Drug: Take c̄ meals to ↓ GI distress. Swallow SR tab whole. **Diet:** Drink 2-3 L fluid/day. Na intake affects renal clearance of drug 30-50 %. Consistent Na intake stabilizes drug levels. Limit xanthine/caffeine, see p 240. Avoid Iodine suppl—↑ risk of hypothyroidism **Nutr:** ↑ THIRST, ↑ WT, anorexia, ↓ wt. **Oral/GI:** DRY MOUTH, metallic taste, N/V, bloating, diarrhea. **S/Cond:** Limit alcohol.[9b] Not c̄ lactation. Syrup precipitates tube feedings.[8] **Other:** FATIGUE, WEAKNESS, CONFUSION, HAND TREMOR, HEADACHE, EDEMA, DIZZINESS, ↑ muscle irritability, goiter, cogwheel rigidity, acne, hypothyroidism.
Blood/Serum: ↑ WHITE BLOOD CELLS, ↑ PLATELETS, ↓ T_4, ↓ T_3, ↑ TSH, ↑ Ca, ↑ P, ↑ PTH, ↑ Mg. **Urinary:** POLYURIA, incontinence, pro.
Monitor: Li levels, thyroid & renal func, Ca, P, Na, WBC c̄ diff.

Lodine — NSAID — See **etodolac p 86**

Loestrin — CONTRACEPTIVE, oral — See **estrogen p 83**

lomefloxacin HCl
Maxaquin

ANTIBIOTIC, Fluoroquinolone — See listing for **ofloxacin p 146**
Tab— lactose — **Other:** Higher incidence of photosensitivity.

Lomotil
diphenoxylate HCl
c̄ **atropine sulfate**
Tab— sucrose, sorbitol

ANTIDIARRHEAL

Drug: May take c̄ food to ↓ GI distress. **Diet:** Diarrhea may ↑ fluid & electrolyte needs. **Nutr:** Anorexia. **Oral/GI:** Dry mouth, sore/swollen gums, N/V, cramps, bloating, constipation, toxic megacolon.
S/Cond: Avoid alcohol. Caution c̄ lactation. Not c̄ pseudomembranous

Liquid— 15% alcohol, 1.8 g sorbitol/5 mL

colitis. Caution $\bar{c}$ children— may mask dehydration or electrolyte imbalance. **Other:** Drowsiness, dizziness, blurred vision, confusion, depression, headache, pancreatitis.
Blood/Serum: ↑ amylase.
Monitor: Fluid & electrolytes.

Loniten ANTIHYPERTENSIVE See **minoxidil p 134**

Lo/Ovral CONTRACEPTIVE, oral See **estrogen p 83**

loperamide HCl
Imodium
Imodium AD
Cap— lactose
Tab— lactose
Liquid— 5.25% alcohol

ANTIDIARRHEAL
Diet: Diarrhea may ↑ fluid & electrolyte needs.
Oral/GI: Dry mouth, N/V, abdominal pains, bloating, constipation.
S/Cond: Caution $\bar{c}$ lactation. Not $\bar{c}$ pseudomembranous colitis. Caution $\bar{c}$ children — may mask dehydration or electrolyte imbalance. 97% serum pro bound.
Other: Drowsiness, dizziness, rash, fatigue.
Monitor: Fluid & electrolytes.

Lopid ANTIHYPERLIPIDEMIC See **gemfibrozil p 98**

Lopressor ANTIHYPERTENSIVE See **metoprolol tartrate p 131**

loracarbef **Lorabid** Susp— sucrose	ANTIBIOTIC, Carbacephem **Drug:** Take on empty stomach 1 hr before or 2 hrs after food. **Nutr:** Anorexia (1% in adults). **Oral/GI:** N/V, abdominal pain, diarrhea. **S/Cond:** Caution c̄ lactation. **Other:** Drowsiness, headache, rash. **Blood/Serum:** <1 % transient dyscrasias, ↑ SGOT, ↑ SGPT, ↑ alk phos, ↑ LDH, ↑ BUN, ↑ crea, ↑ PT.
loratadine **Claritin** Tab - lactose	ANTIHISTAMINE H_1-Receptor Antagonist **Drug:** Take on empty stomach once a day. **Oral/GI:** Dry mouth. **S/Cond:** Not c̄ lactation. **Other:** Headache, drowsiness, fatigue.
lorazepam **Ativan** Tab— lactose Intensol- alcohol free Parenteral— 2 % benzyl alcohol	ANTIANXIETY, Benzodiazepine Oral or Parenteral (IM & IV) **Drug:** May take c̄ food to ↓ GI distress. Dilute intensol in H_2O, juice, soda or semi-solid food. **Diet**: Limit caffeine to < 500 mg/ day,[9b] see p 240. **Oral/GI:** Dry mouth, nausea, constipation. **S/Cond:** Avoid alcohol. Not c̄ lactation. May be habit forming c̄ LT use. **Other:** Sedation, dizziness, weakness, ataxia, blurred vision. **Blood/Serum:** ↑ LDH, ↓ WBC. **Monitor:** CBC c̄ diff & hepatic func c̄ LT use.
Lorcet	ANALGESIC, Narcotic See listing for **oxycodone p 150** **hydrocodone** & **acetaminophen** & **acetaminophen p 17**
losartan **Cozaar** Tab— lactose,	ANTIHYPERTENSIVE, Angiotensin II Receptor Antagonist **Drug:** Take s̄ regard to food. **Diet:** ↓ Na, ↓ cal may be recommended. Avoid natural licorice. **S/Cond:** Not c̄ lactation. > 98% serum pro bound.

starch

Other: Dizziness, leg pain, upper respiratory infection. **Blood/Serum:** Slightly ↓ Hgb, ↓ HCT. < 1% slightly ↑ BUN, ↑ crea, ↑ SGOT, ↑ SGPT, ↑ bil.

Lotensin

ANTIHYPERTENSIVE, ACE Inhibitor

See **benazepril p 32**

lovastatin
Mevacor
Tab— lactose, starch

ANTIHYPERLIPIDEMIC, HMG-CoA Reductase Inhibitor

Drug: Take c̄ meals to ↑ abs. If single dose, take c̄ evening meal. **Diet:** ↓ fat, ↓ chol. (↓ cal if wt loss needed). Separate fiber, pectin or oat bran from drug by several hrs (↓ abs).[33] Not c̄ high dose Nia — possible myopathy. **Oral/GI:** Nausea, dyspepsia, abdominal pain, constipation, flatulence. **S/Cond:** Limit alcohol. Not c̄ lactation. **Other:** Headache, rash, blurred vision, dizziness, muscle pain, insomnia. **Blood/Serum:** ↓ CHOL, ↓ LDL, ↓ VLDL, ↑ HDL, ↓ TG, ↑ CPK, ↑ SGOT, ↑ SGPT. **Monitor:** Chol, CPK, hepatic func.

loxapine HCl
Loxitane
Cap— lactose

ANTIPSYCHOTIC, Dibenzoxazepine — Oral or Parenteral (IM)

Drug: Take c̄ food or 8 oz H_2O or milk to ↓ GI distress. Dilute soln in at least 60 mL orange or grapefruit juice. **Nutr:** ↑ or ↓ wt. **Oral/GI:** Dry mouth, N/V, constipation. **S/Cond:** Avoid alcohol. Not c̄ lactation. ↑ risk of dental problems, see p 9 & 14. **Other:** EPS, drowsiness, blurred vision, ↓ BP, confusion, dizziness. Tardive dyskinesia c̄ LT use. **Blood/Serum:** ↑ alk phos, ↑ SGOT, ↑ SGPT. Rare dyscrasias. **Monitor:** CBC, hepatic func.

Lozol	ANTIHYPERTENSIVE, DIURETIC	See **indapamide p 107**
L-thyroxine	THYROID HORMONE (T4)	See **thyroid p 196**
Lupron	HORMONE	See **leuprolide acetate p 116**
Luride	MINERAL SUPPLEMENT	See **fluoride p 91**
Luvox	ANTI-OCD, SSRI	See **fluvoxamine p 94**
Maalox	ANTACID	See **aluminum hydroxide & magnesium hydroxide p 23**
Maalox Plus plus simethicone	ANTACID, ANTIFLATULENT **S/Cond:** Thickens tube feedings.[8]	See **aluminum hydroxide & magnesium hydroxide p 23**
Macrobid (SR) **Macrodantin**	ANTIBIOTIC, urinary macrocrystals	See **nitrofurantoin p 143**

magnesium — MINERAL SUPPLEMENT, ANTACID, LAXATIVE

Magonate (Mg Gluconate)
27 mg/Tab
54 mg/5 mL Soln
Mag-Ox (MgO)
241 mg/Tab
Slow-Mag (SR MgCl)
64 mg/Tab

Drug: As antacid— take after meals & HS. As Mg suppl— 5 mg/kg/day recommended.[1] **Diet:** Take Fol or Fe suppl separately by 2 hrs. Do not take c̄ high phytate food, see p 242. See Mg sources, p 247. **Nutr:** RDA— Men = 350 mg; Women = 280; Pregnant = 320; Lactation = 355-340. ↓ bone calcification c̄ LT use.[2] **Oral/GI:** Chalky taste, N/V, cramps, diarrhea. **S/Cond:** Not c̄ ESRD. High alcohol intake ↑ Mg need by ↑ excretion.[13] **Blood/Serum:** ↑ Mg, ↓ Ca.[31] **Monitor:** Mg c̄ use as suppl.

Mandelamine ANTIBIOTIC, urinary See **methenamine mandelate p 128**

Mandol ANTIBIOTIC, cefamandole nafate See **cephalosporins p 46**

Marinol ANTIEMETIC See **dronabinol p 78**

Maxaquin ANTIBIOTIC, Fluoroquinolone See listing for **ofloxacin p 146**

Maxzide ANTIHYPERTENSIVE, DIURETIC See **triamterene p 200 & hydrochlorothiazide p 102**

mechlorethamine HCl ANTINEOPLASTIC, Alkylating Agent, Nitrogen Mustard
Mustargen
Parenteral only (IV or Intracavitary)

Diet: Encourage ↑ fluids to ↑ uric acid excretion.
Nutr: Anorexia, dehydration.
Oral/GI: Stomatitis (rare), metallic taste, SEVERE N/V, diarrhea.
S/Cond: Not c̄ lactation. Do dental care cautiously, see p 10 & 14.
Other: BONE MARROW SUPPRESSION, herpes zoster, hearing loss, weakness, headache, drowsiness, dizziness, muscle paralysis, rash. Rare jaundice, nephropathy.
Blood/Serum: ↓ WHITE BLOOD CELLS, ↓ PLATELETS, anemia, ↑ uric acid, ↑ SGOT, ↑ SGPT, ↑ bil, ↑ LDH.
Monitor: Frequent CBC c̄ diff, hepatic func, renal func, uric acid.

meclizine HCl **Antivert** Tab— sucrose, starch	ANTINAUSEANT, ANTIVERTIGO **Drug:** May take c̄ food, H_2O or milk to ↓ GI distress. **Oral/GI:** Dry mouth/throat, constipation. **S/Cond:** Avoid alcohol. Caution c̄ lactation. **Other:** Drowsiness, fatigue, blurred vision.
Medrol	CORTICOSTEROID, methylprednisolone See **corticosteroids p 60**
medroxyprogesterone acetate **Cycrin** Tab— lactose **Provera** (oral) Tab— lactose, sucrose **Depo-Provera** (IM)	HORMONE (Progestin), CONTRACEPTIVE (IM), ANTINEOPLASTIC (IM) Oral or Parenteral (IM) **Drug:** Take s̄ regard to food. May take c̄ food to ↓ GI distress. **Nutr:** ↑ APPETITE, ↑ WEIGHT. **Oral/GI:** Nausea, bloating. **S/Cond:** Caution c̄ lactation. Caution c̄ diabetes— ↑ glucose. **Other:** EDEMA, depression, headache, drowsiness, weakness, insomnia, hot flashes. Rare thromboembolism. **Blood/Serum:** ↑ Na, ↓ HDL, ↑ LDL, ↑ alk phos, ↑ bil, ↑ SGOT, ↑ SGPT.
Mefoxin	ANTIBIOTIC, cefoxitin See **cephalosporins p 46**
megestrol acetate **Megace** Tab— lactose, starch Susp— sucrose, < 0.06% alcohol	ANTINEOPLASTIC, APPETITE STIMULANT for HIV, Hormone (progestin) See listing for **medroxyprogesterone acetate** above
Mellaril	ANTIPSYCHOTIC, Phenothiazine See **thioridazine HCl p 195**

melphalan
Alkeran
Tab— lactose, sucrose
Parenteral— 0.52 mL ethanol/ 10 mL

ANTINEOPLASTIC, Alkylating Agent, Nitrogen Mustard — Oral or Parenteral (IV)

Diet: Encourage ↑ fluids to ↑ uric acid excretion. Food significantly ↓ bioavailability. **Oral/GI:** Stomatitis (rare), mild N/V, diarrhea.
S/Cond: Not c̄ lactation. Do dental care cautiously, see p 10 & 14.
Other: BONE MARROW SUPPRESSION, rash. Rare nephropathy, hepatotoxicity c̄ IV, pulmonary fibrosis. **Blood/Serum:** ↓ WHITE BLOOD CELLS, ↓ PLATELETS, anemia, ↑ uric acid. **Urinary:** ↑ uric acid.
Monitor: Frequent CBC c̄ diff/ platelets, uric acid.

meperidine HCl
Demerol
Tab— starch
Syrup— glucose, saccharin
Generic parenteral— sulfites

ANALGESIC, Narcotic — Oral or Parenteral (IM or IV)

Drug: Dilute syrup in 4 oz H_2O. **Nutr:** Anorexia.
Oral/GI: Dry mouth, N/V, GI pain, constipation.
S/Cond: Avoid alcohol. Not c̄ lactation. May be habit forming c̄ LT use.
Other: Respiratory depression, drowsiness, dizziness, sedation, weakness, ↓ BP, headache, visual changes, confusion, tachycardia.
Blood/Serum: ↑ amylase, ↑ lipase. **Urinary:** Retention.

meprobamate
Equanil
Tab— lactose
Miltown
200 mg Tab— sugar

ANTIANXIETY

Drug: May take c̄ food to ↓ GI distress. **Oral/GI:** Dry mouth, N/V, diarrhea. **S/Cond:** Avoid alcohol. Not c̄ lactation. May be habit forming c̄ LT use. **Other:** Drowsiness, ataxia, dizziness, headache, blurred vision, weakness, edema, rash, paresthesia. **Blood/Serum:** Rare dyscrasias.

Mepron

ANTI-PCP in HIV — See **atovaquone p 30**

mercaptopurine **Purinethol** Tab— lactose	ANTINEOPLASTIC **Diet:** Encourage ↑ fluids to ↑ uric acid excretion. **Nutr:** ANOREXIA. **Oral/GI:** MILD N/V, GI ulcers, diarrhea. **S/Cond:**. Not c̄ lactation. **Other:** BONE MARROW SUPPRESSION, headache, weakness, rash, hepatotoxicity, nephropathy. **Blood/Serum:** ↓ WHITE BLOOD CELLS, ↓ PLATELETS, ANEMIA, ↑ uric acid, ↑ bil, ↑ SGOT, ↑ SGPT, ↑ alk phos. False ↑ glucose c̄ SMA. **Urinary:** ↑ uric acid. **Monitor:** CBC c̄ diff weekly, hepatic func, uric acid.
mesalamine (5 ASA) **Asacol** (SR) Tab— lactose **Pentasa** (SR) Cap— starch, sugar **Rowasa** (rectal) Susp— sulfite	ANTI-INFLAMMATORY (in ulcerative colitis) Oral or Rectal **Drug:** Use rectal form HS. Swallow tab/cap whole c̄ 8 oz H_2O. Do not break or crush. **Nutrition:** Anorexia. **Oral/GI:** N/V, dyspepsia, abdominal cramps, diarrhea, flatulence. **S/Cond:** Not c̄ lactation. **Other:** Headache, weakness, rash, fever. Rare hepatitis, pancreatitis. **Blood/Serum:** ↑ SGOT, ↑ SGPT, ↑ alk phos, ↑ BUN, ↑ crea, ↑ amylase, ↑ lipase.
mesoridazine **Serentil** Conc— 0.6% alcohol, sorbitol Tab— all strengths— lactose, sucrose. 50 & 100 mg— starch	ANTIPSYCHOTIC, Phenothiazine Oral or Parenteral (IM) **Drug:** The active metabolite of thioridazine. See listing for **thioridazine p 195**
Metamucil	LAXATIVE, bulk forming See **psyllium p 171**

metaproterenol sulfate **Alupent** **Metaprel** Syrup— saccharin, sorbitol Tab— lactose	BRONCHODILATOR, Sympathomimetic — Oral or Inhalant **Drug:** May take c̄ food to ↓ GI distress. **Diet:** Limit caffeine, see p 240. **Oral/GI:** Dry mouth/throat, N/V, dyspepsia, diarrhea. **S/Cond:** Caution c̄ lactation. Caution c̄ HTN. **Other:** NERVOUSNESS, tachycardia, tremor, headache, ↑ BP, dizziness, insomnia, muscle cramps, weakness, cough.
metformin **Glucophage**	ORAL HYPOGLYCEMIC, Biguanide **Drug:** Take with meals to ↓ GI distress. **Diet:** Prescribed ADA diet. **Nutr:** Anorexia. Stable or ↓ wt. ↓ Vit B_{12} abs.[9a] **Oral/GI:** Metallic taste, NAUSEA/VOMITING, BLOATING, DIARRHEA, FLATULENCE. **S/Cond:** Limit alcohol. Not c̄ lactation. **Blood/Serum:** ↓ GLUCOSE, ↓ GLY HGB, ↓ CHOL, ↓ LDL, ↓ TG, ↑ HDL, ↓B_{12}. **Monitor:** Glucose, glycosylated Hgb, possibly B_{12}.
methadone HCl **Dolophine** Tab— lactose, sucrose **Methadone** Soln — 8% alcohol, sorbitol	ANALGESIC, Narcotic — Oral or Parenteral (IM or SC) **Drug:** Dissolve dispersible tab in fruit juice or H_2O. Dilute conc c̄ H_2O. **Nutr:** Anorexia. **Oral/GI:** Dry mouth, N/V, cramps, constipation. **S/Cond:** Avoid alcohol. Not c̄ lactation. May be habit forming c̄ LT use. **Other:** RESPIRATORY DEPRESSION, DROWSINESS, dizziness, ↓ BP, headache, confusion, flushing, edema, visual changes, nervousness, rash. **Blood/Serum:** ↑ amylase, ↑ lipase, ↑ T_4, ↑ T_3.[7]

See "Guide to the Use of This Book" inside front cover.

methenamine mandelate
Mandelamine

ANTIBIOTIC, urinary
Drug: Take with food to ↓ GI distress. Swallow tab whole. Maintain urine pH < 5.5.
Diet: Insure adequate fluid intake, but not copious amts. Avoid urinary alkalinizers eg Ca or Mg antacids or suppl.[13]
Nutr: Anorexia. **Oral/GI:** Stomatitis, N/V, dyspepsia, cramps.
S/Cond: Not c̄ lactation.[6] Susp precipitates tube feeding.[8]
Other: Headache.
Urinary: False ↑ VMA. **Monitor:** Urinary pH.

methicillin sodium
Staphcillin
69 mg Na/g pwd

ANTIBIOTIC, Penicillin (penicillinase resistant) Parenteral only (IM or IV)
Oral/GI: N/V, diarrhea. Rare pseudomembranous colitis, oral candidiasis, stomatitis. **S/Cond:** Not c̄ lactation.
Other: Rash, NEPHRITIS, weakness, headache.
Blood/Serum: Dyscrasias, EOSINOPHILIA, ↑ BUN, ↑ crea.
Monitor: CBC c̄ diff, hepatic & renal func.

methocarbamol
Robaxin
Tab— saccharin

MUSCLE RELAXANT Oral or Parenteral (IM or IV)
Drug: Tab may be crushed, mixed c̄ food or liquid. **Nutr:** Anorexia.
Oral/GI: Metallic taste, N/V, GI upset.
S/Cond: Avoid alcohol. Not c̄ lactation.
Other: Drowsiness, dizziness, blurred vision, ↓ BP, fever, headache, rash.
Blood/Serum: ↓ Hgb (IV only). Rare ↓ WBC.
Urinary: Dark color, RBC.

methotrexate
Methotrexate
IV— 50 mg Na/10 mL, 161 mg Na/1g vial, benzyl alcohol
Tab— lactose
Rheumatrex
Tab— lactose

ANTINEOPLASTIC, ANTIPSORIATRIC, ANTIARTHRITIC
Oral or Parenteral (IV)

Diet: Encourage ↑ fluid intake to ↑ urine output. Food delays abs, ↓ peak conc & bioavailability.
Nutr: May ↓ abs of fat, Vit B_{12}, Ca, Fol.[11] ANOREXIA, ↓ wt.
Oral/GI: STOMATITIS, gingivitis, altered taste, N/V, diarrhea, hemorrhagic enteritis. **S/Cond:** Avoid alcohol. Not c̄ lactation. Do dental care cautiously, see p 10 & 14.
Other: BONE MARROW SUPPRESSION, infection, nephropathy, hepatotoxicity, headache, dizziness, drowsiness, rash, pulmonary toxicity.
Blood/Serum: ↓ WHITE BLOOD CELLS, ↓ PLATELETS, ANEMIA, ↑ uric acid, ↑ SGOT, ↑ SGPT, ↑ bil, ↑ BUN.
Urinary: ↑ uric acid.
Monitor: CBC c̄ diff, platelets, alb, hepatic & renal func.

methylcellulose
Citrucel
Pwd— sucrose
Sugar Free Pwd— asparatame

LAXATIVE, Bulk Forming

Drug: Take c̄ 8 oz H_2O or other liquid.Do not swallow dry pwd.
Diet: High fiber c̄ 1500-2000 mL fluid/day to prevent constipation.
Oral/GI: ↑ PERISTALSIS & BOWEL MOTILITY. Rare bowel obstruction.
S/Cond: Not c̄ dysphagia. Use sugar free form with diabetes.

methyldopa
Aldomet
Susp & Parenteral— sulfites
Susp— 1% alcohol, sugar

ANTIHYPERTENSIVE — Oral or Parenteral (IV)

Diet: ↓ Na, ↓ cal may be recommended. Avoid natural licorice. Take Fe suppl separately by 2 hrs (↓ abs of drug).[9b] **Nutr:** ↑ need for Vit B_{12}, & Fol c̄ high dose.[12] **Oral/GI:** Dry mouth, sore/black tongue, N/V, diarrhea. **S/Cond:** Avoid alcohol. Caution c̄ lactation. ↑ risk of dental problems, see p 9 & 14. Caution c̄ G_6PD def— ↑ risk of hemolytic anemia. **Other:** SEDATION, DROWSINESS, headache, peripheral edema, fever, ↓ BP, blurred vision, weakness, rash, Parkinsonism, ↓ mental acuity, lupus-like syndrome. Rare hepatitis or pancreatitis (can be fatal). **Blood/Serum:** ↑ alk phos, ↑ SGOT, ↑ SGPT, ↑ bil, + Coombs test, ↑ uric acid, ↑ BUN, ↑ amylase, ↑ K, ↑ Na, ↑ prolactin, hemolytic anemia, ↑ PT, + ANA. Rare dyscrasias. **Urinary:** ↑ uric acid. **Monitor:** CBC, hepatic, Coombs test.

methylphenidate HCl
Ritalin
Tab— lactose, sucrose, 5 & 10 mg Tab- starch
SR Tab— lactose

ANTI-ADHD, ANTI-NARCOLEPSY, Stimulant

Drug: Take s̄ regard to meals[1,7] no later than 6 PM. Swallow SR tab whole. **Diet:** Insure adequate cal intake. Limit caffeine, see p 240. **Nutr:** ANOREXIA, ↓ wt, ↓ GROWTH c̄ LT USE. **Oral/GI:** Dry throat, nausea, abdominal pain. **S/Cond:** Avoid alcohol. Caution c̄ lactation. Caution c̄ HTN. May be habit forming c̄ LT high dose. **Other:** ↑ BP, NERVOUSNESS, INSOMNIA, tachycardia, rash, dizziness, drowsiness, headache. **Monitor:** CBC c̄ diff & platelets c̄ LT use. BP. Children's growth.

methylprednisolone — CORTICOSTEROID — See **corticosteroids p 60**

metoclopramide HCl
Reglan
Tab 5 mg— lactose
Tab 10 mg— mannitol
Syrup— sorbitol

ANTIEMETIC, ANTI-GERD, Dopamine Antagonist
Oral or Parenteral (IM or IV)

Drug: Take 1/2 hr before meals & HS. **Oral/GI:** Dry mouth, nausea, diarrhea, constipation. **S/Cond:** Avoid alcohol. Caution c̄ lactation. Caution c̄ diabetes—- may alter insulin requirements. Incompatible c̄ some tube feedings.[32] **Other:** Restlessness, drowsiness, fatigue, dizziness, headache, galactorrhea, transient edema.
Rare EPS (↑ incidence in children, young adults).
Rare tardive dyskinesia c̄ LT use (↑ incidence in elderly).
Blood/Serum: ↑ prolactin. Transient ↑ aldosterone.

metolazone
Zaroxolyn

ANTIHYPERTENSIVE, DIURETIC See listing for **hydrochlorothiazide p 102**
Thiazide-like (K-depleting) Generally prescribed c̄ loop diuretic. The combination causes severe K depletion.

metoprolol tartrate
Lopressor
Tab— lactose

ANTIHYPERTENSIVE, ANTIANGINAL, Cardioselective Beta-Blocker
Oral or Parenteral (IV)

Drug: Take c̄ food to ↑ bioavailability. **Diet:** ↓ Na, ↓ cal may be recommended. Avoid natural licorice. **Oral/GI:** Dry mouth, nausea, dyspepsia, flatulence, diarrhea, constipation. **S/Cond:** Caution c̄ lactation. Caution c̄ diabetes— may mask signs of hypoglycemia. **Other:** Confusion, fatigue, dizziness, insomnia, depression, rash, ↓ BP, peripheral edema, bradycardia, headache.
Blood/Serum: ↑ SGOT, ↑ SGPT, ↑ alk phos, ↑ LDH, ↑ K, ↑ TG, ↑ uric acid. **Monitor:** BP.

metronidazole
Flagyl
RTU IV—
322 mg Na/100 mL, mannitol

ANTIBIOTIC, AMEBICIDE, ANTITRICHOMONAL Oral or Parenteral (IV)

Drug: May take c̄ meals to ↓ GI distress. **Diet:** Consider Na content c̄ ↓ Na diet. **Nutr:** Anorexia. **Oral/GI:** Dry mouth, stomatitis, metallic taste, N/V, epigastric distress, diarrhea.

S/Cond: Avoid all alcohol (disulfiram-like reaction). Not c̄ lactation. ↑ risk of dental problems, see p 9, 10 & 14.

Other: Dizziness, headache, ataxia, confusion, rash. Rare peripheral neuropathy, seizures c̄ high dose.

Mevacor

ANTIHYPERLIPIDEMIC, HMG-CoA Reductase Inhibitor See **lovastatin p 121**

mezlocillin
Mezlin

ANTIBIOTIC, Penicillin See listing for **ticarcillin disodium p197**
43 mg Na/g
Parenteral only (IM or IV)

Miacalcin

Ca REGULATOR, Hormone See **calcitonin p 39**

miconazole
Monistat i.v.
Castor Oil

ANTIFUNGAL Parenteral (IV)

Oral/GI: Bitter taste, N/V, diarrhea. **Nutr:** Anorexia. **S/Cond:** Caution c̄ diabetics on sulfonylureas— hypoglycemia.[6] 91-93% serum pro bound.

Other: PHLEBITIS, ITCHING, fever & chills, rash, headache, dizziness, drowsiness, flushing, blurred vision.

Blood/Serum: Transient ↓ HCT, ↑ chol, ↑ TG. Rare ↓ Na, dyscrasias.

Monitor: Hgb, HCT, electrolytes, lipids.

Micro-K

ELECTROLYTE, Potassium Supplement See **potassium chloride p 164**

Micronase — ORAL HYPOGLYCEMIC, Sulfonylurea — See **glyburide p 99**

Midol IB — NSAID — See **ibuprofen p 104**

Milk of Magnesia (MOM)
Philip's MOM
0.12 mg Na/Tab or tsp
Tab— sucrose
Conc— sucrose, sorbitol
Liquid— saccharin, 972 mg Mg/30 mL

LAXATIVE, ANTACID, Magnesium Hydroxide

Drug: Take each dose c̄ 8 oz H_2O or citrus juice (to improve taste). **Diet:** High fiber c̄ 1500-2000 mL fluid/day to prevent constipation. Take Fe suppl separately by 2 hrs. **Nutr:** 15-30% of Mg is abs. **Oral/GI:** Chalky taste, nausea, cramping, diarrhea. Laxative dependence c̄ LT use. **S/Cond:** Caution c̄ ESRD— ↑ Mg. **Monitor:** Electrolytes & Mg c̄ LT use.

Miltown — ANTIANXIETY — See **meprobamate p 125**

mineral oil
Agoral plain
7 mg Na/15 mL, sugar free, egg albumin

LUBRICANT LAXATIVE

Drug: Take on empty stomach 2 hrs away from food. Do not take HS—may cause lipid pneumonitis due to oil aspiration. **Diet:** High fiber c̄ 1500-2000 mL fluid/day to prevent constipation. **Nutr:** May ↓ abs of fat soluble Vits (A, D, E, & K) & Ca, P, K.[27] ↓ wt, anorexia.[14] **Oral/GI:** Belching, nausea, dyspepsia, cramps, flatulence, diarrhea. **S/Cond:** Not c̄ dysphagia. Avoid LT continuous use.

Minipress — ANTIHYPERTENSIVE — See **prazosin HCl p 165**

minocycline HCl
Minocin
Susp— 5% alcohol, Na sulfites saccharin, 6 g sorbitol/5 mL

ANTIBIOTIC, Tetracycline — See listing for **tetracycline HCl p 194**
Oral or Parenteral (IV)

Drug: Unlike tetracycline, may be taken c̄ food or milk.
Other: ↑ CNS effects— dizziness, ataxia, headache, drowsiness.[6]
Blood/Serum: Does not ↑ BUN.[13]

minoxidil
Loniten
Tab— lactose

ANTIHYPERTENSIVE, Arterial Vasodilator
Diet: ↓ Na, ↓ cal may be recommended. Avoid natural licorice.
Oral/GI: N/V, bloating. **S/Cond:** Not c̄ lactation. Caution c̄ diabetes— ↑ glucose.[18] **Other:** TACHYCARDIA, edema, ↓ BP, headache, fatigue. Paresthesia c̄ LT use. **Blood/Serum:** ↑ Na, ↑ alk phos. Transient ↓ HCT, ↓ Hgb, ↓ RBC, ↑ BUN, ↑ crea.
Monitor: Fluid & electrolyte balance, BP, daily wt.

misoprostol
Cytotec

ANTIULCER c̄ NSAID use, Gastric Mucosa Protectant
Drug: Take c̄ meals & HS. **Nutr:** Mg antacids/suppl— ↑ risk of diarrhea.
Oral/GI: ↓ GASTRIC ACID, N/V, dyspepsia, abdominal pain, flatulence, diarrhea, constipation.
S/Cond: Not c̄ lactation. **Other:** Headache.

mitomycin
Mutamycin
5 mg vial— 10 mg mannitol
20 mg vial— 40 mg mannitol

ANTINEOPLASTIC — Parenteral only (IV)
Nutr: Anorexia, ↓ wt. **Oral/GI:** Stomatitis, N/V, diarrhea. **S/Cond:** Not c̄ lactation. Do dental care cautiously, see p 10 & 14. **Other:** BONE MARROW SUPPRESSION, fever, weakness, fatigue, confusion, headache, blurred vision, hemolytic uremic syndrome c̄ high dose. Rare pulmonary toxicity (can be fatal). **Blood/Serum:** ↓ PLATELETS, ↓ WHITE BLOOD CELLS,

40 mg vial—
80 mg mannitol

anemia, ↑ BUN, ↑ crea, ↑ Ca.[48]
Monitor: Frequent CBC c̄ diff, platelets. Renal func. Blood smears for fragmented RBC c̄ LT, high dose.

mitoxantrone
Novantrone
3.2 mg Na/mL

ANTINEOPLASTIC — Parenteral only (IV)
Diet: Encourage ↑ fluids to ↑ uric acid excretion. **Oral/GI:** STOMATITIS, NAUSEA/VOMITING, abdominal pain, GI bleeding, DIARRHEA. **S/Cond:** Not c̄ lactation. Do dental care cautiously, see p 10 & 14. **Other:** BONE MARROW SUPPRESSION, FEVER, headache, cough, jaundice, seizures. **Blood/Serum:** ↓ PLATELETS, ↓ WHITE BLOOD CELLS, anemia, ↑ SGPT, ↑ SGOT, ↑ LDH, ↑ bil, ↑ uric acid. **Urinary:** ↑ uric acid. **Monitor:** CBC, platelets, hepatic func, uric acid.

Moban

ANTIPSYCHOTIC, Dihydroindolone — See **molindone HCl below**

Moduretic
Tab— lactose

ANTIHYPERTENSIVE c̄ DIURETIC — See **amiloride HCl & hydrochlorothiazide p 24**

molindone HCl
Moban
Tab— lactose, calcium
Conc— sulfites, alcohol, sorbitol

ANTIPSYCHOTIC, Dihydroindolone
Drug: Take c̄ food or 8 oz milk or H_2O to ↓ GI distress. Mix conc c̄ ≥ 2 oz beverage. **Nutr:** Anorexia, ↓ wt. **Oral/GI:** Dry mouth, nausea, GI upset, constipation. **S/Cond:** Avoid alcohol. Caution c̄ lactation. ↑ risk of dental problems, see p 9 & 14. **Other:** DROWSINESS, restlessness, headache, blurred vision, EPS, tardive dyskinesia c̄ LT use, depression, dizziness, insomnia. **Blood/Serum:** ↑ or ↓ WBC, ↑ prolactin. **Urinary:** Retention.

Monistat i.v.	ANTIFUNGAL	See **miconazole p 132**
Monocid	ANTIBIOTIC, cefonicid sodium	See **cephalosporins p 46**
Monopril	ANTIHYPERTENSIVE, ACE Inhibitor	See **fosinopril sodium p 95**

morphine sulfate — ANALGESIC, Narcotic — Oral, Parenteral or rectal suppository

MS Contin (SR)
Tab— lactose
MSIR
Conc— sugar, sucrose
Cap— starch, lactose, sucrose

Drug: May take $\bar{c}$ food to ↓ GI distress. Swallow SR tab whole. Insure adequate fluid intake. **Nutr:** Anorexia. **Oral/GI:** Dry mouth, ↓ gastric motility, N/V, CONSTIPATION. **S/Cond:** Avoid alcohol. Not $\bar{c}$ lactation. ↑ risk of dental problems, see p 9 & 14. May be habit forming $\bar{c}$ LT use. **Other:** RESPIRATORY DEPRESSION, ↓ BP, DROWSINESS, sedation, dizziness, weakness, blurred vision, headache, confusion, rash, edema. **Blood/Serum:** ↑ amylase, ↑ lipase. **Urinary:** Retention.

Motrin	NSAID	See **ibuprofen p 104**
MS Contin	ANALGESIC, Narcotic	See **morphine above**
Mustargen	ANTINEOPLASTIC	See **mechlorethamine HCl p 123**
Mutamycin	ANTINEOPLASTIC	See **mitomycin p 134**
Myambutol	ANTITUBERCULAR	See **ethambutol HCl p 84**
Mycelex	ANTIFUNGAL	See **clotrimazole p 57**

Mycobutin ANTIBIOTIC, ANTI-MAC in HIV See **rifabutin p 176**

Mycostatin ANTIFUNGAL See **nystatin p 146**

Mylanta
Mylanta Double Strength ANTACID, ANTIFLATULENT See **aluminum hydroxide & magnesium hydroxide p 23**
contain simethicone
S/Cond: Mylanta Double Strength thickens some tube feedings.[8]

Mylanta Gas ANTIFLATULENT See **simethicone p 182**

Myleran ANTINEOPLASTIC See **busulfan p 38**

Mylicon ANTIFLATULENT See **simethicone p 182**

Myotonachol CHOLINERGIC STIMULANT See **bethanechol Cl p 34**

nabumetone
Relafen NSAID, ANALGESIC, ANTIARTHRITIC
Drug: Take c̄ food or milk to ↓ GI irritation & ↑ abs.
Diet: Caution c̄ GI irritants eg K suppl (↑ risk of GI irritation).
Oral/GI: Dry mouth, stomatitis, N/V, dyspepsia, gastritis, abdominal cramps, flatulence, diarrhea, constipation. Rare GI ulcers & bleeding (may be sudden & serious). **S/Cond:** Avoid alcohol. Not c̄ lactation. > 99% serum pro bound. **Other:** Headache, dizziness, edema, rash, drowsiness, insomnia, nervousness, photosensitivity. Rare-jaundice & hepatitis. **Blood/Serum:** ↑ SGOT, ↑ SGPT.
Monitor: Hepatic func LT use.

nadolol
Corgard

ANTIHYPERTENSIVE, ANTIANGINAL, Non-selective Beta-Blocker
Drug: May take s̄ regard to meals. **Diet:** ↓ Na, ↓ cal may be recommended. Avoid natural licorice. **S/Cond:** Limit alcohol. Not c̄ lactation. Caution c̄ diabetes— may mask symptoms of & prolong hypoglycemia. May inhibit insulin response to hyperglycemia.
Other: Dizziness, fatigue, depression. **Monitor:** BP.

nafcillin sodium
Parenteral— 67 mg Na/g
Nafcil (Parenteral)
Unipen
(Oral or Parenteral)
Tab— lactose

ANTIBIOTIC, Penicillin — Oral or Parenteral (IM or IV)
Drug: Take c̄ 8 oz H_2O 1 hr before or 2 hrs after food.
Diet: Consider Na content c̄ ↓ Na diet. **Oral/GI:** N/V, epigastric distress, diarrhea, flatulence. Rare pseudomembranous colitis.
S/Cond: Caution c̄ lactation. 90% serum pro bound. **Other:** Rash.
Blood/Serum: Eosinophilia, ↓ WBC c̄ LT use (> 10 days). False ↑ pro (method dependent). Transient c̄ IV— ↑ SGOT, ↑ SGPT, ↑ alk phos.
Urinary: False + pro (method dependent).
Monitor: Renal & hepatic func, CBC c̄ diff.

naltrexone HCl
ReVia
Tab— sugar

ALCOHOL ABUSE DETERRENT, NARCOTIC ANTAGONIST
Drug: May take c̄ food to ↓ GI distress. **Nutr:** Anorexia, ↓ wt, ↑ thirst.
Oral/GI: N/V, abdominal pain, cramps, constipation, diarrhea.
S/Cond: Caution c̄ lactation. **Other:** Insomnia, anxiety, muscle/joint pain, fatigue, headache, chills, rash, depression, drowsiness, dizziness.
Blood/Serum: ↑ SGOT, ↑ SGPT, ↑ LDH, ↑ LH, ↑ ACTH, ↑ cortisol.
Monitor: Hepatic func.

naproxen
Naprosyn
Susp— 8 mg Na/mL, sorbitol, sucrose, NaCl
naproxen sodium
Anaprox
275 mg tab— lactose, 25 mg Na
550 mg tab— 50 mg Na
Aleve— 20 mg Na

NSAID, ANTIARTHRITIC, ANALGESIC

Drug: Take c̄ food or milk to ↓ GI irritation. **Diet:** Consider Na content c̄ ↓ Na diet. Caution c̄ GI irritants eg K suppl (↑ risk of GI irritation).
Nutr: ↑ thirst. **Oral/GI:** Stomatitis, dry mouth, nausea, dyspepsia, GI pain, constipation, diarrhea. GI ulcers & bleeding (may be sudden & serious).
S/Cond: Avoid alcohol. Not c̄ lactation. 99% serum pro bound.
Other: Dizziness, drowsiness, headache, peripheral edema, blurred vision, rash. Rare jaundice & hepatitis. **Blood/Serum:** ↑ SGPT, ↑ SGOT, ↑ alk phos, ↑ BUN, ↑ crea, ↑ K. Rare dyscrasias.
Monitor: CBC, hepatic & renal func c̄ LT use.

Nardil	ANTIDEPRESSANT	See **phenelzine sulfate p 158**
Nasalcrom	ANTIASTHMA	See **cromolyn sodium p 61**
Navane	ANTIPSYCHOTIC	See **thiothixene p 196**
Navelbine	ANTINEOPLASTIC	See **vinorelbine tartrate p 208**
Nebcin	ANTIBIOTIC, Aminoglycoside	See **tobramycin sulfate p 197**
NebuPent	ANTIPROTOZOAL, aerosol	See **pentamidine isethionate p 156**

nefazodone
Serzone

ANTIDEPRESSANT
Drug: Food ↓ rate of abs & ↓ bioavailability 20%.
Nutr: ↑ appetite, ↑ thirst.
Oral/GI: Dry mouth, taste changes, N/V, dyspepsia, constipation, diarrhea.
S/Cond: Avoid alcohol. Caution $\bar{c}$ lactation. 99% serum pro bound.
Other: Weakness, drowsiness, dizziness, confusion, blurred vision, ↓ BP, headache, insomnia, edema, chills, fever, rash.

Neupogen — COLONY STIMULATING FACTOR — See **filgrastim p 89**

Neurontin — ANTICONVULSANT — See **gabapentin p 96**

Neutra-Phos — ACIDIFIER, PHOSPHOROUS SUPPLEMENT — See **phosphates p 162**

Neutrexin — ANTI-PCP in HIV, Folate Antagonist — See **trimetrexate glucuronate p 203**

niacin
nicotinic acid
Nicobid (SR)
Nicolar
Tab— tartrazine

niacinamide
(nicotinamide)

ANTIHYPERLIPIDEMIC, ANTIPELLAGRA, B Complex Vitamin
Drug: Only nicotinic acid form (1- 9 g/day) will ↓ lipids. Take $\bar{c}$ food or milk to ↓ GI distress. Swallow SR tab whole.
Diet: Antipellagra dose— 300-500 mg daily + 5 mg each Thi, Rib, Pyr. Both forms are vitamin suppls. As antihyperlipidemic— ↓ fat, ↓ chol diet.
Nutr: Adult RDA = 13-19 mg.
Lactation = 20 mg. 60 mg dietary tryptophan = 1 mg niacin.
Oral/GI: Dry mouth, N/V, peptic ulcer, dyspepsia, cramps,

Generic brands	diarrhea, flatulence. **S/Cond:** Not c̄ lactation in high doses. Caution c̄ diabetes— ↑ glucose. **Other:** FLUSHING, HEADACHE (nicotinic acid only). ITCHING, dizziness, arrhythmias, muscle pain, gout, jaundice & hepatotoxicity (↑ c̄ SR form at dose as low as 500 mg daily). **Blood/Serum:** High dose— ↑ glucose, ↑ glycosylated Hgb,[18] ↑ alk phos, ↑ SGOT, ↑ SGPT, ↑ bil, ↑ LDH, ↑ uric acid, ↑ CPK. Rare ↓ alb. Nicotinic acid only— ↓ CHOL, ↓ TG, ↓ VLDL, ↓ LDL, ↑ HDL. **Urinary:** False + glucose ($CuSO_4$).[13] **Monitor:** c̄ high dose— hepatic func, glucose, lipids, uric acid.
nicardipine **Cardene** **Cardene SR** Cap— lactose, starch	ANTIHYPERTENSIVE, ANTIANGINAL, Ca Channel Blocker **Drug:** Take on empty stomach. Swallow SR cap whole. **Diet:** High fat meal ↓ abs by 20-30%.[6] ↓ Na, ↓ cal may be recommended. Avoid natural licorice. Caution c̄ grapefruit juice— may ↑ drug effect.[50] **Oral/GI:** Dry mouth nausea, dyspepsia. **S/Cond:** Not c̄ lactation. > 95% pro bound. **Other:** ↓ BP, peripheral edema, flushing, dizziness, headache, weakness, drowsiness, palpitations. **Monitor:** BP.
Nicobid **Nicolar**	ANTIHYPERLIPIDEMIC — See **niacin above**
Nicoderm	SMOKING DETERRENT, skin patch — See **nicotine transdermal p 142**

nicotine polacrilex **Nicorette** Sugar free, sorbitol	SMOKING DETERRENT, gum **Drug:** Chew slowly & intermittently over 30 minutes. Do not swallow gum. Do not eat or drink within 15 minutes. May damage dental work. **Diet:** Limit caffeine. **Nutr:** ↓ appetite. **Oral/GI:** Unpleasant taste, ↑ salivation, mouth or throat irritation/ulcers, HICCUPS, N/V, dyspepsia, belching, diarrhea. **S/Cond:** Caution $\bar{c}$ lactation. Caution $\bar{c}$ insulin-dependent diabetes—↑ subcutaneous insulin abs. May be habit forming $\bar{c}$ LT use. Avoid all smoking. **Other:** Dizziness, headache, tremor, paresthesia, muscle pain. Rare arrhythmias.
nicotine transdermal system **Habitrol** **Nicoderm** **Nicotrol** **ProStep**	SMOKING DETERRENT, skin patch **Diet:** Limit caffeine. **Oral/GI:** Abdominal pain. **S/Cond:** Caution $\bar{c}$ lactation. Caution $\bar{c}$ insulin-dependent diabetes—↑ subcutaneous insulin abs. Avoid all smoking. **Other:** Drowsiness, rash, sweating.
nicotinic acid	ANTIHYPERLIPIDEMIC, B Complex Vitamin See **niacin p 140**
Nicotrol	SMOKING DETERRENT, skin patch See **nicotine transdermal above**

nifedipine **Adalat** 10 mg Cap— saccharin **Adalat CC** (SR) Tab— lactose **Procardia** 10 mg Cap— saccharin **Procardia XL** (SR) Tab— NaCl	ANTIANGINAL, ANTIHYPERTENSIVE (SR form), Ca Channel Blocker **Drug:** Swallow SR tab whole. Food may ↓ rate but not extent of abs of SR form.[13] **Diet:** ↓ Na, ↓ cal may be recommended. Avoid natural licorice. Grapefruit juice slightly ↑ bioavailability of drug (not clinically significant).[3, 50] **Oral/GI:** Sore throat, nausea, dyspepsia, constipation, flatulence. **S/Cond:** Avoid alcohol.[9b] Not c̄ lactation. **Other:** ↓ BP, flushing, edema, cough, dizziness, headache, weakness, tremor, palpitations, fatigue, blurred vision. Rare transient blindness at peak conc.[1] **Blood/Serum:** Rare dyscrasias, ↑ alk phos, ↑ SGOT, ↑ SGPT, ↑ LDH, + ANA. **Monitor:** BP.
nitrofurantoin **Macrobid** (SR) Cap— lactose **Macrodantin** Cap— lactose, starch	ANTIBIOTIC, urinary **Drug:** Take c̄ food or milk (ideally c̄ breakfast & dinner) to ↓ GI distress & ↑ bioavailability. Swallow SR cap whole. **Diet:** Adequate cal, pro, Vit B complex.[30] Mg suppl ↓ abs— take separately by 2 hrs. **Nutr:** Anorexia. **Oral/GI:** N/V, dyspepsia, abdominal pain, diarrhea, flatulence. **S/Cond:** Not c̄ lactation. Caution c̄ G6PD def— risk of hemolytic anemia. Not c̄ ESRD. **Other:** Headache. Rare hepatitis, peripheral neuropathy or pulmonary reactions (can be fatal). **Blood/Serum:** ↑ SGOT, ↑ SGPT, ↑ P. Rare ↓ Hgb, dyscrasias. **Urinary:** False + glucose ($CuSO_4$), dark color. **Monitor:** Pulmonary & hepatic func.

nitroglycerin ANTIANGINAL Oral, Parenteral (IV), patch, spray, ointment

Parenteral forms— alcohol
Nitro-Bid IV- parenteral
Nitro-Dur- patch
Nitrostat- sublingual
Tab— lactose, sucrose
Transderm-Nitro- patch

Drug: Consult pharmacist for proper administration. Take regular oral forms on empty stomach 1 hr before or 2 hrs after meals. Swallow SR forms whole. **Oral/GI:** N/V, abdominal pain.
S/Cond: Avoid alcohol. Caution c̄ lactation.
Other: HEADACHE, dizziness, ↓ BP, blurred vision, flushing, tachycardia.
Monitor: BP & heart rate.

nizatidine ANTIULCER, ANTIGERD, Antisecretory, Histamine H_2 Antagonist

Axid
Cap— starch

Drug: Take HS if once a day. **Diet:** Bland diet may be recommended. Limit caffeine/ xanthine, see p 240. **Nutr:** May ↓ Vit B12 abs.[74]
Oral/GI: ↓ GASTRIC ACID SECRETIONS, ↑ GASTRIC pH.
S/Cond: Avoid alcohol. Not c̄ lactation. Avoid or limit smoking.
Blood/Serum: Possible ↓ Vit B_{12} c̄ LT use. <1% ↑ SGOT, ↑ SGPT, ↑ alk phos ↑ uric acid, anemia. **Monitor:** Hepatic func.

Nizoral	ANTIFUNGAL	See **ketoconazole p 112**
NoDoz	STIMULANT	See **caffeine p 38**
Nolvadex	ANTINEOPLASTIC	See **tamoxifen citrate p 191**
Nordette	ORAL CONTRACEPTIVE	See **estrogen p 83**
Norinyl	ORAL CONTRACEPTIVE	See **estrogen p 83**

Normodyne ANTIHYPERTENSIVE See **labetalol HCl p 114**

Norpace ANTIARRHYTHMIC See **disopyramide p 75**

Norpramin ANTIDEPRESSANT See **desipramine HCl p 67**

nortriptyline HCl ANTIDEPRESSANT, Tricyclic See listing for **amitriptyline HCl p 25**
Pamelor Soln— 4% alcohol, 2 mg/mL sorbitol. Cap— benzyl alcohol, starch, 50 mg—sulfite

Nortriptyline is the metabolite of amitriptyline, but is less sedating & has lower anticholinergic effects.

Norvasc ANTIHYPERTENSIVE, Ca Channel Blocker See **amlodipine p 25**

Novantrone ANTINEOPLASTIC See **mitoxantrone p 135**

Novolin ANTIDIABETIC, HYPOGLYCEMIC See **insulin p 108**

NPH Insulin ANTIDIABETIC, HYPOGLYCEMIC See **insulin p 108**

Nydrazid ANTITUBERCULOSIS See **isoniazid p 110**

nystatin
Mycostatin
Susp— 1% alcohol, 2.5 g sucrose/5 mL
Pastille— sucrose, anise & cinnamon oils

ANTI-CANDIDIASIS, Antifungal
Drug: Take oral susp as directed. Retain oral drug in mouth as long as possible. Dissolve pastille slowly in mouth— do not chew.
Oral/GI: GI distress, N/V, stomach pain, diarrhea.
S/Cond: Do dental care cautiously, see p 10 & 14.

Nytol

SLEEP AID See **diphenhydramine HCl p 74**

octreotide acetate
Sandostatin

ANTIDIARRHEAL, ANTI-GROWTH HORMONE
ANTI-PITUITARY TUMOR — Parenteral only (SC or IV)
Drug: Inject between meals & HS to ↓ GI effects. **Nutr:** May cause fat & fat soluble vit malabsorption & delay gallbladder emptying. Alters insulin, growth hormone, thyroid hormone & glucagon levels. **Oral/GI:** N/V, abdominal pain, diarrhea, steatorrhea, constipation, flatulence.
S/Cond: Caution c̄ lactation. Caution c̄ diabetes— ↑ or ↓ glucose.
Other: GALLBLADDER ABNORMALITIES, hypothyroidism, goiter, headache, dizziness, edema, fatigue, flushing, weakness. **Blood/Serum:** ↓ T_4, ↑ or ↓ glucose, ↓ Vit B_{12}.[7] **Monitor:** c̄ LT use— Gallbladder by ultrasound, fecal fat & carotene, glucose, thyroid func, vit B_{12}.

ofloxacin
Floxin
Tab— lactose

ANTIBIOTIC, Fluoroquinolone — Oral or Parenteral (IV)
Drug: May take s̄ regard to food.[6] Take c̄ 8 oz H_2O. **Diet:** Insure liberal fluid intake. Take antacids, Mg, Ca, Fe or Zn suppl or MVI c̄ minerals separately by 2 hrs.[10] **Nutr:** ↓ appetite. **Oral/GI:** Dry mouth, taste loss, N/V, diarrhea, flatulence. Rare pseudomembranous colitis.

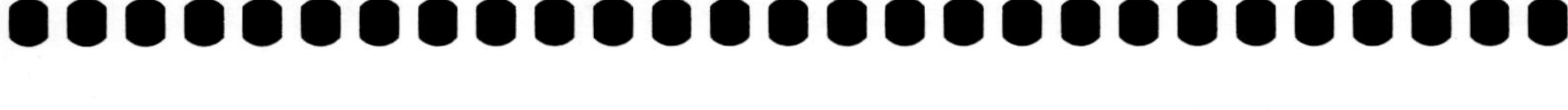

S/Cond: Not c̄ lactation. Caution c̄ diabetes— ↑ or ↓ glucose.[6]
Other: Headache, insomnia, dizziness, fatigue, visual changes, rash.
Blood/Serum: ↑ SGOT, ↑ SGPT, dyscrasias.
<1%— ↑ LDH, ↑ alk phos, ↑ bil, ↑ GGT, ↑ BUN, ↑ crea.
Urinary: < 1% ↑ pH, + glucose, pro, hematuria.
Monitor: Hepatic & renal func & CBC c̄ diff c̄ LT use.

Ogen — HORMONE — See **estrogen p 83**

olsalazine sodium
Dipentum — ANTI-INFLAMMATORY — See listing for **mesalamine p 126**
Drug: Take c̄ food.

omeprazole
Prilosec
Cap (delayed release)
lactose,
mannitol

ANTISECRETORY, ANTIGERD, Proton Pump Inhibitor
Drug: Take just before a meal, usually AM. Swallow whole. Do not open, chew or crush. **Diet:** May ↓ abs of Fe.[13] ↓ Vit B_{12} abs.[3] **Oral/GI:** ↓ GASTRIC ACID SECRETION, ↑ GASTRIC pH, constipation, diarrhea. **S/Cond:** Not c̄ lactation. 95% serum pro bound. **Other:** Headache, dizziness, cough, rash, back pain. Rare hepatitis, pancreatitis. **Blood/Serum:** Possible ↓ Vit B_{12}. < 1% ↑ SGOT, ↑ SGPT, ↑ alk phos, ↑ bil, ↑ crea, ↓ glucose.

Oncaspar — ANTINEOPLASTIC — See **pegaspargase p 153**

Oncovin — ANTINEOPLASTIC — See **vincristine sulfate p 207**

ondansetron HCl ANTIEMETIC Oral or Parenteral (IV)
Zofran
Tab— lactose, starch

Oral/GI: Dry mouth, abdominal pain, constipation, diarrhea.
S/Cond: Caution c̄ lactation. **Other:** Headache, weakness, fever/chills, rash, drowsiness. **Blood/Serum:** Transient ↑ SGOT, ↑ SGPT, ↑ bil. Rare ↓ K.

Oretic ANTIHYPERTENSIVE, DIURETIC See **hydrochlorothiazide p 102**

Organidin NR EXPECTORANT See **guaifenesin p 100**

Orinase ORAL HYPOGLYCEMIC See **tolbutamide p 198**

Ornade (SR) ANTIHISTAMINE DECONGESTANT See **chlorpheniramine maleate p 49 & phenylpropanolamine p 160**
Cap— lactose, starch, benzyl alcohol

Ortho-Cept ORAL CONTRACEPTIVE See **estrogen p 83**

Ortho-Cyclen ORAL CONTRACEPTIVE See **estrogen p 83**

Ortho-Novum ORAL CONTRACEPTIVE See **estrogen p 83**

Os-Cal CALCIUM SUPPLEMENT See **calcium carbonate p 40**

oxaprozin
Daypro
Tab— starch

NSAID, ANTIARTHRITIC

Drug: Take c̄ food or milk to ↓ GI irritation. **Diet:** Caution c̄ GI irritants eg K suppl (↑ risk of GI irritation).[13]

Nutr: Anorexia.

Oral/GI: N/V, dyspepsia, abdominal pain, constipation, diarrhea, flatulence, GI ulcers & bleeding (may be sudden & serious).

S/Cond: Avoid alcohol. Caution c̄ lactation. 99.9% serum albumin bound.

Other: Depression, drowsiness, sedation, confusion, insomnia, rash.

Blood/Serum: ↑ SGOT, ↑ SGPT, ↓ HGB, ↓ HCT, ↑ BUN, ↑ crea, ↓ uric acid.[13]

Urinary: Dysuria, ↑ frequency, ↑ uric acid.[13]

oxazepam
Serax
Cap— lactose
Tab— tartrazine, lactose

ANTIANXIETY, Benzodiazepine

Drug: May take c̄ food to ↓ GI effects. **Oral/GI:** Dry mouth (rare), nausea, constipation.

S/Cond: Avoid alcohol. Not c̄ lactation. May be habit forming c̄ LT use. 97% serum pro bound. Hypoalbuminemia (< 3 g/dL) may ↑ drug effects.[13] **Other:** Drowsiness, sedation, dizziness, ataxia. Rare jaundice & hepatitis.

Blood/Serum: Rare dyscrasias, anemia, ↑ LDH, ↑ alk phos, ↑ SGOT, ↑ SGPT.

Monitor: CBC c̄ diff & hepatic func c̄ LT use.

oxybutynin chloride
Ditropan
Tab— lactose
Syrup— sorbitol, sucrose

ANTISPASMODIC, ANTICHOLINERGIC, urinary
Drug: May take c̄ food or milk to ↓ GI distress. **Oral/GI:** DRY MOUTH & throat, dysphagia, N/V, constipation. **S/Cond:** Avoid alcohol. Caution c̄ lactation.↑ risk of dental problems, see p 9 & 14.
Other: Drowsiness, dizziness, palpitations, tachycardia, blurred vision, weakness, rash, insomnia, headache, flushing.
Urinary: ↓ URGENCY, ↓ FREQUENCY, RETENTION.

oxycodone
Roxicodone
Soln— 7-9% alcohol, sorbitol

ANALGESIC, Narcotic
Drug: May take c̄ food or milk to ↓ GI distress. **Oral/GI:** Dry mouth, N/V, constipation. **S/Cond:** Avoid alcohol. Caution c̄ lactation. May be habit forming c̄ LT use. **Other:** Sedation, drowsiness, fatigue, ↓ BP, dizziness, respiratory depression, headache, nervousness, rash.
Blood/Serum: ↑ amylase, ↑ lipase. **Urinary:** Retention.

paclitaxel
Taxol
castor oil, 50 % dehydrated alcohol

ANTINEOPLASTIC, Antimicrotubule Agent — Parenteral only (IV)
Oral/GI: MUCOSITIS, NAUSEA/VOMITING, DIARRHEA.
S/Cond: Not c̄ lactation. Do dental care cautiously, see p 10 & 14. 89-98 % serum pro bound.
Other: BONE MARROW SUPPRESSION, PERIPHERAL NEUROPATHY, EDEMA, INFECTION, ALLERGIC REACTION, MUSCLE PAIN, ↓ BP, fatigue, rash, itching, bradycardia.
Blood/Serum: ↓ WHITE BLOOD CELLS, ANEMIA, ↓ PLATELETS, ↑ ALK PHOS, ↑ SGOT, ↑ bil. Transient ↑ TG.
Monitor: Frequent CBC c̄ diff, platelets.

Pamelor ANTIDEPRESSANT, Tricyclic See **nortriptyline p 145**

pamidronate disodium
Aredia
mannitol

ANTIHYPERCALCEMIA, Ca Regulator, Bisphosphonate
Parenteral only (IV)

Drug: Insure adequate fluid intake for urine output of 2 L/day.[1]
Diet: Maintain well balanced diet, adequate in Ca & Vit D. May need ↑ P or P suppl.[7] Avoid Ca or Vit D suppl.
Nutr: Anorexia.
Oral/GI: N/V, abdominal pain, GI bleeding, constipation.
S/Cond: Caution c̄ lactation.
Other: FEVER, bone pain, ↑ BP, fatigue, headache, hypothyroidism.
Blood/Serum: ↓ Ca, ↓ Phosphate, ↓ Mg, ↓ K, anemia, ↑ BUN, ↑ crea.
Monitor: Ca, P, electrolytes, Mg,
CBC c̄ diff, renal func.

Panadol ANALGESIC, ANTIPYRETIC See **acetaminophen p 17**

Paraflex MUSCLE RELAXANT See **chlorzoxazone p 51**

Parafon Forte DSC MUSCLE RELAXANT See **chlorzoxazone p 51**

Paraplatin ANTINEOPLASTIC See **carboplatin p 42**

Parlodel ANTIPARKINSON See **bromocriptine p 36**

Parnate — ANTIDEPRESSANT, MAOI — See **tranylcypromine sulfate p 199**

paroxetine
Paxil

ANTIDEPRESSANT, SSRI

Diet: Take s̄ regard to food. Not c̄ tryptophan suppl.
Nutr: ↓ appetite, ↓ or ↑ wt.
Oral/GI: Dry mouth, taste changes, nausea, dyspepsia, constipation, diarrhea, flatulence.
S/Cond: Avoid alcohol. Caution c̄ lactation. 93-95% serum pro bound. Caution c̄ elderly— ↑ drug conc.
Other: Weakness, insomnia, drowsiness, dizziness, sweating, tremor, blurred vision, nervousness, confusion, paresthesia, palpitations.
Urinary: ↑ frequency, hesitancy.

PCE — ANTIBIOTIC — See **erythromycin p 82**

Pediaflor — MINERAL SUPPLEMENT — See **fluoride p 91**

Pediazole
Susp— sucrose

ANTIBIOTIC, Sulfonamide, Macrolide
S/Cond: Caution c̄ G6PD def.

See **erythromycin p 82 & sulfisoxazole p 189**

pegaspargase
Oncaspar

ANTINEOPLASTIC, Anti-leukemia

Nutr: Anorexia. **Oral/GI:** Lip edema, N/V, abdominal pain, diarrhea.
S/Cond: Not c̄ lactation. Caution c̄ diabetes— ↑ or ↓ glucose.
Other: ALLERGIC REACTION, fever, weakness, headache, ↓ BP, chills, tachycardia, muscle pain, peripheral edema, ascites, paresthesia, convulsions, jaundice, pancreatitis, rash.
Blood/Serum: ↑ SGPT, ↑ or ↓ glucose, ↑ SGOT, ↑ bil, ↑ PT, ↑ PTT, ↓ alb, ↑ uric acid, dyscrasias, ↑ amylase, ↑ lipase.
Urinary: Pro.
Monitor: CBC c̄ diff, amylase, glucose.
Possibly bone marrow, hepatic func, PT, PTT, fibrinogen.

pemoline
Cylert
Tab— lactose
Chew Tab— mannitol

ANTI-ADHD, Stimulant

Drug: Take in AM. Chew chewable tab well.
Diet: Limit caffeine.[17]
Nutr: Transient anorexia, ↓ wt. **Oral/GI:** Nausea, stomach pain, diarrhea.
S/Cond: Caution c̄ lactation. Avoid alcohol.[17]
Other: INSOMNIA (usually transient), dyskinesia, dizziness, headache, drowsiness, depression, convulsions, ↑ irritability, rash.
Blood/Serum: LT use— ↑ SGOT, ↑ SGPT, ↑ LDH, ↑ alk phos.
Rare aplastic anemia.
Monitor: Children's growth (ht/wt gain), hepatic func.

See "Guide to the Use of This Book" inside front cover.

penicillamine
Cuprimine
Cap— lactose
Depen
Tab— lactose

ANTIARTHRITIC, CHELATING AGENT, Heavy Metal Antagonist
(Used to treat Wilson's disease & cystinuria)

Drug: Take 1 hr before or 2 hrs after food (food ↓ abs 60%). Take HS dose at least 3 hrs after supper. May mix c̄ juice or fruit.

Diet: Take Fe or Zn suppl separately by 2 hrs. Avoid other mineral suppl. ↑ Pyr need— add 25-50 mg/day.

For Wilson's disease— ↓ Cu diet (1-2 mg Cu/day). Distilled H_2O if local H_2O Cu ≥ 100 ug/L.

For lead poisoning— ↓ Ca diet.[1]

For cystinuria— Copious fluids to maintain alkaline urine (pH 7.5). ↓ methionine diet, except for children or pregnancy.

Nutr: Possible Fe or Zn def. ↓ appetite.

Oral/GI: Stomatitis, ↓ taste acuity, metallic taste, N/V, epigastric pain, diarrhea.

S/Cond: Limit alcohol.[11c] Not c̄ lactation. Do dental care cautiously, see p 10 & 14.

Other: ALLERGIC REACTION, RASH, fever, bone marrow suppression, lupus-like syndrome.

Blood/Serum: Dyscrasias, ↓ WBC, ↓ platelets, + ANA. Rare aplastic or hemolytic anemia, ↑ SGOT, ↑ SGPT, ↑ alk phos, ↑ LDH.

Urinary: Pro, hematuria, ↑ Cu, ↑ Zn, ↑ Fe, ↑ Pyr.

Monitor: CBC c̄ diff, platelets, hepatic & renal func. Urinalysis.

penicillin ANTIBIOTIC Oral or Parenteral

Drug: Pen VK— Take s̄ regard to food. **Diet:** Caution c̄ K suppl c̄ K forms. **Nutr:** Anorexia.
Oral/GI: Black hairy tongue, dry mouth, taste changes, oral candidiasis, N/V, epigastric distress, diarrhea, flatulence. Rare pseudomembranous colitis.
S/Cond: Caution c̄ lactation.
Other: Allergic reaction, rash. Neuropathy or nephropathy c̄ high dose parenteral.
Blood/Serum: Dyscrasias. ↑ K (especially c̄ pen G K IV). ↑ Na (pen G Na IV).
Urinary: False + glucose ($CuSO_4$) or false ↑ steroids (method dependent) c̄ pen G.
Monitor: c̄ LT or high dose IV— CBC c̄ diff, renal func, electrolytes. K or Na especially c̄ pen G.

Oral forms—
penicillin V potassium
101 mg K/g
Betapen VK Tab— lactose.
Pwd— sucrose, saccharin.
Beepen VK Tab- lactose.
Pwd- saccharin, sucrose.
Ledercillin 250 mg Tab— lactose. Pwd— saccharin.
Pen Vee K Tab - lactose. Pwd- saccharin, sucrose.
Veetids Tab- lactose. Pwd- saccharin, sucrose.
V-Cillin K Tab - lactose. Pwd- saccharin, sucrose.

Parenteral forms—
penicillin G benzathine (IM only)
Bicillin
10 mg Na/5 mL Susp
penicillin G sodium (IV)
46 mg Na/1 million unit
penicillin G potassium (IV)
7 mg Na/1 million units
66 mg K/1 million units
penicillin G procaine (IM only)

See "Guide to the Use of This Book" inside front cover.

pentamidine isethionate
NebuPent
Aerosol
Pentam 300
Parenteral

ANTI-PCP IN HIV, ANTI-PROTOZOAL

Parenteral (IM or IV) or Aerosol

Nutr: Anorexia, ↑ thirst. **Oral/GI:** Metallic taste, N/V, abdominal pain, diarrhea. Aerosol— oral ulcers, pharyngitis, dysphagia.

S/Cond: Avoid alcohol. Not c̄ lactation. May cause or aggravate diabetes— may cause severe ↓ glucose.

Other: NEPHROTOXICITY, hepatotoxicity, fever/chills, ↓ BP, headache, confusion, muscle pain, edema, allergic reaction, rash, pancreatitis, arrhythmia, tachycardia. Aerosol— COUGH, RASH, DIZZINESS, FATIGUE, CHEST PAIN.

Blood/Serum: Parenteral— ↓ WBC, ↓ platelets, anemia, ↑ SGOT, ↑ SGPT, ↑ bil, ↑ alk phos, ↑ BUN, ↑ CREA, ↑ or ↓ glucose. <1%— ↑ K, ↓ Ca, ↓ Mg.

Monitor: BUN, crea & glucose daily. BP. CBC, platelets, hepatic func, Ca, Mg, ECG.

Pentasa

ANTI-INFLAMMATORY

See **mesalamine p 126**

pentoxifylline
Trental
SR Tab—
benzyl alcohol

ANTI-PERIPHERAL VASCULAR DISEASE

Drug: Take c̄ meals to ↓ GI irritation. Swallow whole. Do NOT crush, break or chew. **Diet:** ↓ cal, ↓ chol may be recommended. Limit xanthine/caffeine, see p 240. **Oral/GI:** N/V, dyspepsia.

S/Cond: Not c̄ lactation. Avoid smoking. **Other**: Dizziness, headache.

Blood/Serum: ↓ VISCOSITY, IMPROVED CAPILLARY FLOW.

Pepcid

ANTIULCER

See **famotidine p 87**

Pepto-Bismol — ANTIDIARRHEAL — See **bismuth subsalicylate p 35**

Percocet
Tab— starch
ANALGESIC, Narcotic — See **oxycodone p 150 & acetaminophen p 17**

Percodan
Tab— starch
ANALGESIC, Narcotic — See **oxycodone p 150 & acetylsalicylic acid p 18**

Perdiem, plain — LAXATIVE — See **psyllium p 171**

Peri-Colace
casanthranol &
docusate sodium
syrup— 10% alcohol, sorbitol, sucrose

LAXATIVE, STOOL SOFTENER
Drug: Take HS c̄ 8 oz H_2O or other liquid.
Diet: High fiber c̄ 1500-2000 mL fluid/day to prevent constipation.
Nutr: Alters abs of H_2O & electrolytes.
Oral/GI: Bitter taste, nausea, abdominal cramps, <u>diarrhea</u>.
Laxative dependence c̄ LT use.
Other: Rash.
Blood/Serum: LT use—↑ glucose, ↓ K.

Periactin — ANTIHISTAMINE, Appetite Stimulant — See **cyproheptadine HCl p 63**

perphenazine
Trilafon
IV— Na bisulfite
Tab— lactose, sugar
Conc— 0.1% alcohol, sugar, sorbitol

ANTIPSYCHOTIC, ANTINAUSEANT, Phenothiazine

Oral or Parenteral (IM or IV)

Drug: Take c̄ food to ↓ GI irritation. Do NOT mix conc c̄ caffeinated beverages, tannins (tea) or pectinate (eg apple juice). **Nutr:** ↑ need for Rib.[41] ↑ appetite, ↑ wt. **Oral/GI:** DRY MOUTH, dysphagia, N/V, CONSTIPATION. **S/Cond:** Avoid alcohol. Not c̄ lactation. ↑ risk of dental problems, see p 9 & 14. Caution c̄ ESRD. 90% serum pro bound.
Other: EPS, drowsiness, dizziness, ↑ or ↓ BP, mild photosensitivity, tachycardia, jaundice. Tardive dyskinesia c̄ LT use.
Blood/Serum: ↑ or ↓ glucose, ↑ SGOT, ↑ SGPT, ↑ bil, ↑ alk phos, ↑ prolactin. Rare ↓ WBC, dyscrasias.
Urinary: ↑ Rib, + glucose, false ↑ bil, dark color.
Monitor: CBC c̄ diff, hepatic & renal func.

Persantine ANTIPLATELET See **dipyridamole p 74**

Phazyme ANTIFLATULENT See **simethicone p 182**

phenelzine sulfate
Nardil
Tab— mannitol, sucrose, wheat flour

ANTIDEPRESSANT, MAOI

Drug: Do not take in the evening to avoid insomnia. **Diet:** Avoid foods ↑ in tyramine & other pressor amines to prevent hypertensive crisis, see p 243. Limit caffeine, see p 240. Avoid tryptophan suppl. May need Pyr suppl.[4]
Nutr: Possible Pyr def. ↑ appetite, ↑ wt. **Oral/GI:** Dry mouth, N/V, constipation. **S/Cond:** Avoid alcohol. Not c̄ lactation. Caution c̄ diabetes—

↓ glucose. **Other:** <u>INSOMNIA</u>, ↑ <u>or</u> ↓ <u>BP</u>, <u>dizziness</u>, <u>drowsiness</u>, <u>blurred vision</u>,[7] tremor, hyperexcitability, headache, edema, SIADH, muscle pain, weakness. Rare rash, hepatotoxicity, peripheral neuropathy.
Blood/Serum: ↑ SGOT, ↑ SGPT, ↓ glucose in diabetes. Rare dyscrasias.
Urinary: Retention.
Monitor: BP, CBC, hepatic func.

Phenergan ANTIHISTAMINE, ANTIVERTIGO, ANTIEMETIC See **promethazine HCl p 167**

phenobarbital
Phenobarbital
Elixir—
14% alcohol,
0.63 g sucrose/5 mL
Tab— lactose

SEDATIVE, HYPNOTIC, ANTICONVULSANT, Barbiturate
Oral or Parenteral (IM or IV)

Diet: ↑ Vit D & Ca intake. Limit xanthine/caffeine, see p 240. 80-400 mg Pyr may ↓ drug effects. May need Vit D, Vit B_{12} & Fol suppls c̄ LT use.
Nutr: ↑ Vit C requirements. ↑ rate of metabolism of Vit D & Vit K.[4]
Oral/GI: N/V, constipation.
S/Cond: Avoid alcohol. Not c̄ lactation. May be habit forming c̄ LT use.
Other: <u>Dizziness</u>, <u>drowsiness</u>, <u>ataxia</u>, <u>depression</u>, <u>hyperactivity</u> (especially in children), headache, confusion, rash, osteomalacia. <u>Mild respiratory depression</u> c̄ IV.
Blood/Serum: ↓ <u>BIL</u>, ↓ Fol, ↑ chol,[39] ↑ NH_3, ↓ Ca,[4] ↓ Mg.[27] Rare ↓ B_{12}, dyscrasias or megaloblastic anemia.
Monitor: c̄ LT use— Fol, B_{12}, CBC c̄ diff, hepatic & renal func, drug levels.

phenolphthalein
Ex-Lax
Tab— sucrose, starch
Chew Tab— cocoa, sugar, non-fat dry milk

LAXATIVE, Stimulant

Drug: Take HS c̄ 8 oz H_2O or juice. Chew chew tab well.
Diet: High fiber c̄ 1500-2000 mL fluid/day to prevent constipation.
Oral/GI: Belching, N/V, cramps. LT use— laxative dependence, malabsorption, steatorrhea. **S/Cond:** Caution c̄ lactation.
Other: Osteomalacia c̄ LT use. **Blood/Serum:** c̄ LT use— ↓ K, ↓ N,[27] ↓ Ca,[6] ↑ glucose. **Urinary:** Pink to red color.

phentermine HCl
Fastin
Cap— sucrose, invert sugar, starch
phentermine resin
Ionamin (SR)
Cap— lactose

APPETITE SUPPRESSANT

Drug: Do not take HS. Take HCl form 2 hrs after breakfast. Swallow resin form whole 1/2 hr before breakfast. May mask taste c̄ fruit juice.
Diet: Adjunct to ↓ cal. Avoid caffeine, see p 240.
Nutr: ANOREXIA, ↓ WT. **Oral/GI:** Dry mouth, unpleasant taste, N/V, N/V, diarrhea, constipation. **S/Cond:** Avoid alcohol. Caution c̄ lactation. Caution c̄ diabetes— may alter insulin or sulfonylurea effects. May be habit forming c̄ LT use. **Other:** INSOMNIA, restlessness, ↑ BP, tremor, tachycardia, dizziness, headache, rash.

phenylpropanolamine
Acutrim (SR)
Dexatrim
SR Cap— lactose

APPETITE SUPPRESSANT, DECONGESTANT

Drug: Take c̄ 8 oz H_2O mid-morning (SR) or 1/2 hr before meals. Swallow SR form whole. **Diet:** Adjunct to ↓ cal. Avoid caffeine, see p 240.
Nutr: ↓ APPETITE, ↓ WT. **Oral/GI:** DRY MOUTH, nausea, abdominal pain.
S/Cond: Caution c̄ alcohol. Caution c̄ lactation. Caution c̄ diabetes—↑ glucose. **Other:** Insomnia, tachycardia, ↑ BP, nervousness, dizziness, headache.

phenytoin
Dilantin
Cap— 8 mg Na/100 mg
Susp— < 0.6% alcohol, sucrose
Extended-release cap— lactose, sucrose
Infatab (chew tab)— saccharin, sucrose

ANTICONVULSANT, Hydantoin — Oral or Parenteral (IV or IM)

Drug: Oral— Take c̄ food or milk to ↓ GI irritation. Chew chew tab well. Swallow SR cap whole— do not crush or chew.
Diet: May need Vit D or Fol suppl. Take Ca or Mg suppl or antacids separately by 2 hrs.
Nutr: High Fol intake (>5 mg/week)[3] ↓ drug bioavailability. ↑ metabolism of Vit D & K, especially in children.[11] May cause rickets or osteomalacia.
Oral/GI: GUM HYPERPLASIA, altered taste, N/V, constipation.
S/Cond: Avoid alcohol. Not c̄ lactation. Caution c̄ diabetes— ↑ glucose. Do dental care cautiously. Tube feedings ↓ bioavailability of drug— stop TF for 2 hrs before & after drug. > 90% serum pro bound. Hypoalbuminemia (<3 g/dL) may ↑ drug effects.[44]
Other: ATAXIA, rash, drowsiness, dizziness, confusion, headache, visual changes, edema. Rare hepatitis, jaundice. Peripheral neuropathy c̄ LT use.
Blood/Serum: ↓ Fol, ↓ Vit D, ↓ Ca, ↓ P, ↓ T_4, ↑ glucose, ↑ alk phos, ↑ GGT, ↓ chol. Rare-dyscrasias or megaloblastic anemia.
Urinary: ↓ Rib.[41]
Monitor: CBC c̄ diff, hepatic func, Ca, thyroid func.

Philip's MOM — LAXATIVE, ANTACID — See **Milk of Magnesia (MOM) p 133**

Phos-Lo — PHOSPHATE BINDER — See **calcium acetate p 39**

phosphates URINARY ACIDIFIER, PHOSPHORUS SUPPLEMENT

Drug: Take at meals & HS to ↓ GI irritation & laxative action. Dissolve Neutra-Phos pwd in 75 mL H_2O or juice. Dissolve K-Phos tab in 8 oz H_2O. **Diet:** Consider Na &/or K content. Avoid Ca or Vit D suppl or salt subs. Caution c̄ K suppl. Take Fe, Mg or Zn suppl separately by 2 hrs. Do not take c̄ high oxalate, see p 241 or high phytate, see p 242, foods— ↓ abs. Insure adequate fluid intake. **Nutr:** ↑ thirst, ↑ wt.
Oral/GI: N/V, stomach pain, diarrhea. **S/Cond:** Caution c̄ lactation. **Other:** Edema, dizziness, headache, confusion, fatigue, muscle cramps, osteomalacia c̄ LT use. **Blood/Serum:** ↓ Ca, ↑ P, ↑ K, ↑ Na.
Urinary: ↓ output. **Monitor:** Electrolytes, Ca, P, renal func.

potassium phosphate

K-Phos Original	114 mg P,	144 mg K,	0 mg Na/tab
Neutra-Phos K	250 mg P,	556 mg K,	0 mg Na/pkt

sodium phosphate & potassium phosphate

K-Phos Neutral	250 mg P,	45 mg K,	298 mg Na/tab
K-Phos MF	126 mg P,	45 mg K,	67 mg Na/tab
K-Phos No 2	250 mg P,	88 mg K,	134 mg Na/tab
Neutra-Phos	250 mg P,	278 mg K,	164 mg Na/pkt

pilocarpine HCl ANTI-XEROSTOMIA, Cholinergic for radiation induced dry mouth
Salagen

Diet: Insure adequate fluid intake. **Oral/GI:** ↑ SALIVATION, dysphagia, N/V, dyspepsia, diarrhea. **S/Cond:** Not c̄ lactation.
Other: ↑ SWEATING, flushing, chills, dizziness, weakness, headache, edema, ↑ BP, tachycardia, tremor.
Urinary: ↑ frequency.

piperacillin sodium ANTIBIOTIC, penicillin — See listing for **ticarcillin disodium p 197**
Pipracil 43 mg Na/g — Parenteral only (IM or IV)

piroxicam
Feldene
Cap— lactose, starch

NSAID, ANTIARTHRITIC
Drug: Take c̄ food or milk to ↓ GI irritation.
Diet: Caution c̄ GI irritants eg K suppl (↑ risk of GI irritation).
Nutr: Anorexia.
Oral/GI: Stomatitis, dyspepsia, nausea, cramps, constipation, diarrhea, flatulence. GI ulcers & bleeding (may be sudden & serious).
S/Cond: Avoid alcohol. Not c̄ lactation. 99.3% serum pro bound.
Other: Dizziness, drowsiness, headache, rash, peripheral edema, photosensitivity.
Blood/Serum: Dyscrasias, ↑ BUN, ↑ crea, ↓ HCT, ↓ Hgb.
<1%— ↑ SGOT, ↑ SGPT.

Plaquenil ANTIARTHRITIC, ANTIMALARIAL — See **hydroxychloroquine sulfate p 103**

Platinol ANTINEOPLASTIC — See **cisplatin p 54**

Plendil ANTIHYPERTENSIVE, Ca Channel Blocker — See **felodipine p 87**

Pondimin APPETITE SUPPRESSANT — See **fenfluramine HCl p 88**

potassium chloride (KCl)   ELECTROLYTE, Mineral Supplement
Drug: Take c̄ meals & 8 oz liquid. Mix liquid, pwd, granule or effervescent tab in 4 oz H_2O or other liquid. Swallow SR form whole, do not crush or chew. **Diet:** Not c̄ salt subs.[13] See potassium sources, p 249.
Nutr: No RDA. Minimum adult K requirement = 1600 - 2000 mg (40-50 mEq). Children = 78 mg (2 mEq)/100 cal.[47] **Oral/GI:** GI irritation, N/V, abdominal pain, diarrhea, flatulence.
S/Cond: Some liquid/syrup forms precipitate tube feedings.[8]
Blood/Serum: ↑ K, ↑ Cl. **Urinary:** ↑ K, ↓ Mg. **Monitor:** Serum K, Cl, Mg.

K-Dur (SR) 10 mEq Tab— 390 mg K/Tab. 20 mEq Tab— 780 mg K/tab
K-Lor Pwd 15 mEq pkt— 585 mg K/dose. 20 mEq pkt— 780 mg K/dose
Klor-Con Pwd 780 mg K/pkt saccharin. **Klor-Con 8** (SR) 312 mg K/Tab. **Klor-Con 10** (SR) 390 mg K/Tab
Klorvess 780 mg K/pkt or Tab, saccharin. Liquid— 780 mg K/15 mL, 0.75% alcohol, saccharin, sucrose.
Klotrix (SR) Tab 390 mg K/Tab
K-Lyte/Cl 25 mEq Tab— 975 mg K/Tab- saccharin. DS- 1950 mg K/Tab- saccharin, lactose.
K-Tab (SR) 10 mEq Tab— 390 mg K/dose
Micro-K (SR) 8 mEq Cap— 312 mg K/Cap. **Micro-K 10** (SR) 390 mg K/Cap
Slow-K (SR) 8 mEq Tab— 312 mg K/Tab— sucrose, starch.
Ten-K (SR) 10 mEq Tab— 390 mg K/Tab

potassium gluconate   ELECTROLYTE, Mineral Supplement   See **potassium chloride above**
0.17 mg K/g

potassium phosphate   URINARY ACIDIFIER   See **phosphates p 162**
K-Phos Original   PHOSPHORUS SUPPLEMENT

pravastatin sodium
Pravachol
Tab— lactose

ANTIHYPERLIPIDEMIC, HMG CoA Reductase Inhibitor
Drug: Take s̄ regard to food. Take single dose HS. **Diet:** ↓ fat, ↓ chol. (↓ cal if needed). Not c̄ high dose Nia— possible myopathy.
Oral/GI: N/V, dyspepsia, diarrhea.
S/Cond: Limit alcohol. Not c̄ lactation.
Other: Headache, muscle pain, rash.
Blood/Serum: ↓ chol, ↓ LDL, ↓ VLDL, ↑ HDL, ↓ TG. Rare dyscrasias. Transient— ↑ SGOT, ↑ SGPT, ↑ CPK.
Monitor: Chol, LDL, CPK, hepatic func.

prazosin HCl
Minipress
Cap— sucrose

ANTIHYPERTENSIVE, $Alpha_1$-Adrenergic Blocker
Diet: ↓ Na, ↓ cal diet may be recommended. Avoid natural licorice.
Oral/GI: Dry mouth, N/V, diarrhea, constipation. **S/Cond:** Caution c̄ alcohol. Caution c̄ lactation. 97 % serum pro bound.
Other: Dizziness, drowsiness, fatigue, weakness, headache, ↓ BP, edema, blurred vision, depression, nervousness, paresthesia, rash.
Blood/Serum: + ANA. Transient ↓ WBC, ↑ uric acid, ↑ BUN.[6]
Urinary: ↑ frequency, incontinence. ↑ VMA. **Monitor:** BP.

prednisolone CORTICOSTEROID See **corticosteroids p 60**

prednisone CORTICOSTEROID See **corticosteroids p 60**

Premarin HORMONE See **estrogen p 83**

Premphase HORMONES See **estrogen p 83 & medroxyprogesterone acetate p 124**
Prempro
estrogen Tab— lactose, sucrose
progesterone Tab— lactose

Prevacid ANTIULCER, ANTISECRETORY See **lansoprazole p 115**

Prilosec ANTIULCER, ANTISECRETORY See **omeprazole p 147**

Primaxin ANTIBIOTIC See **imipenem & cilastatin p 106**

Prinivil ANTIHYPERTENSIVE See **lisinopril p 117**

procainamide HCl ANTIARRHYTHMIC Oral or Parenteral (IM or IV)
Procan SR
500 mg— sucrose
Pronestyl
Tab— tartrazine
250 & 375 Cap— lactose
Parenteral— benzyl alcohol, Na bisulfite

Drug: Take c̄ 8 oz H_2O on empty stomach to ↑ rate of abs, but may take c̄ food or milk to ↓ GI irritation. Swallow SR tab whole— do not crush or chew. **Nutr:** Anorexia. **Oral/GI:** Bitter taste, N/V, abdominal pain, diarrhea. **S/Cond:** Caution c̄ alcohol. Not c̄ lactation.
Other: LUPUS-LIKE SYNDROME, ↓ BP, tachycardia.
Blood/Serum: + ANA, ↑ SGOT, ↑ SGPT, ↑ alk phos, ↑ LDH, ↑ bil. Rare— dyscrasias, anemias, ↑ amylase.[6]
Monitor: CBC c̄ diff & platelets weekly x 3 months, then periodically. ANA. BP & ECG.

Procardia ANTIANGINA See **nifedipine p 142**

prochlorperazine ANTIEMETIC, ANTIPSYCHOTIC, Phenothiazine

Compazine Oral, Parenteral (IM or IV), Suppository

5 & 10 mg Tab— lactose, starch
25 mg Tab— sucrose, starch
Cap (SR)— sucrose, starch, benzyl alcohol
Parenteral— benzyl alcohol
Syrup— sucrose

Drug: If possible, take c̄ food, milk or 8 oz H_2O. Swallow SR cap whole. **Diet:** Limit caffeine, see p 240. **Nutr:** ↑ need for Rib.[41] ↑ appetite, ↑ wt. **Oral/GI:** Dry mouth, constipation. **S/Cond:** Avoid alcohol. Not c̄ lactation. ↑ risk of dental problems, see p 9 & 14. > 90% serum pro bound. **Other:** EXTRAPYRAMIDAL SYMPTOMS, dizziness, drowsiness. Rare jaundice. Tardive dyskinesia c̄ LT use. **Blood/Serum:** ↑ SGOT, ↑ SGPT, ↑ LDH, ↑ alk phos, ↑ bil, ↑ or ↓ glucose, ↑ prolactin. Rare dyscrasias. Transient ↓ WBC. **Urinary:** ↑ Rib, + glucose. **Monitor:** CBC c̄ diff & hepatic func c̄ LT use.

Prolixin ANTIPSYCHOTIC, Phenothiazine See **fluphenazine HCl p 93**

promethazine HCl ANTIHISTAMINE, ANTIVERTIGO, ANTIEMETIC, SEDATIVE

Phenergan Phenothiazine derivative Oral or Parenteral (IM or IV)

Syrups— saccharin, plain— 7% alcohol, fortis—- 1.5% alcohol
Parenteral ampule— 0.25 mg Na metabisulfite/mL
Tab— lactose 12.5 & 25 mg— saccharin

Drug: Take with meals or HS c̄ 8 oz H_2O or milk to ↓ GI irritation. **Nutr:** ↑ need for Rib.[41] **Oral/GI:** Dry mouth, taste changes,[37] N/V, constipation. **S/Cond:** Avoid alcohol. Not c̄ lactation. ↑ risk of dental problems, see p 9 & 14. 76-93% serum pro bound.[6] **Other:** DROWSINESS, SEDATION, blurred vision, confusion, photosensitivity, rash. Rare EPS, jaundice. **Blood/Serum:** ↑ glucose. Rare dyscrasias. **Urinary:** ↑ Rib.

Pronestyl ANTIARRHYTHMIC See **procainamide HCl p 166**

Propacet — ANALGESIC, Narcotic — See **propoxyphene napsylate below & acetaminophen p 17**

propoxyphene HCl
Darvon
Tab— starch
propoxyphene napsylate
Darvon-N
Tab— acetaminophen, lactose
Susp— glucose, saccharin, sucrose

ANALGESIC, Narcotic

Drug: May take c̄ food to ↓ GI distress.
Oral/GI: Dry mouth, N/V, abdominal pain, constipation.
S/Cond: Limit alcohol. Caution c̄ lactation.[6] ↑ risk of dental problems, see p 9 & 14. May be habit forming c̄ high dose & LT use.
Other: Dizziness, drowsiness, ↓ BP, weakness, headache, blurred vision. Rare jaundice.
Blood/Serum: ↑ SGOT, ↑ SGPT, ↑ alk phos, ↑ bil, ↑ LDH.
Monitor: Hepatic func c̄ LT use.

propranolol HCl
Inderal
Tab— lactose
Inderal LA (SR)

ANTIARRHYTHMIC, ANTIANGINAL, ANTIHYPERTENSIVE
Non-selective Beta-Blocker — Oral or Parenteral (IV)

Drug: Take c̄ food to enhance bioavailability.[7] Swallow SR (LA) form whole. Mix conc c̄ liquid or semi-solid food. **Diet:** ↓ Na, ↓ cal may be recommended. Avoid natural licorice. Ca suppl may ↓ abs.[9b]
Oral/GI: Dry mouth, N/V, epigastric distress, diarrhea, constipation, flatulence.
S/Cond: Avoid alcohol. Caution c̄ lactation.
Caution c̄ diabetes— may mask symptoms of & prolong hypoglycemia. May inhibit insulin response to hyperglycemia. 93% serum pro bound. Hypoalbuminemia (< 3 g/dL) may ↑ drug effects.
Smoking ↓ drug effect.

Other: Dizziness, drowsiness, fatigue, ↓ BP, insomnia, weakness, depression, bradycardia, ataxia, confusion.
Blood/Serum: ↑ SGOT, ↑ SGPT, ↑ alk phos, ↑ LDH, ↓ T_4, ↓ T_3, ↑ K. Rare dyscrasias.
Monitor: BP, hepatic & renal func.

Propulsid — ANTIGERD — See **cisapride p 53**

propylthiouracil (PTU) **Propyl-Thyracil** — ANTITHYROID, ANTIHYPERTHYROIDISM

Drug: Take c̄ food. **Oral/GI:** N/V, gastric pain.
S/Cond: Not c̄ lactation— monitor infant's thyroid func if used c̄ lactation.[1]
Other: Rash, fever, dizziness, drowsiness, headache, edema, joint pain, peripheral neuropathy. Rare jaundice or hepatitis.
Blood/Serum: ↑ LDH, ↑ SGPT, ↑ SGOT, ↑ alk phos, ↑ bil, ↑ PT. Rare ↓ WBC, ↓ platelets, aplastic anemia.
Monitor: Thyroid func, CBC c̄ diff if sore throat or infection.

Proscar — ANDROGEN HORMONE INHIBITOR — See **finasteride p 89**

ProStep — SMOKING DETERRENT — See **nicotine transdermal system p 142**

protriptyline HCl
Vivactil
Tab— lactose, starch

ANTIDEPRESSANT, Anti-Narcolepsy, Tricyclic

Drug: May take c̄ food to ↓ GI irritation. Do not take late in the day to avoid insomnia. **Diet:** ↑ fiber may ↓ drug effect.[3] Avoid caffeine, see p 240. **Nutr:** ↑ APPETITE especially for sweets, ↑ WT. **Oral/GI:** DRY MOUTH, taste changes, N/V, constipation, diarrhea, flatulence. **S/Cond:** Avoid alcohol. Not c̄ lactation. 92% serum pro bound. ↑ risk of dental problems, see p 9 & 14. **Other:** INSOMNIA, RESTLESSNESS, TACHYCARDIA, POSTURAL ↓ BP, dizziness, blurred vision, sweating, tremor, headache, fatigue, confusion, rash. Rare sedation, drowsiness, jaundice, SIADH. **Blood/Serum:** ↑ or ↓ glucose, ↑ prolactin. Rare dyscrasias, ↑ SGOT, ↑ SGPT, ↑ alk phos. **Urinary:** Retention.

Proventil — BRONCHODILATOR — See **albuterol sulfate p 20**

Provera — HORMONE — See **medroxyprogesterone acetate p 124**

Prozac — ANTIDEPRESSANT, SSRI — See **fluoxetine p 92**

pseudoephedrine HCl
Sudafed
Syrup— 2.4% alcohol, sucrose
60 mg Tab— sucrose
Liquid— sorbitol, sucrose

DECONGESTANT

Drug: Take last dose a few hrs before bedtime. Swallow SR forms whole. SR cap contents may be mixed c̄ jam or jelly, do not chew.[13]
Nutr: Anorexia. **Oral/GI:** Dry mouth, N/V c̄ large dose.
S/Cond: Not c̄ lactation. Caution c̄ diabetes. Syrup precipitates some tube feedings.[8] **Other:** Nervousness, insomnia, restlessness, tachycardia, dizziness, tremor, headache, drowsiness, weakness.

psyllium
hydrophilic mucilloid
Fiberall-Pwd-10 mg Na, 60 mg K, 6 cal/dose, wheat bran
Metamucil-Pwd-5 mg Na, 30 mg K, 14 cal/dose, sucrose or dextrose
Sugar-Free— aspartame
Perdiem plain- 2 mg Na, 35 mg K, 4 cal/tsp

LAXATIVE, bulk-forming

Drug: Dissolve pwd in ≥ 8 oz H_2O, milk or juice. Do <u>not</u> swallow or inhale dry pwd. Drink ≥ 8 oz fluid with wafer.
Diet: Appropriate for ↓ Na diet. ↓ Rib abs.[11] High fiber c̄ 1500-2000 mL fluid/day to prevent constipation.
Nutr: ↓ appetite.
Oral/GI: N/V, abdominal cramps, bloating, diarrhea, flatulence.
S/Cond: Not c̄ dysphagia. Caution c̄ diabetes— some forms contain sugar.
Blood/Serum: ↓ <u>CHOL</u>, ↓ <u>LDL</u>.

Pulmozyme — ANTI CYSTIC FIBROSIS — See **dornase alfa p 77**

Purinethol — ANTINEOPLASTIC — See **mercaptopurine p 126**

pyrazinamide

ANTITUBERCULOSIS

Nutr: Anorexia. **Oral/GI:** N/V.
S/Cond: Not c̄ lactation.
Other: <u>Hepatotoxicity</u>, jaundice, muscle and/or joint pain, gout.
Blood/Serum: ↑ <u>URIC ACID</u>, ↑ <u>SGOT</u>, ↑ <u>SGPT</u>.
Urinary: ↓ <u>URIC ACID</u>.
Monitor: Hepatic func, uric acid.

pyridoxine Some Parenteral brands— benzyl alcohol	VITAMIN B_6 — Oral or Parenteral (IM or IV) **Drug:** 2.5-10 mg/day to treat Pyr def.[6] Swallow SR cap whole. **Nutr:** ↑ Pyr req c̄ ↑ pro intake. Adult RDA— Men = 2.0 mg; Women = 1.6; Pregnancy = 2.2; Lactation = 2.1. Doses ≥ 200 mg/day for > 30 days may create Pyr dependency.[13] ↑ requirement c̄ HIV. **Oral/GI:** Nausea c̄ high dose. **S/Cond:** High dose (>200 mg/day) inhibits lactation.[2] Active form, pyridoxal phosphate, is 100% serum pro bound. **Other:** Headache, drowsiness, mild flushing, paresthesia. LT use of megadose (≥2 g/day) causes chronic toxicity c̄ severe sensory <u>neuropathy</u> & <u>ataxia</u>. **Blood/Serum:** High dose— ↑ SGOT, ↓ Fol, ↓ prolactin.
quazepam **Doral** Tab— lactose	SEDATIVE, HYPNOTIC, Sleep Aid, Benzodiazepine **Drug:** May take c̄ food if GI distress. **Oral/GI:** Dry mouth, dyspepsia. **S/Cond:** Avoid alcohol. Not c̄ lactation. May be habit forming c̄ LT use > 6 wks. > 95% serum pro bound. **Other:** <u>Drowsiness</u>, dizziness, headache, fatigue.
Questran	ANTIHYPERLIPIDEMIC — See **cholestyramine p 52**
quinapril **Accupril** Tab— lactose, $MgCO_3$, Mg stearate	ANTIHYPERTENSIVE, ACE Inhibitor **Drug:** Rate & extent of abs ↓ 25-30% c̄ high fat meal. (Research meal = 58 g fat, 59% of cal from fat.) **Diet:** ↓ Na, ↓ cal may be recommended. Avoid natural licorice. Avoid salt subs. Caution c̄ K or Mg suppl. **Nutr:** Drug has significant Mg content. **Oral/GI:** N/V. **S/Cond:** Limit alcohol. Caution c̄ lactation. Consider Mg content c̄ ESRD. 5 mg Tab - 18 mg Mg, 10 mg Tab -

37 mg Mg, 20 mg Tab - 50 mg Mg, 40 mg Tab - 100 mg Mg. 97% serum pro bound. **Other:** Cough, ↓ BP, dizziness, fatigue. Rare angioedema. **Blood/Serum:** ↑ K, ↓ Na. Transient ↑ BUN, ↑ crea. <1%— ↓ Hgb, ↓ HCT, ↑ alk phos, ↑ bil, ↑ SGOT, ↑ SGPT. **Monitor:** BP, K, CBC c̄ diff, renal func.

quinidine gluconate
Quinaglute Dura-Tabs (SR)
Tab— sugar
quinidine sulfate
Quinidex (SR)
Tab— sucrose
Quinora

ANTIARRHYTHMIC — Oral or Parenteral (IM or IV)

Drug: ↑ abs on empty stomach. May take c̄ food or milk to ↓ GI irritation. Insure adequate fluid intake. Maintain urinary pH 6-7. Swallow SR tab whole. **Diet:** Caution c̄ K suppl. Avoid high dose Ca suppl (↑ urinary pH) or high dose Vit C (↓ urinary pH). **Nutr:** Anorexia. ↑ K may ↑ drug effects.[13] **Oral/GI:** Bitter taste, esophagitis, N/V, abdominal pain, diarrhea. **S/Cond:** Extreme caution c̄ lactation.[6] Caution c̄ hypokalemia— ↓ drug effects. 70-90% serum pro bound. Hypoalbuminemia (< 3 g/dL) may ↑ drug effects.[6] **Other:** Cardiotoxicity,[4] hepatotoxicity, ↓ BP, headache, confusion, fever, visual disturbances. Rare angioedema. **Blood/Serum:** ↑ SGOT, ↑ CPK (sulfate form). Rare ↓ platelets, anemia, ↓ glucose.[18] **Monitor:** BP. CBC c̄ diff, hepatic & renal func.

quinine sulfate
Quinamm
Tab— sucrose
Quinine

ANTIMALARIAL

Drug: Take c̄ or after meals to ↓ GI irritation. Do not crush (↑ GI irritation). **Oral/GI:** N/V, epigastric distress, cramps, diarrhea. **S/Cond:** Caution c̄ lactation. Not c̄ G6PD def. 85-90% serum pro bound in malaria patients.[13] **Other:** Headache, visual disturbances, confusion. Rare hepatitis, allergic reaction. **Blood/Serum:** Rare dyscrasias, ↑ insulin, ↓ glucose.

ramipril
Altace
Cap— starch

ANTIHYPERTENSIVE, ACE Inhibitor

Drug: Take s̄ regard to food. May open cap & mix contents c̄ 4 oz applesauce, apple juice or H_2O.
Diet: ↓ Na, ↓ cal may be recommended. Avoid natural licorice. Avoid salt subs. Caution c̄ K suppl.
S/Cond: Limit alcohol. Not c̄ lactation.
Other: COUGH, ↓ BP, dizziness, fatigue. Rare angioedema.
Blood/Serum: ↑ K, ↓ Na, ↑ BUN, ↑ crea. <1%— ↓ Hgb, ↓ HCT, ↑ alk phos, ↑ bil, ↑ SGOT, ↑ SGPT, ↑ glucose, ↑ uric acid.
Urinary: Rare pro.
Monitor: BP, K, CBC c̄ diff, renal func.

ranitidine
Zantac
Syrup— 7.5% alcohol, saccharin, sorbitol
Cap— sorbitol, coconut oil
Granules— aspartame, 174 mg Na/pkt

ANTISECRETORY, ANTIULCER, ANTI-GERD — Histamine H_2-antagonist
Oral or Parenteral (IM or IV)

Drug: Take c̄ meal(s) &/or HS. **Diet:** Bland diet may be recommended. Limit caffeine/xanthine, see p 240. **Nutr:** ↓ Vit B_{12} abs.[74]
Oral/GI: N/V, abdominal pain, diarrhea, constipation.
S/Cond: Caution c̄ alcohol. Caution c̄ lactation. Avoid smoking.
Other: Headache, dizziness, drowsiness, rash. Rare blurred vision.
Blood/Serum: ↑ SGPT, ↑ SGOT, ↑ GGT, ↑ crea. Possible ↓ Vit B_{12} c̄ LT use.
Urinary: False + pro c̄ Multistix. **Monitor:** Hepatic func.

Reglan — ANTIEMETIC, ANTI-GERD — See **metoclopramide HCl p 131**

Relafen — NSAID — See **nabumetone p 137**

reserpine — ANTIHYPERTENSIVE, rauwolfia alkaloid

Drug: Take c̄ food or milk to ↓ GI distress. **Diet:** ↓ Na, ↓ cal may be recommended. Avoid natural licorice. **Nutr:** Anorexia, ↑ appetite, ↑ wt. **Oral/GI:** Dry mouth, N/V, stomach cramps, black tarry stools, diarrhea, GI bleeding. **S/Cond:** Avoid alcohol. Not c̄ lactation. ↑ risk of dental problems, see p 9 & 14.

Other: Dizziness, nasal congestion, drowsiness, headache, peripheral edema, rash, depression (may be severe), arrhythmias, bradycardia, anxiety, weakness, blurred vision, muscle aches, EPS c̄ large doses.

Blood/Serum: ↑ prolactin.

Monitor: BP.

Restoril — SEDATIVE, Sleep Aid, Benzodiazepine — See **temazepam p 191**

Retrovir — ANTIVIRAL — See **zidovudine p 215**

ReVia — ANTI ALCOHOLISM — See **naltrexone HCl p 138**

Rheumatrex — ANTIARTHRITIC — See **methotrexate p 129**

ribavirin
Virazole — ANTIVIRAL, Aerosol only — (Oral or IV— investigational)

S/Cond: Not c̄ lactation. **Other:** Bradycardia, ↓ BP, conjunctivitis, rash. (Oral or IV— Fatigue, insomnia, anorexia, headache, nausea.)

Blood/Serum: Anemia. Oral or IV— ↑ bil, ↑ SGOT, ↑ SGPT.[6]

rifabutin
Mycobutin

ANTIBIOTIC, ANTIMAC in HIV

Drug: Take on empty stomach or c̄ food to ↓ GI distress. **Diet:** ↑ fat meals ↓ the rate, but not the extent of abs. **Oral/GI:** Taste changes, N/V, abdominal pain, dyspepsia, flatulence. **S/Cond:** Not c̄ lactation.
Other: Red/orange body fluids, muscle pain, fever, rash.
Blood/Serum: ↓ WBC, ↓ platelets.
Urinary: RED/ORANGE URINE. **Monitor:** WBC & platelets.

Rifamate

ANTIBIOTIC, ANTITUBERCULOSIS — See **isoniazid p 110** & **rifampin below**

rifampin
Rifadin

ANTIBIOTIC, ANTITUBERCULOSIS — Oral or Parenteral (IV)

Drug: Take c̄ 8 oz H_2O 1 hr before or 2 hrs after food. May take c̄ meal to ↓ GI irritation. May mix cap contents c̄ applesauce or jelly.
Nutr: Anorexia. May affect Vit D metabolism.
Oral/GI: Oral candidiasis, dyspepsia, N/V, cramps, diarrhea, flatulence. Rare pseudomembranous colitis. **S/Cond:** Avoid alcohol. Not c̄ lactation. Caution c̄ diabetics on sulfonylureas— ↑ glucose. 84-91% serum pro bound.[6]
Other: Red/orange body fluids, rash, flu-like syndrome, allergic reaction, dizziness, drowsiness, confusion, visual changes, headache, ataxia, flushing, itching, facial & peripheral edema. Rare jaundice and hepatitis.
Blood/Serum: ↑ SGOT, ↑ SGPT, ↑ alk phos, ↑ bil, ↓ Vit D, ↑ PTH, ↑ BUN, ↑ crea, ↑ uric acid. Rare dyscrasias. Inaccurate micorbiological Fol & Vit B_{12} assays. **Urinary:** RED/ORANGE URINE. **Monitor:** CBC, hepatic func.

Rifater
Tab— sucrose

ANTITUBERCULOSIS — See **rifampin above, isoniazid p 110** & **pyrazinamide p 171**

rimantadine
Flumadine
Syrup— saccharin, sorbitol

ANTIVIRAL, ANTI-INFLUENZA A

Drug: Take s̄ regard to food. **Oral/GI:** Dry mouth, nausea. **S/Cond:** Not c̄ lactation. **Other:** Insomnia, nervousness.

Riopan
magaldrate
Riopan Plus
+ simethicone
sorbitol, saccharin, Na free

ANTACID, ANTIFLATULENT c̄ simethicone

Drug: Take between meals & HS. Follow c̄ 8 oz H_2O. **Diet:** Take Fe or F suppl or MVI + minerals separately by ≥ 2 hrs. **Nutr:** ↓ abs Fe, F.
Oral/GI: Chalky taste. **S/Cond:** Thickens some tube feedings.[8]
Blood/Serum: ↓ P & ↓ K c̄ LT use of high doses.
Urinary: ↓ pH.

risperidone
Risperdal
Tab— lactose

ANTIPSYCHOTIC

Drug: Take s̄ regard to food. **Nutr:** ↑ appetite, ↑ wt.
Oral/GI: ↑ salivation, N/V, dyspepsia, abdominal pain, constipation, diarrhea.
S/Cond: Avoid alcohol. Not c̄ lactation. 90% serum pro bound.
Other: Drowsiness, insomnia, anxiety, weakness, EPS at high dose, dizziness, rash, muscle pain, tachycardia. **Blood/Serum:** ↑ prolactin. < 1% ↓ Na, ↑ CPK, ↑ SGOT, ↑ SGPT, ↓ Hgb, ↓ HCT.

Ritalin

PSYCHOSTIMULANT, ANTI-ADHD — See **methylphenidate HCl p 130**

Robaxin — MUSCLE RELAXANT — See **methocarbamol p 128**

Robitussin — EXPECTORANT — See **guaifenesin p 100**

Rocaltrol — Ca REGULATOR, Active Vit D_3 — See **calcitriol p 39**

Rocephin — ANTIBIOTIC, ceftriaxone — See **cephalosporins p 46**

Roferon-A — ANTINEOPLASTIC — See **interferon alfa 2a p 108**

Rolaids Calcium Rich/ Sodium Free — ANTACID, Ca SUPPLEMENT — See **calcium carbonate p 40**

Rondec/ Rondec TR (SR)
carbinoxamine maleate,
pseudoephedrine HCl
Tab— lactose
Rondec DM
+ **dextromethorphan hydrobromide**
All liquid forms— sorbitol

ANTIHISTAMINE, DECONGESTANT + ANTITUSSIVE (**Rondec DM** only)
Drug: Take c̄ food, H_2O, or milk to ↓ GI distress. Drink 8 oz H_2O after each dose. Swallow SR tab whole. **Nutr:** Anorexia. **Oral/GI:** Dry mouth, N/V, dyspepsia, diarrhea. **S/Cond:** Avoid alcohol. Caution c̄ lactation. Pseudoephedrine syrup precipitates some tube feedings.[8]
Other: Drowsiness, dizziness, headache, tremor, nervousness, arrhythmias.
Blood/Serum: Dyscrasias.

Roxicet — ANALGESIC, Narcotic — See **oxycodone p 150 & acetaminophen p 17**
Soln— 0.4% alcohol, sorbitol

Roxicodone — ANALGESIC, Narcotic — See **oxycodone p 150**

Rowasa ANTI-INFLAMMATORY See **mesalamine p 126**

Salagen ANTI-XEROSTOMIA, Cholinergic See **pilocarpine HCl p 162**

salmeterol xinafoate
Serevent
ANTIASTHMA Inhalation Aerosol
Oral/GI: N/V, stomachache, diarrhea. **S/Cond:** Caution c̄ lactation.
Other: <u>Headache</u>, tachycardia, palpitations, tremor, nervousness, rash, cough.

salsalate
(salicylsalicylic acid)
Disalcid
500 mg Cap— starch
NSAID, ANTIARTHRITIC, Analgesic
Drug: Take c̄ food or 8 oz H_2O or milk.
Diet: Limit caffeine, see p 240. **Oral/GI:** <u>N</u>/V, dyspepsia.
S/Cond: Limit alcohol. Caution c̄ lactation or not c̄ lactation if LT use of high doses.[6] Caution c̄ diabetes— ↓ glucose.
Other: <u>Dizziness</u>, <u>rash</u>. Rare hepatitis, Reye's syndrome. No effect on platelet aggregation.
Blood/Serum: ↓ T_3, ↓ T_4, ↑ or ↓ uric acid, ↓ K, ↑ SGOT, ↑ SGPT, ↑ alk phos.
Urinary: False ↑ or ↓ glucose (method dependent). pH change affects drug excretion & blood levels.

Sandimmune IMMUNOSUPPRESSANT See **cyclosporine p 63**

Sandostatin ANTIDIARRHEAL See **octreotide acetate p 146**

scopolamine
Transderm-Scop

ANTIEMETIC, ANTIVERTIGO — transdermal patch

S/Cond: Avoid alcohol. Caution c̄ lactation. **Oral/GI:** DRY MOUTH, constipation. **Other:** Drowsiness, blurred vision, confusion, dizziness, rash, toxic psychosis.[1] **Urinary:** Retention.

secobarbital sodium
Seconal Sodium
9 mg Na/
100 mg Cap

SLEEP AID (short term), Hypnotic, Barbiturate — Oral or Parenteral (IM or IV)

Diet: ↑ Vit D intake or suppl c̄ LT use. Pyr suppl ↓ drug effects.[9b] Limit caffeine/ xanthine, see p 240. **Nutr:** ↑ rate of metabolism of Vit D & Vit K.[4] **Oral/GI:** N/V, constipation. **S/Cond:** Avoid alcohol. Not c̄ lactation. May be habit forming c̄ LT use. **Other:** DROWSINESS, dizziness. **Blood/Serum:** ↓ bil, ↓ Ca,[4] ↑ NH_3,[6] ↓ T_4. Rare dyscrasias. **Monitor:** CBC, renal & hepatic func c̄ LT use.

Seldane

ANTIHISTAMINE — See **terfenadine p 193**

Seldane-D
Tab— lactose

ANTIHISTAMINE, DECONGESTANT — See **terfenadine p 193 & pseudoephedrine HCl p 170**

selegiline
Eldepryl
Tab— lactose

ANTIPARKINSON (adjunct to carbidopa/levodopa)

Drug: Take c̄ breakfast & lunch. **Diet:** If dose > 10 mg/day, avoid high tyramine foods, see p 243. **Oral/GI:** Dry mouth, dysphagia, nausea, abdominal pain. **S/Cond:** Not c̄ lactation.[10] ↑ risk of dental problems, see p 9 & 14. **Other:** Dizziness, confusion, hallucinations, headache, insomnia, EPS, tardive dyskinesia, peripheral edema, arrhythmias, ↑ or ↓ BP. **Blood/Serum:** Transient ↑ SGOT, ↑ SGPT.

selenium (Se)

MINERAL SUPPLEMENT

Drug: 50 to 100 ug/day maximum suppl to treat def. Suppl recommended c̄ HIV or TPN. **Diet:** Large dose Vit C ↓ abs.[73] **Nutr:** Se antioxidant action is synergistic c̄ Vit E. RDA— Men = 70 ug; Women = 55; Children = 20-50; Pregnancy = 65; Lactation = 75. ↑ need c̄ HIV.
Oral/GI: Toxicity— metallic or sour milk taste, garlic breadth odor, dysphagia, N/V, abdominal pain, diarrhea.
S/Cond: Def symptoms— Kashen disease, cardiomyopathy, CHF, muscle weakness. **Other:** Toxicity reported c̄ dose ≥ 1 mg/day. Toxicity— Muscle weakness, fatigue, dermatitis, nail & hair changes/loss, garlic body odor, irritability, growth retardation, hepatic necrosis. **Monitor:** Se c̄ LT TPN.[75]

senna
Senokot
Syrup— 7% alcohol, sucrose
Granules— cocoa, sucrose
Tab— lactose

STIMULANT LAXATIVE

Drug: Take HS c̄ 8 oz H_2O or juice. Dissolve granules in 8 oz H_2O or other liquid.[13] **Diet:** High fiber c̄ 1500-2000 mL fluid/day to prevent constipation. **Nutr:** Electrolyte imbalance c̄ excessive use.
Oral/GI: N/V, cramps, diarrhea, laxative dependence & loss of normal bowel func c̄ LT use.
Blood/Serum: LT or excess— ↑ glucose, ↓ K, ↓ Ca.

Senokot-S
Tab— lactose

STIMULANT LAXATIVE, STOOL SOFTENER

See **senna above & docusate sodium p 76**

Septra

ANTIBIOTIC
Susp— 0.26% alcohol, sorbitol, saccharin

See **trimethoprim c̄ sulfamethoxazole p 202**

Serax — ANTIANXIETY, Benzodiazepine — See **oxazepam p 149**

Serentil — ANTIPSYCHOTIC, Phenothiazine — See **mesoridazine p 126**

Serevent — ANTIASTHMA — See **salmeterol xinafoate p 179**

sertraline HCl
Zoloft

ANTIDEPRESSANT, SSRI
Drug: Take consistently c̄ or s̄ food (food ↑ abs). **Nutr:** Anorexia, ↓ wt.
Oral/GI: Dry mouth, N/V, dyspepsia, diarrhea, constipation.
S/Cond: Avoid alcohol. Caution c̄ lactation.
Caution c̄ elderly— ↓ plasma clearance of drug.[10] 98% serum pro bound.
Other: Insomnia, dizziness, drowsiness, tremor, headache, palpitations, agitation, anxiety, visual disturbances.
Blood/Serum: Slight ↑ chol & TG, ↓ uric acid. <1% ↑ SGOT, ↑ SGPT.

Serzone — ANTIDEPRESSANT — See **nefazodone p 140**

simethicone
Mylanta Gas
Chew Tab— sorbitol
Mylicon
Drops— saccharin
Phazyme
Tab— lactose
Drops— saccharin

ANTIFLATULENT
Drug: Take after meals &/or HS. Chew chewable tab well.
May mix drops c̄ 1 oz cool H_2O or other liquid.
Diet: Proper diet and exercise important.[13] Avoid carbonated beverages & gas-forming foods to prevent flatulence.
Oral/GI: Belching. Not absorbed from GI tract.

simvastatin
Zocor
Tab— lactose, starch

ANTIHYPERLIPIDEMIC, HMG-CoA reductase inhibitor

Drug: Take s̄ regard to food. Take single dose HS. **Diet:** ↓ fat, ↓ chol, (↓ cal if needed). Not c̄ high dose Nia — possible myopathy.
Oral/GI: Dyspepsia, constipation.
S/Cond: Limit alcohol. Not c̄ lactation. 95% serum pro bound.
Other: Muscle pain, insomnia.
Blood/Serum: ↓ CHOL, ↓ LDL, ↓ VLDL, ↑ HDL, ↓ TG.
Transient— ↑ CPK, ↑ SGOT, ↑ SGPT.
Monitor: Chol, LDL, CPK, hepatic func.

Sinemet	ANTIPARKINSON	See **levodopa & carbidopa p 117**
Sinequan	ANTIDEPRESSANT	See **doxepin HCl p 77**
Slo-Bid	BRONCHODILATOR	See **theophylline p 194**
Slo-Phyllin	BRONCHODILATOR	See **theophylline p 194**
Slow-K	ELECTROLYTE, MINERAL SUPPLEMENT	See **potassium chloride p 164**
Slow-Mag	MINERAL SUPPLEMENT	See **magnesium p 122**

sodium bicarbonate
Sodium Bicarbonate
($NaHCO_3$)
27% Na
90 mg Na/325 mg Tab
23 mg Na/vial Parenteral
972 mg Na/tsp Pwd

ANTACID, ALKALINIZING AGENT Oral or Parenteral (IV)
Drug: As antacid—take after meals c̄ 8 oz H_2O.
Diet: Consider the Na content c̄ ↓ Na diet. Take Fe suppl separately, 1 hr before or 2 hrs after drug. Caution c̄ Ca suppl & limit milk c̄ LT use—may cause milk-alkali syndrome.
Nutr: ↑ thirst, ↑ wt (edema).
Oral/GI: Belching, gastric distention, cramps, flatulence.
S/Cond: Caution c̄ ESRD.
Other: Peripheral edema. **Blood/Serum:** ↑ Na. ↓ K, ↓ Ca c̄ IV.
Urinary: ↑ pH.

sodium phosphate
Fleet
Phospho-soda
2,200 mg Na/4 tsp

LAXATIVE, Saline See also listing for **phosphates p 162**
Drug: Take on empty stomach. Dilute in 4 oz cool H_2O, follow c̄ 8 oz H_2O or fruit juice. **Diet:** Encourage ↑ fluids unless otherwise directed.
Oral/GI: N/V, abdominal cramps, diarrhea. **S/Cond:** Caution c̄ lactation. Not c̄ ↓ Na diet or ESRD. Thickens some tube feedings.
Other: Dehydration.
Blood/Serum: ↓ K, ↑ Na, ↑ glucose c̄ LT or excessive use. ↓ Ca, ↑ P, in ESRD.

sodium polystyrene sulfonate
Kayexalate
Pwd— 100 mg Na/g

ANTIHYPERKALEMIA, Cation Exchange Resin
Drug: Mix pwd c̄ 20-100 mL cool H_2O or 70% sorbitol syrup. May mix pwd or susp c̄ cool food. DO NOT HEAT.
Diet: ↓ K. Avoid K suppl. Take Ca suppl or antacids separately by

Sodium Polystyrene Sulfonate
Susp—14 g sorbitol, 1500 mg Na/60 mL, saccharin, 0.1% alcohol

several hrs.
Nutr: Anorexia. 33% of Na is abs = 33 mg Na/g drug; 500 mg Na/dose.
Oral/GI: N/V, CONSTIPATION, fecal impaction especially in elderly, diarrhea.
S/Cond: Caution c̄ lactation. Caution c̄ those on ↓ Na diet.
Other: Edema, hypokalemia, hypocalcemia, confusion, weakness, irritability, irregular heart beat.
Blood/Serum: ↓ POTASSIUM, ↓ Mg, ↓ Ca.
Monitor: Electrolytes, Mg, Ca.

Solu-Cortef — CORTICOSTEROID, hydrocortisone — See **corticosteroids p 60**

Solu-Medrol — CORTICOSTEROID, methylprednisolone — See **corticosteroids p 60**

Soma — MUSCLE RELAXANT — See **carisoprodol p 43**

sorbitol — LAXATIVE, Hyperosmotic — Oral or Rectal Suppository
Drug: Take HS.
Diet: High fiber c̄ 1500-2000 mL fluid/day to prevent constipation.
Nutr: Not absorbed.
Oral/GI: SWEET TASTE, bloating, flatulence, diarrhea.

Sorbitrate — ANTIANGINAL — See **isosorbide dinitrate p 110**

sotalol HCl
Betapace
Tab— lactose, starch

ANTIARRHYTHMIC, Non-Selective Beta-Blocker
Drug: Food ↓ abs 20%. Take consistently c̄ or s̄ food. **Nutr:** Wt changes.
Oral/GI: N/V, dyspepsia, abdominal pain, diarrhea, flatulence.
S/Cond: Avoid alcohol. Not c̄ lactation. Caution c̄ diabetes— may mask symptoms of & prolong hypoglycemia. May inhibit insulin response to hyperglycemia. Not c̄ hypokalemia or hypomagnesemia.[7]
Other: DIZZINESS, FATIGUE, weakness, headache, edema, ↓ BP, rash.
Blood/Serum: Rare ↑ SGOT, ↑ SGPT, dyscrasias.
Monitor: BP. CBC, hepatic & renal func.[13]

spironolactone
Aldactone

ANTIHYPERTENSIVE, DIURETIC, K-Sparing
Drug: Take c̄ food to ↓ GI irritation & ↑ abs.
Diet: Avoid excessive K intake, K suppl, salt subs. ↓ Na, ↓ cal may be recommended. Avoid natural licorice.
Nutr: Anorexia, ↑ thirst.
Oral/GI: Dry mouth, N/V, gastritis, rare gastric bleeding, cramps, diarrhea.
S/Cond: Not c̄ lactation. Caution c̄ ESRD. > 90% serum pro bound.
Other: Headache, dizziness, ataxia, confusion, dehydration.
Blood/Serum: ↑ K, ↓ Na, ↓ Cl, ↑ BUN, ↑ crea, ↑ Mg.
Urinary: ↑ Na, ↑ Cl, ↓ K, ↑ Ca.
Monitor: BP, electrolytes, renal func.

Sporanox ANTIFUNGAL, ANTI-CANDIDIASIS See **itraconazole p 112**

Staphcillin ANTIBIOTIC, penicillin See **methicillin sodium p 128**

stavudine (d4T)
Zerit
Cap— lactose

ANTIVIRAL, ANTI-HIV
Drug: Take s̄ regard to meals. **Nutr:** Anorexia, ↓ wt.
Oral/GI: Stomatitis, N/V, abdominal pain, diarrhea.
S/Cond: Limit alcohol. Not c̄ lactation.
Other: PERIPHERAL NEUROPATHY, chills/fever, headache, weakness, muscle pain, dementia, insomnia, rash, pancreatitis (can be fatal).
Blood/Serum: ↑ SGOT, ↑ SGPT, ↑ alk phos, ↑ bil, ↑ amylase, ↑ lipase, anemia, ↓ platelets, ↓ neutrophils. **Monitor:** Hepatic func, amylase, lipase.

Stelazine
Tab— lactose
Conc— Na bisulfite, sucrose

ANTIPSYCHOTIC, Phenothiazine
trifluoperazine HCl
Parenteral— benzyl alcohol

Oral or Parenteral (IM)
See listing for **perphenazine p 158**

Stilphostrol

ANTINEOPLASTIC, Hormone

See **diethylstilbestrol p 71**

succimer
Chemet
Cap— sucrose, starch

ANTI-LEAD (Pb) POISONING, Chelating Agent
Drug: Insure adequate fluid intake. May take c̄ juice or mix contents of cap c̄ soft food. **Nutr:** Anorexia. **Oral/GI:** Metallic taste, N/V, cramps, diarrhea. **S/Cond:** Discourage lactation.
Other: Drowsiness, dizziness, headache, muscle pain, paresthesia, sensory neuropathy.
Blood/Serum: ↓ Pb, ↓ Zn, ↑ SGOT, ↑ SGPT, ↑ alk phos, ↑ chol, ↓ WBC, ↑ platelets. False ↓ uric acid & CPK.
Urinary: ↑ Pb, ↑ Zn, pro. False + ketones.
Monitor: Weekly CBC c̄ diff, platelets, & hepatic func.

sucralfate
Carafate
Tab— starch
Susp— sorbitol

ANTIULCER, Gastric Mucosa Protectant

Drug: Take c̄ H_2O on empty stomach 1 hr before meals & HS. May suspend tab in flavored syrup or other liquid. **Diet:** Bland diet may be recommended. Take Ca or Mg suppl separately by 30 minutes.
Oral/GI: ↓ pepsin activity by 32%, constipation, cramps.
S/Cond: Avoid or limit alcohol. Caution c̄ lactation. Avoid or limit smoking. Caution c̄ ESRD— high Al content.

Sudafed

DECONGESTANT See **pseudoephedrine HCl p 170**

sulfamethoxazole
Gantanol

ANTIBIOTIC, Sulfonamide

Drug: Take c̄ 8 oz H_2O. **Diet:** Insure adequate fluid intake. to insure output of ≥ 1500 cc/day.[1] **Nutr:** Anorexia. **Oral/GI:** Stomatitis, N/V, diarrhea. Rare pseudomembranous colitis. **S/Cond:** Limit alcohol. Not c̄ lactation. Caution c̄ diabetics on sulfonylurea — ↓ glucose. Caution c̄ G6PD def— ↑ risk of hemolytic anemia.
Other: Allergic reaction, rash, photosensitivity, fatigue, dizziness, headache, depression, edema, insomnia. Rare hepatitis, jaundice, Stevens-Johnson syndrome, pancreatitis.
Blood/Serum: ↑ SGOT, ↑ SGPT, ↑ bil, ↑ BUN, ↑ crea, dyscrasias. Rare hemolytic or aplastic anemia (can be fatal).
Urinary: False + glucose ($CuSO_4$). Rare crystalluria.
Monitor: CBC, urinalysis & renal func c̄ LT use.

sulfasalazine
Azulfidine
Azulfidine EN
enteric-coated

ANTI-INFLAMMATORY, Sulfonamide (anti-ulcerative colitis, Crohn's)

Drug: Take c̄ 8 oz H_2O after meals or c̄ food to ↓ GI irritation. Swallow EN tab whole. **Diet:** Insure adequate fluid intake to insure output of ≥ 1500 cc/day.[1] Fol suppl (1 mg/day) recommended.[1] ↑ Fol intake. **Nutr:** ANOREXIA. ↓ abs & metabolism of Fol. **Oral/GI:** NAUSEA/VOMITING, GI DISTRESS, diarrhea. **S/Cond:** Not c̄ lactation. Caution c̄ G6PD def— ↑ risk of hemolytic anemia. Caution c̄ diabetics on sulfonylurea— ↓ glucose.[9b] 99% serum pro bound.
Other: HEADACHE, dizziness, rash, photosensitivity, orange/yellow skin.
Blood/Serum: ↓ Fol. Dyscrasias. Rare aplastic anemia (can be fatal).
Urinary: Orange/yellow color. **Monitor:** CBC c̄ diff.

sulfisoxazole
Gantrisin

ANTIBIOTIC, sulfonamide See listing for **sulfamethoxazole p 188**

Tab— lactose Syrup— 3.5 g sucrose/5 mL, 0.9% alcohol

sulindac
Clinoril
Tab— starch

NSAID, ANTIARTHRITIC

Drug: Take c̄ food & 8 oz milk or H_2O to ↓ GI irritation.
Diet: Caution c̄ GI irritants eg K suppl (↑ risk of GI irritation).
Nutr: ↓ appetite. **Oral/GI:** Pain, dyspepsia, N/V, constipation, diarrhea, flatulence, bloating, GI ulcers & bleeding (may be sudden & serious).
S/Cond: Avoid alcohol. Not c̄ lactation. 93-98% serum pro bound.
Other: Dizziness, headache, rash, nervousness, edema.
Blood/Serum: ↑ alk phos, ↑ SGOT, ↑ SGPT. <1% dyscrasias, ↑ K, ↑ BUN, ↑ amylase.
Urinary: <1% pro, hematuria. **Monitor:** Hepatic & renal func c̄ LT use.

sumatriptan succinate ANTIMIGRAINE Oral or Parenteral (SC)
Imitrex
Parenteral— 7 mg NaCl/mL
Tab— lactose

Drug: Swallow tab whole, do not break, crush or chew.
Oral/GI: Jaw, mouth & throat discomfort, dysphagia.
S/Cond: Avoid alcohol. Caution c̄ lactation.
Other: ATYPICAL SENSATIONS (eg tingling, flushing), dizziness, flushing, headache, vision changes, weakness, muscle cramps, mildly ↑ BP.

Sumycin ANTIBIOTIC See **tetracycline HCl p 194**

Suprax ANTIBIOTIC, Cephalosporin See **cefixime p 44**

Surfak STOOL SOFTENER See **docusate calcium p 76**

Symmetrel ANTIPARKINSON, ANTIVIRAL See **amantadine HCl p 23**

Synthroid THYROID HORMONE (T_4) See **thyroid p 196**
levothyroxine sodium
Tab— lactose, sugar

tacrine ANTI-ALZHEIMER'S, Cholinesterase Inhibitor
Cognex
Cap— lactose

Drug: Take 1 hr before or 2 hrs after meals. Food ↓ bioavailability 30-40%. May take c̄ food to ↓ GI irritation. **Nutr:** Anorexia, ↓ wt.
Oral/GI: May ↑ gastric acid secretion, N/V, dyspepsia, diarrhea, constipation, flatulence. **S/Cond:** Plasma drug conc ↓ 67% in smokers.
Other: HEPATOTOXICITY, dizziness, ataxia, insomnia, fatigue, muscle pain, rash, peripheral edema, tremor. **Blood/Serum:** ↑ SGPT, ↑ SGOT. <1%- -dyscrasias. **Monitor:** SGPT, SGOT weekly x 18 wks, then q 3 mos.

Tagamet — ANTIULCER — See **cimetidine p 52**

tamoxifen citrate
Nolvadex
Tab— mannitol, starch
Nolvadex-D (enteric-coat) (Canada only)

ANTINEOPLASTIC, Estrogen Antagonist

Drug: Swallow enteric-coated tab whole.
Diet: Take Ca or Mg suppl separately from enteric coated tab by 2 hrs.
Nutr: Anorexia, ↓ wt.
Oral/GI: N/V. **S/Cond:** Not c̄ lactation.
Other: Hot flashes, peripheral edema, cough, headache, fatigue, rash.
Blood/Serum: ↑ Ca, ↑ SGOT, ↑ bil, ↑ alk phos,↓ chol,[76] ↓ LDL,[76] ↑ BUN, ↑ crea, ↓ WBC, ↓ platelets. Rare ↑ chol, ↑ TG, ↓ T_4.
Monitor: CBC c̄ diff, platelets, hepatic func.

Tavist — ANTIHISTAMINE — See **clemastine fumarate p 55**

Tavist-D
Tab— lactose
— ANTIHISTAMINE, DECONGESTANT — See **clemastine fumarate p 55 & phenylpropanolamine p 160**

Taxol — ANTINEOPLASTIC — See **paclitaxel p 150**

Tazidime — ANTIBIOTIC, ceftazidime — See **cephalosporins p 46**

Tegretol — ANTICONVULSANT — See **carbamazepine p 42**

Teldrin — ANTIHISTAMINE — See **chlorpheniramine maleate p 49**

temazepam
Restoril
Cap— lactose, benzyl alcohol

SLEEP AID, Sedative, Hypnotic, Benzodiazepine

Drug: Take 30 to 60 minutes before bed. **S/Cond:** Avoid alcohol. Caution c̄ lactation. May be habit forming c̄ LT use. 96% serum pro bound.
Other: Drowsiness, dizziness, confusion
Blood/Serum: Possible ↑ SGOT, ↑ SGPT, ↑ alk phos, ↑ bil, ↑ LDH. Rare dyscrasias.
Monitor: CBC c̄ diff, hepatic func c̄ LT routine use.

Tempra — ANALGESIC — See **acetaminophen p 17**

Tenex — ANTIHYPERTENSIVE — See **guanfacine HCl p 100**

Ten-K — ELECTROLYTE, Mineral Supplement — See **potassium chloride p 164**

Tenoretic — ANTIHYPERTENSIVE — See **atenolol p 29 & chlorthalidone p 51**

Tenormin — ANTIHYPERTENSIVE — See **atenolol p 29**

terazosin HCl
Hytrin
Tab— lactose

ANTIHYPERTENSIVE, ANTI-BPH (Benign Prostatic Hyperplasia)
$Alpha_1$ Adrenergic Blocker

Drug: Take HS.
Diet: ↓ Na, ↓ cal diet may be recommended. Avoid natural licorice.
Nutr: ↑ wt.
Oral/GI: Dry mouth, nausea.
S/Cond: Caution c̄ alcohol. Caution c̄ lactation.

90-94 % serum pro bound.
Other: Dizziness, weakness, ↓ BP, blurred vision, drowsiness, peripheral edema, palpitations, paresthesia, back pain, rash. **Blood/Serum:** ↓ HCT, ↓ Hgb, ↓ WBC, ↓ alb, ↓ TP, ↓ chol, ↓ LDL, ↓ VLDL. **Monitor:** BP.

terbutaline sulfate
Brethine
Tab— lactose, starch
Bricanyl
Tab— lactose

BRONCHODILATOR, Sympathomimetic   Oral, Inhalant or Parenteral (SC)
Drug: Take oral form on empty stomach. Food ↓ abs 33 %.[13]
Diet: Limit caffeine/xanthine, see p 240.
Oral/GI: Dry mouth/throat & unusual taste (inhalant), N/V, dyspepsia.
S/Cond: Caution c̄ lactation.
Caution c̄ diabetes— ↑ glucose. Caution c̄ hypertension.
Other: TREMOR, nervousness, headache, palpitations, tachycardia, ↑ BP, dizziness, drowsiness, insomnia, sweating, muscle cramps, weakness.
Blood/Serum: ↓ K c̄ high dose.[13]

terfenadine
Seldane
Tab— lactose

ANTIHISTAMINE
Drug: May take c̄ food to ↓ GI distress.
Nutr: ↑ appetite, ↑ wt.
Oral/GI: Dry mouth/throat, N/V, GI distress, diarrhea.
S/Cond: Not c̄ lactation. 97 % serum pro bound.
Other: Headache, drowsiness, fatigue.
Blood/Serum: Rare ↑ SGOT, ↑ SGPT, ↑ alk phos, ↑ bil.

tetracycline HCl
Achromycin-V
Cap— lactose
Sumycin
Tab/Cap— lactose
Tetracycline

ANTIBIOTIC

Drug: Take c̄ 8 oz H_2O 1 hr before or 2 hrs after food/milk.
Diet: Take Ca, Fe, Mg, Zn or MVI c̄ minerals separately by 3 hrs. Not c̄ Al, Ca, or Mg suppl or antacids. **Nutr:** Forms chelates c̄ Ca, Fe, Mg, or Zn & ↓ both drug & mineral abs. ↓ abs amino acids.[11] Possible ↓ Vit K due to ↓ bacterial synthesis in intestine. Possible B Vit def c̄ LT use.[6] Anorexia.
Oral/GI: Stomatitis, oral candidiasis, dysphagia, N/V, cramps, diarrhea. Rare pseudomembranous colitis.
S/Cond: Not c̄ lactation. Caution c̄ diabetes— ↓ glucose.[18] Caution c̄ tube feeding— chelation c̄ minerals may ↓ both drug & mineral abs.[8] **Other:** Ataxia, dizziness, photosensitivity, headache. Rare hepatotoxicity c̄ high dose.
Blood/Serum: ↑ alk phos, ↑ bil, ↑ SGOT, ↑ SGPT, ↑ BUN, ↑ amylase. ↓ Pyr, ↓ Vit B_{12}, ↓ pantothenic acid. **Urinary:** ↑ Rib, ↑ Fol.

theophylline
Elixophyllin
Elixir— 20% alcohol
Slo-Bid
Slo-Phyllin
Theobid
Theo-Dur
Theolair
Theo-24
Uniphyl

BRONCHODILATOR, Methylxanthine Oral or Parenteral (IV)

Drug: Follow manufacturer's recommendations about taking with food. Food affects abs in some SR forms. Swallow enteric-coated & SR forms whole, do not crush or chew.
Diet: Consistent intake of CHO & pro for consistent drug levels. Limit charcoal-broiled foods. Avoid drastic changes in caffeine intake,[3] see p 240.
Nutr: Anorexia. ↑ pro, ↓ CHO — ↑ metabolism of drug & ↓ blood level.
Oral/GI: Bitter aftertaste, gastro-esophageal reflux, N/V, epigastric pain.
S/Cond: Not c̄ lactation. Caution c̄ diabetes— ↑ glucose c̄ high dose. Smoking ↑ metabolism of drug & ↓ blood level.

Check brand for— lactose, sucrose, starch &/or sorbitol

Other: Nervousness, insomnia, dizziness, headache, rash, seizures, SIADH. **Blood/Serum:** ↑ glucose, ↑ SGOT.[6] False ↑ uric acid, c̄ some methods. **Urinary:** Pro, diuresis (↑ Na, ↑ output), ↑ frequency. **Monitor:** Serum theophylline level.

thiamine
thiamin
vitamin B_1

B COMPLEX VITAMIN, ANTI-BERIBERI

Drug: Anti-beriberi dose is 5-10 mg TID.[1, 13] **Nutr:** ↑ cal &/or CHO intake ↑ Thi requirement. 0.5 mg/1000 cal recommended.

RDA- Men = 1.5 mg, Women = 1.1; Pregnancy = 1.5, Lactation = 1.6.

Oral/GI: IV — Nausea, diarrhea, GI bleeding.

S/Cond: Fol or pro def ↓ abs of Thi. Alcohol inhibits abs.[13] Impaired utilization in elderly—possible ↑ requirements. **Other:** IV— feeling of warmth, weakness, angioedema, allergic reaction, rash.

thioridazine HCl
Mellaril
Conc 30— 3% alcohol, sorbitol
100— 4.2% alcohol, sorbitol
Susp— 3 g sucrose/5 mL
Tab— lactose, sucrose, starch

ANTIPSYCHOTIC, Phenothiazine

Drug: Take c̄ food or 8 oz milk or H_2O. Liquid— dilute in orange or grapefruit juice. **Nutr:** ↑ need for Rib.[41] ↑ APPETITE, ↑ WT.

Oral/GI: DRY MOUTH, N/V, CONSTIPATION. **S/Cond:** Avoid alcohol. Not c̄ lactation. ↑ risk of dental problems, see p 9 & 14. Liquid forms precipitate tube feeding.[8] > 90% serum pro bound. **Other:** Drowsiness, dizziness, ↓ BP, blurred vision, weakness, rash, peripheral edema, tachycardia, EPS. Tardive dyskinesia c̄ LT use. **Blood/Serum:** ↑ bil, ↑ alk phos, ↑ SGOT, ↑ SGPT, ↑ prolactin, ↑ chol, ↑ glucose. <1%- dyscrasias.

Urinary: Retention, ↑ Rib. + glucose. False + bil.

Monitor: CBC c̄ diff, hepatic func.

See "Guide to the Use of This Book" inside front cover.

thiothixene **Navane** Conc— 7% alcohol, dextrose, sorbitol Cap— lactose, starch Parenteral—benzyl alcohol, dextrose	ANTIPSYCHOTIC **Drug:** Take c̄ food or H_2O. **Nutr:** ↑ need for Rib.[11] ↑ APPETITE, ↑ WT. **Oral/GI:** Dry mouth, N/V, constipation. **S/Cond:** Avoid alcohol. Caution c̄ lactation. ↑ risk of dental problems, see p 9 & 14. **Other:** EXTRAPYRAMIDAL SYMPTOMS, DROWSINESS, restlessness, ↓ BP, dizziness, photosensitivity, tachycardia, insomnia, rash, seizures. Tardive dyskinesia c̄ LT use. **Blood/Serum:** ↑ alk phos, ↑ SGOT, ↑ SGPT, ↓ uric acid, ↓ WBC, ↓ PT. **Urinary:** Retention. **Monitor:** CBC c̄ diff c̄ high dose or LT use.[13]	Oral or Parenteral (IM)
Thorazine	ANTIPSYCHOTIC, Phenothiazine	See **chlorpromazine HCl p 50**
thyroid **levothyroxine sodium** **Synthroid** (T_4) Tab— lactose, sugar **Levoxyl** **Levothroid**	THYROID PREPARATION **Drug:** Take on empty stomach before breakfast to ↑ abs. **Diet:** Take Fe suppl separately by 4 hrs (may ↓ abs).[9b] **Nutr:** Appetite changes, ↓ wt. **Oral/GI:** Nausea, diarrhea. **S/Cond:** Caution c̄ lactation. Caution c̄ diabetics on insulin or sulfonylurea— ↑ glucose. 99% serum pro bound. **Other:** Headache, tremor, nervousness, insomnia, ↑ BP, ↑ pulse, palpitations. **Blood/Serum:** ↑ T_4, ↑ T_3, ↓ TSH, ↑ glucose, ↓ chol. **Monitor:** Thyroid func, eg free T_4 index or free T_4, TSH.	Oral or Parenteral (IV or IM)

ticarcillin disodium
Ticar
Pwd—120-150 mg Na/g

ANTIBIOTIC, penicillin — Parenteral only (IM or IV)

Diet: Consider Na content c̄ ↓ Na diet. **Oral/GI:** Oral candidiasis, altered taste, N/V, diarrhea. Rare pseudomembranous colitis.
S/Cond: Caution c̄ lactation.
Other: Headache, fatigue, rash.
Blood/Serum: Dyscrasias, ↑ PT, ↑ SGOT, ↑ SGPT, ↑ bil, ↑ alk phos, ↑ LDH, ↑ crea, ↑ BUN, ↓ K, ↑ Na, ↑ PTT. Rare ↓ glucose.
Urinary: False + pro. False + glucose ($CuSO_4$).
Monitor: K, CBC c̄ diff, renal & hepatic func c̄ LT use.

Tigan

ANTINAUSEANT, ANTIEMETIC — See **trimethobenzamide HCl p 202**

Timentin
ticarcillin disodium
& **clavulanate K**

ANTIBIOTIC, penicillin — See **ticarcillin disodium above**
Pwd— 109 mg Na/g & 60 mg K/100 mg — Parenteral only (IM or IV)
Soln— 430 mg Na/100 mL

tobramycin sulfate
Nebcin
Na bisulfite

ANTIBIOTIC, Aminoglycoside — Parenteral only (IM or IV)
See listing for **gentamicin sulfate p 98**

Tofranil

ANTIDEPRESSANT, Tricyclic — See **imipramine HCl p 106**

tolazamide
Tolinase

ORAL HYPOGLYCEMIC, Sulfonylurea — See listing for **tolbutamide p 198**

tolbutamide
Orinase
Tab— lactose

ORAL HYPOGLYCEMIC, Sulfonylurea

Drug: Take in AM or divided doses. **Diet:** Prescribed diet compliance important. **Nutr:** ↑ or ↓ appetite. **Oral/GI:** Altered taste, N/V, dyspepsia, epigastric fullness, constipation, diarrhea. **S/Cond:** Limit alcohol. Not c̄ lactation. 95% serum pro bound. Hypoalbuminemia (<3 g/dL) may ↑ drug effects. **Other:** Headache, dizziness, drowsiness, rash, photosensitivity. Rare SIADH, jaundice, hepatitis.

Blood/Serum: ↓ GLUCOSE, ↑ alk phos, ↑ SGOT, ↑ SGPT, ↑ LDH, ↑ BUN, ↑ crea. Rare ↓ Na, dyscrasias **Urinary:** ↓ GLUCOSE.

Monitor: Glucose, possibly glycosylated Hgb.

Toradol NSAID See **ketorolac tromethamine p 113**

tramadol
Ultram
Tab— lactose

ANALGESIC

Drug: Take s̄ regard to food. **Nutr:** Anorexia. **Oral/GI:** Dry mouth, dyspepsia, NAUSEA/vomiting, abdominal pain, CONSTIPATION, flatulence.

S/Cond: Caution c̄ alcohol. Not c̄ lactation.

Other: DIZZINESS, HEADACHE, DROWSINESS, itching, weakness, sweating, rash, visual changes, anxiety, confusion, ataxia, vasodilation.

Blood/Serum: ↑ crea, ↑ SGOT, ↑ SGPT, ↓ Hgb. **Urinary:** Pro. Retention.

Transderm-Nitro ANTIANGINAL See **nitroglycerin p 144**

Transderm-Scop ANTIEMETIC See **scopolamine p 180**

Tranxene ANTIANXIETY, Benzodiazepine See **listing for chlordiazepoxide p 48**

tranylcypromine sulfate
Parnate
Tab— lactose, starch

ANTIDEPRESSANT, MAOI

Diet: Avoid foods ↑ tyramine & other pressor amines to prevent hypertensive crisis, see p 243. Limit caffeine, see p 240. Avoid tryptophan suppl.
Nutr: ↑ appetite, ↑ wt, anorexia. **Oral/GI:** Dry mouth, nausea, constipation, diarrhea. **S/Cond:** Avoid alcohol. Not c̄ lactation. Caution c̄ diabetics on insulin or sulfonylurea— ↓ glucose.
Other: ↑ or ↓ BP, drowsiness, dizziness, tremor, headache, blurred vision, insomnia, edema. Rare SIADH, hepatotoxicity.
Blood/Serum: ↑ SGOT, ↑ SGPT, ↑ Na. Rare ↑ CPK, dyscrasias.
Monitor: BP, hepatic func, CBC.

trazodone HCl
Desyrel
50 & 100 mg
Tabs— lactose
150 & 300 mg
Tabs— starch

ANTIDEPRESSANT

Drug: Take c̄ meals or snack to ↓ dizziness. **Nutr:** ↑ or ↓ appetite, ↑ or ↓ wt. **Oral/GI:** Unpleasant taste, DRY MOUTH, N/V, constipation. **S/Cond:** Avoid alcohol. Caution c̄ lactation. ↑ risk of dental problems, see p 9 & 14. 89-95% serum pro bound. **Other:** DROWSINESS, dizziness, blurred vision, ataxia, headache, tremor, ↑ or ↓ BP, edema, paresthesia, allergic reaction. **Blood/Serum:** Mildly ↑ SGOT, ↑ SGPT, ↑ alk phos. <1% ↓ WBC, ↓ neutrophils, anemia.

Trecator-SC ANTITUBERCULAR See **ethionamide p 84**

Trental HEMORRHEOLOGIC See **pentoxifylline p 156**

triamcinolone
Aristocort
Tab— lactose
Kenalog— Parenteral
benzyl alcohol

CORTICOSTEROID — See **corticosteroids p 60**
Oral or Parenteral

Nutr: Anorexia, unlike other corticosteroids, which may ↑ appetite.[13]

triamcinolone acetonide
Azmacort
1% dehydrated alcohol

ANTIASTHMA, Corticosteroid, inhalant, aerosol

Drug: Moisten throat c̄ H_2O before use. Rinse mouth after use. Do not swallow rinse water. **Oral/GI:** Oral candidiasis,[7] dry mouth, sore throat, nausea. **S/Cond:** Caution c̄ lactation. Good oral hygiene essential.
Other: Headache, cough, facial edema.

Triaminic

ANTIHISTAMINE, DECONGESTANT See **chlorpheniramine maleate p 49** & **phenylpropanolamine HCl p 160**

triamterene
Dyrenium
Cap- lactose,
benzyl alcohol

DIURETIC, K sparing (adjunct to antihypertensive therapy)

Drug: Take after meals or c̄ milk to ↓ GI irritation.
Diet: Avoid excessive K intake, K suppl, salt subs. ↓ Na, ↓ cal may be recommended. Avoid natural licorice.
Nutr: Chemically related to Fol (weak dihydro-folate reductase antagonist). ↓ utilization of Fol.
Oral/GI: N/V, diarrhea.
S/Cond: Not c̄ lactation. Caution c̄ diabetes & ESRD.
Other: Dizziness, headache, photosensitivity.
Blood/Serum: ↑ K, ↓ Mg, ↓ bicarb, ↑ uric acid, ↓ Fol.

Rare ↓ platelets, anemia, ↑ BUN, ↑ crea, ↓ Na, ↑ Cl.[6]
Urinary: ↑ Na, ↑ Cl, slight ↓ K, ↑ Ca, ↑ Mg, ↑ bicarb, ↑ pH.
Monitor: Electrolytes, Mg, renal func, BP, CBC c̄ diff, platelets.

trifluoperazine HCl
Stelazine
Tab— lactose

ANTIPSYCHOTIC, Phenothiazine
Conc— Na bisulfite, sucrose
Parenteral— benzyl alcohol

Oral or Parenteral (IM)
See listing for **perphenazine p 158**

trihexyphenidyl HCl
Artane
Elixir— 5% alcohol, NaCl, sorbitol
Sequel (SR)— sucrose
Tab— starch

ANTIPARKINSON, ANTI-EPS, Anticholinergic
Drug: Take c̄ meals to ↓ GI distress. Swallow Sequel (SR cap) whole.
Oral/GI: DRY MOUTH, MILD NAUSEA/vomiting, constipation.
S/Cond: Avoid alcohol. May inhibit lactation. ↑ risk of dental problems, see p 9 & 14. May aggravate tardive dyskinesia.
Other: DIZZINESS, BLURRED VISION, drowsiness, weakness, nervousness, ↓ sweating, headache, tachycardia. **Urinary:** Retention.

Trilafon
ANTIPSYCHOTIC, Phenothiazine
See **perphenazine p 158**

Tri-Levlen
ORAL CONTRACEPTIVE
See **estrogen p 83**

Trilisate
Liquid— high fructose corn syrup

NSAID
choline salicylate & **magnesium salicylate**
See listing for **salsalate p 158**

trimethobenzamide HCl
Tigan
Cap— lactose, starch

ANTIEMETIC, ANTINAUSEANT — Oral, Parenteral (IM) or Suppository

Oral/GI: Diarrhea. **S/Cond:** Avoid alcohol. Not c̄ lactation.
Other: Drowsiness, dizziness, blurred vision, headache, muscle cramps, rash. Rare hepatotoxicity (jaundice), Reye's syndrome, seizures, EPS.
Blood/Serum: Rare dyscrasias.

trimethoprim c sulfamethoxazole
Bactrim
Susp— 2.5 mg sucrose/5 mL, 0.3% alcohol, saccharin, sorbitol
Tab— starch
Parenteral— 1% benzyl alcohol, Na metabisulfite
Rare anemias, dyscrasias.
Cotrim
Septra
Susp— 0.26% alcohol, saccharin, sorbitol

ANTIBIOTIC, Sulfonamide — Oral or Parenteral (IV)

Drug: Take c̄ food & 8 oz H_2O. **Diet:** Insure adequate fluid intake to insure output of ≥ 1500 cc/day.[1] May need Fol suppl. **Nutr:** Anorexia. Interferes c̄ Fol metabolism. **Oral/GI:** Stomatitis, N/V, diarrhea. Rare pseudomembranous colitis.
S/Cond: Not c̄ lactation. Caution c̄ diabetics on sulfonylurea— ↓ glucose. Caution c̄ G6PD def — ↑ risk of hemolytic anemia.
Other: Allergic reaction, rash, photosensitivity, fatigue, dizziness, headache, ataxia, depression, edema, insomnia. Rare hepatitis, jaundice, pancreatitis.
Blood/Serum: ↑ SGOT, ↑ SGPT, ↑ bil, dyscrasias, ↑ BUN, ↑ crea, ↓ Fol.
Urinary: False + glucose ($CuSO_4$). Crystalluria.
Monitor: CBC, urinalysis, renal func c̄ LT use.

trimetrexate glucuronate ANTI-PCP in HIV, Dihydrofolate Reductase Inhibitor Parenteral only (IV)
Neutrexin
preservative free

Drug: Leucovorin (folinic acid) must be taken to prevent bone marrow suppression. **Oral/GI:** N/V. **S/Cond:** Not $\bar{c}$ lactation. 95% serum pro bound. **Other:** Fatigue, confusion. **Blood/Serum:** ↓ neutrophils, ↑ SGOT, ↑ SGPT, ↑ alk phos, ↑ BUN, ↑ crea, ↓ Ca. Rare ↓ RBC, ↓ platelets.
Monitor: 2X/week— CBC $\bar{c}$ diff, platelets, hepatic & renal func.

Trimox	ANTIBIOTIC	See **amoxicillin p 26**
Tri-Norinyl	ORAL CONTRACEPTIVE	See **estrogen p 83**
Triphasil	ORAL CONTRACEPTIVE	See **estrogen p 83**
triprolidine HCl & pseudoephedrine HCl	ANTIHISTAMINE, DECONGESTANT	See **Actifed p 19**
Tums	ANTACID	See **calcium carbonate p 40**
Tylenol	ANALGESIC	See **acetaminophen p 17**
Tylox Cap— Na metabisulfite	ANALGESIC, NARCOTIC	See **oxycodone HCl p 150 & acetaminophen p 17**
Ultram	ANALGESIC	See **tramadol p 198**

Unasyn ANTIBIOTIC See **ampicillin & sulbactam p 27**

Unipen ANTIBIOTIC See **nafcillin sodium p 138**

Uniphyl BRONCHODILATOR See **theophylline p 194**

Urecholine CHOLINERGIC STIMULANT, ANTI-GERD See **bethanechol Cl p 34**

Valium ANTIANXIETY See **diazepam p 69**

valproic acid ANTICONVULSANT

Depakene
Syrup— sorbitol, sucrose
Depakote
(divalproex Na)
Tab—Delayed Release
Sprinkle Cap

Drug: Take c̄ meals to ↓ GI irritation. Swallow cap/tab whole c̄ H_2O. Do not take tab c̄ milk. Do not take syrup c̄ carbonated beverages— will liberate drug & may cause mouth/throat irritation or unpleasant taste.[6] May mix contents of sprinkle cap c̄ semi-solid food (do not chew).
Nutr: Anorexia, ↓ wt, ↑ appetite, ↑ wt. **Oral/GI:** N/V, indigestion, cramps, diarrhea, constipation. **S/Cond:** Avoid alcohol. Extreme caution c̄ lactation. Not c̄ hepatic disease. 90-95% serum pro bound. Hypoalbuminemia (< 3.0 g/dL) may ↑ drug effects.[13] **Other:** HAND TREMOR, sedation, dizziness, peripheral edema. Rare pancreatitis, hepatotoxicity (can be fatal).
Blood/Serum: ↑ alk phos, ↑ SGOT, ↑ SGPT, ↑ LDH, ↑ bil, ↑ NH_3, ↑ chol,[39] ↑ HDL,[39] ↓ WHITE BLOOD CELLS, ↓ NEUTROPHILS, ↓ T_3, ↓ T_4, ↓ platelets, ↑ coagulation time. Rare ↑ glycine, ↑ amylase. **Urinary:** False + ketones.
Monitor: Hepatic func, CBC c̄ diff, platelets, NH_3, coagulation time, drug level, possibly amylase.

Vancenase
Vanceril
ANTIASTHMA, ADRENOCORTICOID — Nasal Inhalant
See **beclomethasone dipropionate p 32**

vancomycin HCl
Vancocin
ANTIBIOTIC — Oral or Parenteral (IV)

Drug: For oral soln— Flavoring syrup may be added to each dose.
Oral/GI: Bitter taste, nausea. **S/Cond:** Not c̄ lactation.
Other: Allergic reaction, rash, IV — "red man syndrome", nephrotoxicity, ototoxicity. **Blood/Serum:** ↓ neutrophils, ↓ eosinophils, ↑ BUN, ↑ crea. Rare. ↓ platelets. **Monitor:** Renal func, urinalysis, drug level.

Vasotec
ANTIHYPERTENSIVE
See **enalapril maleate p 80**

Veetids
ANTIBIOTIC, penicillin V potassium
See **penicillin p 155**

Velban
ANTINEOPLASTIC
See **vinblastine sulfate p 207**

Velosef
ANTIBIOTIC, Cephalosporin
See **cephradine p 47**

venlafaxine
Effexor
Tab— lactose
ANTIDEPRESSANT, SSRI

Drug: Take s̄ regard to food. **Nutr:** Anorexia, ↓ wt. **Oral/GI:** Dry mouth, taste changes, N/V, dyspepsia, constipation, diarrhea, flatulence.
S/Cond: Avoid alcohol. Caution c̄ lactation.
Other: Drowsiness, dizziness, weakness, insomnia, nervousness, anxiety, tremor, headache, sweating, ↑ BP, blurred vision, rash. **Monitor:** BP.

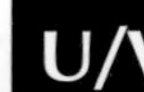

Ventolin BRONCHODILATOR See **albuterol sulfate p 20**

VePesid (VP-16) ANTINEOPLASTIC See **etoposide p 86**

verapamil HCl
Calan
Tab— lactose
Isoptin
Tab— lactose
Verelan
Cap— sugar

ANTIARRHYTHMIC, ANTIANGINA, ANTIHYPERTENSIVE,
Ca Channel Blocker Oral or Parenteral (IV)

Drug: Swallow SR tab whole c̄ food or milk. Take other forms s̄ regard to food. **Diet:** ↓ Na, ↓ cal may be recommended. Avoid natural licorice. Limit caffeine, see p 240. Caution c̄ Ca &/or Vit D suppl— hypercalcemia ↓ effect of drug. **Oral/GI:** Gingival hyperplasia (rare), nausea, constipation. **S/Cond:** Avoid or limit alcohol. Not c̄ lactation. 90% serum pro bound. **Other:** Headache, dizziness, fatigue, weakness, ↓ BP, rash, peripheral &/or pulmonary edema, bradycardia, tachycardia. Rare hepatitis. **Blood/Serum:** ↑ SGOT, ↑ SGPT. **Monitor:** BP. Hepatic func c̄ LT use.

Vibramycin ANTIBIOTIC See **doxycycline p 78**

Vicodin ANALGESIC, Narcotic
hydrocodone bitartrate & acetaminophen
See listing for **oxycodone p 150** & **acetaminophen p 17**

Videx ANTIVIRAL, ANTI-HIV See **didanosine (ddI) p 71**

vinblastine sulfate
Velban

ANTINEOPLASTIC, Vinca Alkaloid — Parenteral only (IV)

Diet: Insure adequate fluid intake. **Nutr:** Anorexia, possible ↓ wt.
Oral/GI: Stomatitis, pharyngitis, sore throat, NAUSEA/VOMITING, abdominal pain, ileus, CONSTIPATION, diarrhea. Rare GI bleeding.
S/Cond: Not $\bar{c}$ lactation. Do dental care cautiously, see p 10 & 14.
Other: BONE MARROW SUPPRESSION, ↑ BP, jaw & bone pain, neurotoxicity, peripheral neuritis, weakness, dizziness, headache, skin lesions, depression.
Blood/Serum: ↓ WHITE BLOOD CELLS, ↓ platelets, ↑ uric acid.[13] Rare anemia
Urinary: ↑ uric acid.[13] **Monitor:** Weekly CBC $\bar{c}$ diff, platelets, hepatic func.

vincristine sulfate
Oncovin
Parenteral— mannitol

ANTINEOPLASTIC, Vinca Alkaloid — Parenteral only (IV)

Diet: Insure adequate fluid intake. **Nutr:** Anorexia, ↓ wt.
Oral/GI: Altered taste, rare stomatitis, dysphagia, mild N/V, bloating, cramps, ileus, severe CONSTIPATION, impaction, diarrhea.
S/Cond: Not $\bar{c}$ lactation.
Other: NEUROTOXICITY (PERIPHERAL NEUROPATHY, PARESTHESIA, ATAXIA, NEURITIC PAIN), acute uric acid nephropathy, jaw & bone pain, muscle pain, ↑ or ↓ BP, headache., rash. Rare SIADH.
Blood/Serum: ↑ URIC ACID, ↑ K. Rare ↓ Na, ↓ WBC, anemia, ↓ platelets.
Urinary: ↑ URIC ACID, retention.
Monitor: Uric acid. Weekly CBC $\bar{c}$ diff, platelets, hepatic func.

vinorelbine tartrate
Navelbine
preservative free

ANTINEOPLASTIC, Vinca Alkaloid — Parenteral only (IV)

Diet: Insure adequate fluid intake. **Nutr:** Anorexia, possible ↓ wt.
Oral/GI: Stomatitis, NAUSEA/VOMITING, CONSTIPATION, diarrhea, paralytic ileus.
S/Cond: Not c̄ lactation. **Other:** BONE MARROW SUPPRESSION, PERIPHERAL NEUROPATHY, PARESTHESIA, WEAKNESS, FATIGUE, jaw, muscle or bone pain, rash, cough, pulmonary reactions.
Monitor: CBC c̄ diff before each dose, hepatic func frequently.

Virazole — ANTIVIRAL — See **ribavirin p 175**

Vistaril — ANTIANXIETY — See **hydroxyzine p 104**

vitamin A
Aquasol A
H_2O miscible retinol form

VITAMIN, Fat Soluble, Antioxidant — Oral or Parenteral (IM)

1 IU = 1 USP = 0.3 RE (retinol equivalent). 1 RE = 1 ug retinol = 6 ug beta carotene = 12 ug other provitamin A carotenoids = 3.33 IU.

Drug: May mix soln c̄ food or juice. H_2O miscible form ↑ abs.
Diet: Adequate fat, pro, Vit E needed for proper abs; Vit E & Zn for proper utilization. Avoid MVI. Avoid high dose Vit E suppl— depletes Vit A stores.
Nutr: RDA— Men = 1000 RE; Women = 800; Lactation = 1300; children = 400-700. Malnutrition or ↓ pro intake ↓ abs of Vit A. Anorexia c̄ toxicity.
Oral/GI: Toxicity causes stomatitis, N/V, abdominal discomfort.
S/Cond: ↓ abs c̄ chronic diarrhea, steatorrhea, cystic fibrosis, hepatic, &/or pancreatic disease. Def symptoms— xerophthalmia (night blindness, dry corneas & conjunctiva, corneal lesions), anorexia, hyperkeratosis, ↑ infection.

Other: Intakes ≥ 25,000 IU for 8 months cause hypervitaminosis A (chronic toxicity).[73] Fetal toxicity occurs c̄ maternal dose of > 6000 IU. Acute toxicity c̄ single dose of ≥ 660,000 IU[77] in adults or 75,000-350,000[13] in children, can be fatal.
Signs of chronic toxicity— Dry skin, nails, lips & mucous membranes, itching, conjunctivitis, hair loss, headache, ataxia, dizziness, visual changes, bone & muscle pain, fatigue, irritability, depression, schizophrenia, fever, hepatotoxicity (can be fatal).
Blood/Serum: Toxicity— ↑ BUN, ↑ crea, ↑ chol, ↑ TG, ↑ Ca, ↑ SGOT, ↑ SGPT, ↓ WBC, ↓ RBC, ↓ platelets, ↓ prothrombin.
Urinary: ↑ frequency c̄ toxicity.

vitamin B_6 B COMPLEX VITAMIN See **pyridoxine p 172**

vitamin B_{12}
cyanocobalamin
hydroxocobalamin
Many Parenteral brands—
benzyl alcohol

VITAMIN, ANTIANEMIC — Oral or Parenteral (IM or SC)

Drug: Parenteral preferred to treat pernicious anemia. **Diet:** Take high dose Vit C separately by 1 hr. Caution c̄ Fol suppl—may mask pernicious anemia & result in progression of neurologic damage. **Nutr:** RDA—Adult = 2.0 ug; Pregnancy = 2.2; Lactation = 2.6. Intrinsic factor & adequate Ca needed for proper abs of oral Vit B_{12}.
Oral/GI: Mild transient diarrhea.
S/Cond: Limit alcohol. ↓ abs of Vit B_{12} c̄ gastric achlorhydria (common in elderly), gastrectomy, HIV, antiulcer drugs. Def symptoms—paresthesia, ↓ sense of vibration or position, unsteadiness, ataxia, mood changes, confusion, memory loss, depression, visual changes, delusions, hallucinations, psychosis, paranoia, dementia, ↑ MCV, ↑ MCH, ↓ Hgb, ↓ HCT, pernicious anemia (macrocytic, megaloblastic).
Neuropsychiatric damage due to low grade def is not accompanied by anemia in 30% of cases.
Other: Hypokalemia in first 48 hrs of parenteral treatment (may be fatal), itching. Rare anaphylactic shock. **Blood/Serum:** ↓ K, ↑ $\underline{B_{12}}$.
Monitor: CBC, B_{12}, Fol, K (for first 48 hrs of parenteral treatment).

vitamin C
ascorbic acid
Ca ascorbate
Na ascorbate—
115 mg Na/g

VITAMIN, ANTISCURVY, Urinary Acidifier — Oral or Parenteral (IV, IM, SC)
Water Soluble, Antioxidant

Drug: 100-250 mg/day to treat scurvy.[6] Do <u>not</u> stop high dose abruptly — taper slowly. May mix oral soln c̄ food or fruit juice.
Diet: Take Vit B_{12} suppl separately by 1 hr. Take c̄ Fe suppl to ↑ Fe abs.
Nutr: RDA— Adult = 60 mg; Pregnancy = 70; Lactation = 95;

Smoker = 100. ↓ Cu abs c̄ ≥ 1.5 g Vit c̄/day.[73] Systemic conditioning c̄ LT high dose causes dependency, rebound scurvy if ↓ abruptly.
Oral/GI: N/V, gastric cramps, diarrhea c̄ > 1 g/day. Excess use of chewable tabs will break down tooth enamel & ↑ caries.
S/Cond: Tobacco smoking & chewing ↑ requirements.[80] Caution c̄ G6PD def— risk of hemolytic anemia. Def symptoms— (scurvy) gum inflammation/bleeding, slow wound healing, joint pain, hyperkeratosis, petechiae & other hemorrhagic effects, weakness, fatigue, depression, hysteria. **Other:** Fatigue, flushing, headache, insomnia.
Rare oxalate kidney stones c̄ > 1 g/day.[13]
Blood/Serum: ↓ bil.[13] **Urinary:** ↓ pH c̄ high dose Vit C (4-12 g), ↑ oxalate, ↑ Ca, ↓ Na, ↑ or ↓ uric acid (dose dependent), false - Hgb c̄ dipstick, false + glucose ($CuSO_4$), false - glucose (glucose oxidase).

vitamin D
ergocalciferol

VITAMIN, Ca REGULATOR, ANTIRICKETS — See listing for **calcitriol p 39**
Fat Soluble Vitamin — Oral or Parenteral (IM)
Drug: Toxic effects are dose dependent. **Nutr:** RDA— Adult = 5-10 ug (200-400 IU); Pregnancy & Lactation = 10 ug (400 IU).
Other: 1.25-2.4 mg/day in adults or 25-45 ug/day in children causes hypervitaminosis D.[47] LT use of 125 ug (5000 IU)/day may cause renal & cardiac damage.[53] **Blood/Serum:** Ergocalciferol induced hypercalcemia persists longer than c̄ calcitriol. **Monitor:** Ca, P, renal func.

vitamin E	VITAMIN, Fat Soluble, Antioxidant 1 USP = 1 IU 1 alpha tocopherol equivalent = 1.5 IU **Drug:** H_2O miscible form ↑ abs. Swallow cap whole— do not crush or chew.[7] Mix soln c̄ food or juice. **Diet:** High PUFA intake ↑ Vit E requirements. Caution c̄ Fe suppl— ↑ Vit E requirement. High dose Vit E ↓ hematologic response to Fe in children c̄ Fe def anemia.[6] **Nutr:** Adult RDA— Men = 15 IU; Women = 12; Pregnancy = 15 Lactation = 18. Excessive intake ↓ Vit A stores. **Oral/GI:** Toxicity causes nausea, diarrhea, flatulence. **S/Cond:** Tobacco smoking & chewing ↑ requirements.[80] Steatorrhea ↓ abs. **Other:** LT intakes ≥ 400-800 IU/day cause hypervitaminosis E[13] & fatigue, weakness, headache, blurred vision. **Blood/Serum:** Toxicity— ↑ CPK, ↑ chol, ↑ TG. **Urinary:** ↑ crea c̄ toxicity.
vitamin K **phytonadione (K_1)** **Aqua MEPHYTON** Parenteral— benzyl alcohol **Mephyton** Tab— lactose, starch	VITAMIN, ANTIHYPOPROTHROMBINEMIA, Fat Soluble Oral or Parenteral (IM or SC preferred) **Diet:** Caution c̄ high dose Vit A, D or E suppl— relative def of Vit K.[1] See Vit K sources, p 249. **Nutr:** RDA— Men = 70-80 ug; Women = 60-65; children = 15-45. **S/Cond:** Caution c̄ lactation. **Other:** Parenteral— Rare anaphylactic reaction (especially c̄ IV), flushing, dizziness, rash. **Blood/Serum:** ↓ PT, ↑ clotting factors. Rare hemolytic anemia, ↑ bil in neonate c̄ ↑ dose.[6] **Monitor:** PT.
Vivactil	ANTIDEPRESSANT, Tricyclic See **protriptyline HCl p 170**

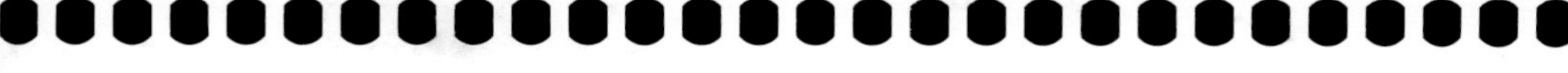

Vivarin STIMULANT See **caffeine p 38**

Voltaren NSAID See **diclofenac sodium p 70**

VP-16 (VePesid) ANTINEOPLASTIC See **etoposide p 86**

warfarin sodium
Coumadin
Tab— lactose, starch

ANTICOAGULANT

Diet: Consistent intake of Vit K essential, see p 249. ↑ Vit K ↓ drug effect & ↓ Vit K ↑ drug effect. Caution $\bar{c}$ Vit K or MVI suppl— changes in intake will ↑ or ↓ PT. Avoid high dose Vit A, E (≥ 400 IU/day) — alters PT.[3, 9b] Caution $\bar{c}$ Vit C (≥ 5 g/day)— may ↓ drug abs.[3] Caution $\bar{c}$ ≥ 60 g raw, fried or boiled onions— ↑ fibrinolytic activity.[51] Avoid or limit some herbs & herbal teas, see p 244.
Oral/GI: N/V, cramps, diarrhea.
S/Cond: Caution $\bar{c}$ alcohol—- chronic alcohol abuse ↑ metabolism of drug & ↓ PT; acute intoxication ↓ metabolism of drug & ↑ PT. Caution $\bar{c}$ lactation. Do dental care cautiously, ↑ risk of bleeding. 99% serum pro bound. Hypoalbuminemia (< 3g/dL)— may ↑ drug effects.
Other: Hemorrhage, fever, rash, skin necrosis. Rare hepatitis or jaundice.
Blood/Serum: ↑ PT, ↓ CLOTTING FACTORS. Rare ↓ WBC, ↑ SGOT, ↑ SGPT, ↑ alk phos, ↑ bil. **Monitor:** PT &/or INR frequently.

Wellbutrin ANTIDEPRESSANT See **bupropion HCl p 37**

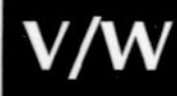

Wygesic ANALGESIC See **acetaminophen p 17 & propoxyphene HCl p 168**

Wymox ANTIBIOTIC See **amoxicillin p 26**

Xanax ANTIANXIETY See **alprazolam p 22**

zalcitabine (DDC) ANTIVIRAL, ANTI-HIV
Hivid
Tab— lactose

Drug: Take on empty stomach if possible.[6] Food ↓ abs. **Nutr:** Anorexia, ↓ wt. **Oral/GI:** Oral ulcers, glossitis, dry mouth, dysphagia, pharyngitis, N/V, dyspepsia, abdominal pain, diarrhea. **S/Cond:** Avoid alcohol. Not c̄ lactation. Do dental care cautiously, see p 10 & 14.
Other: PERIPHERAL NEUROPATHY, headache, fatigue, rash, cough, fever, dizziness, confusion, muscle pain, pancreatitis (can be fatal).
Blood/Serum: Dyscrasias, ↓ WBC, anemia, ↑ SGOT, ↑ SGPT, ↑ bil, ↑ GGT, ↑ alk phos, ↑ amylase, ↑ lipase, ↑ or ↓ glucose, ↑ or ↓ Na, ↓ Mg, ↓ Ca, ↓ P. **Monitor:** CBC c̄ diff, blood chemistry.

Zantac ANTIULCER See **ranitidine p 174**

Zarontin ANTICONVULSANT See **ethosuximide p 85**

Zaroxolyn DIURETIC See **metolazone p 131**

Zefazone ANTIBIOTIC, cefmetazole See **cephalosporins p 46**

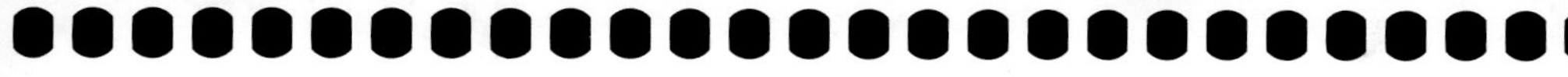

Zerit ANTIVIRAL, ANTI-HIV See **stavudine p 187**

Zestril ANTIHYPERTENSIVE See **lisinopril p 117**

zidovudine
Retrovir
(AZT)

ANTIVIRAL, ANTI-HIV Oral or Parenteral (IV)

Nutr: ANOREXIA. **Oral/GI:** NAUSEA/vomiting, dyspepsia, pain, constipation. **S/Cond:** Not c̄ lactation.

Other: BONE MARROW SUPPRESSION, headache, weakness, fatigue, dizziness, paresthesia, fever, muscle pain, insomnia, rash.

Blood/Serum: Severe ANEMIA, ↓ WHITE BLOOD CELLS, ↑ or ↓ platelets, other dyscrasias. Rare ↑ SGOT, ↑ SGPT, ↑ alk phos, ↑ bil.

Monitor: CBC c̄ diff monthly x 3 months, then q 3 months, hepatic func.

Zinacef ANTIBIOTIC, Cephalosporin See **cefuroxime sodium p 45**

zinc

Zn gluconate— 14.3% zinc

Zn sulfate— 23% zinc

Zn chloride— 48% zinc

MINERAL SUPPLEMENT

Drug: Take 1 hr before or 2 hrs after meals. **Diet:** Take Cu, Fe, P, Ca, Fol suppl separately by 2 hrs. Take 2 hrs apart from food high in Ca, P, bran fiber or phytate, see p 242, to avoid nonabsorbable complexes.
Nutr: ↑ bioavailability from animal protein sources. Excess intake may cause Cu &/or Fe def.[1] RDA— Men = 15 mg; Women = 12; Pregnancy = 15; Lactation = 19; children = 10.
Oral/GI: Intake > 25 mg/day— metallic taste, N/V, abdominal pain.
S/Cond: $ZnSO_4$ precipitates tube feedings.[8] ↑ need in HIV.
Other: LT intake of 100-300 mg/day causes chronic toxicity— Cu &/or Fe def, ↓ immune response, headache, chills, fever, fatigue. Acute toxicity occurs c̄ single dose of ≥ 2 g. Def symptoms— suboptimal growth, delayed wound healing, ↓ taste acuity, anorexia, hypogonadism, rash, skin/ eye lesions, night blindness, hair loss, nail dystrophy.
Blood/Serum: ↑ Zn, ↓ Cu, ↑ alk phos. ↓ HDL c̄ excessive intake. Rare dyscrasias.

Zithromax ANTIBIOTIC See **azithromycin p 31**

Zocor ANTIHYPERLIPIDEMIC, HMG-CoA reductase Inhibitor See **simvastatin p 183**

Zofran ANTIEMETIC See **ondansetron HCl p 148**

Zoloft ANTIDEPRESSANT, SSRI See **sertraline HCl p 182**

zolpidem tartrate
Ambien
Tab— lactose

SLEEP AID
Drug: Take HS. Do not take immediately after a meal.[7] Food ↓ abs & delays onset of drug action. **Oral/GI:** Dry mouth, diarrhea, constipation.
S/Cond: Avoid alcohol. Not $\bar{c}$ lactation.
Other: <u>Daytime</u> <u>drowsiness</u>, drugged feeling, dizziness, headache, rash.

Zonalan
topical cream

TRICYCLIC (Antihistamine effect) See **doxepin p 77**

Zosyn

ANTIBIOTIC Parenteral only (IV) See listing for **ticarcillin disodium p 197**
piperacillin sodium
& tazobactam sodium

Zovirax

ANTIVIRAL See **acyclovir p 19**

Zyloprim

ANTIGOUT See **allopurinol p 21**

LABORATORY TESTS

"Normal ranges" depend on analytical method; values vary among laboratories. Values are for **blood/serum** unless otherwise stated.

Many factors influence results. Interpretation of nutritionally significant abnormalities <u>must</u> be in conjunction c̄ supportive clinical evidence.

*These tests indicate possible blood dyscrasia (any abnormal or pathological condition of the blood).

CONSTITUENT	NORMAL RANGE	CAUSE/SIGNIFICANCE OF ABNORMAL VALUES
Activated Partial Thromboplastin Time APTT	16-25 seconds	Screen for coagulation/clotting disorders and to monitor heparin therapy. ↑ c̄ Vit K def, hemophilia, hepatic disease, DIC (disseminated intravascular coagulation). Antibiotic therapy. ↓ c̄ extensive cancer (except c̄ hepatic involvement), acute hemorrhage, early DIC.
Albumin Alb	3.5-5.0 gm/dL	↑ c̄ dehydration. ↓ c̄ edema, hepatic disease, malabsorption, diarrhea, burns, eclampsia, hypocalcemia, ESRD, malnutrition, stress, over-hydration, cancer, ↓ values normal in pregnancy. ↓ values normal c̄ aging. <u>Depletion c̄ protein malnutrition:</u> <u>Mild</u> = 3-3.4 gm/dL, <u>Moderate</u> = 2.1-3 gm/dL, <u>Severe</u> < 2.1 gm/dL. < 3 gm/dL ↓ binding of acidic drugs, ↑ free drug level = increased effects.

*Alkaline Phosphatase alk phos or ALP	Adult: 20-70 U/L Child: 20-150 U/L	Marked ↑ $\bar{c}$ hepatic disease or metastasis, Paget's diseas of bone, metastatic bone disease. Moderate ↑ $\bar{c}$ hypercalcemia (indicates possible hyperparathyroidism), pancreatitis, hepatitis. Also ↑ $\bar{c}$ bone growth (children/pregnancy), rickets, osteomalacia. ↓ $\bar{c}$ hypophosphatasia, malnutrition, cretinism, hypothyroidism, pernicious anemia, Vit C def/scurvy, Milk-alkali syndrome.
Ammonia NH_3	10-80 ug/dL	↑ $\bar{c}$ hepatic disease or coma (cirrhosis or severe hepatitis), severe heart failure, azotemia, pericarditis, pulmonary emphysema, acute bronchitis, Reye's syndrome. Also ↑ $\bar{c}$ high protein diet, vigorous exercise.
Amylase	53-123 U/L	↑ $\bar{c}$ acute (or exacerbation of chronic) pancreatitis, mumps, perforated peptic ulcer, alcohol poisoning, renal insufficiency, acute cholecystitis. ↓ $\bar{c}$ hepatitis, cirrhosis, pancreatic insufficiency, toxemia of pregnancy, severe burns.
Apolipoprotein A-1	120 mg% ± 20	Correlate of HDL-CHOL: ↑ values indicate ↓ CHD risk.
Apolipoprotein B	85 mg% ± 15	Correlate of LDL-CHOL: ↑ values indicate ↑ CHD risk.
Ascorbic acid Vit C	0.4-1.5 mg/dL	↑ $\bar{c}$ oxalate stones, ↑ uric acid, ↓ Vit B_{12} abs. ↓ $\bar{c}$ anemia, alcoholism, chronic inflammatory disease, cigarette smoking, stress, OC use, scurvy, high aspirin use, ↓ Fe abs, duodenal ulcer, postpartum.

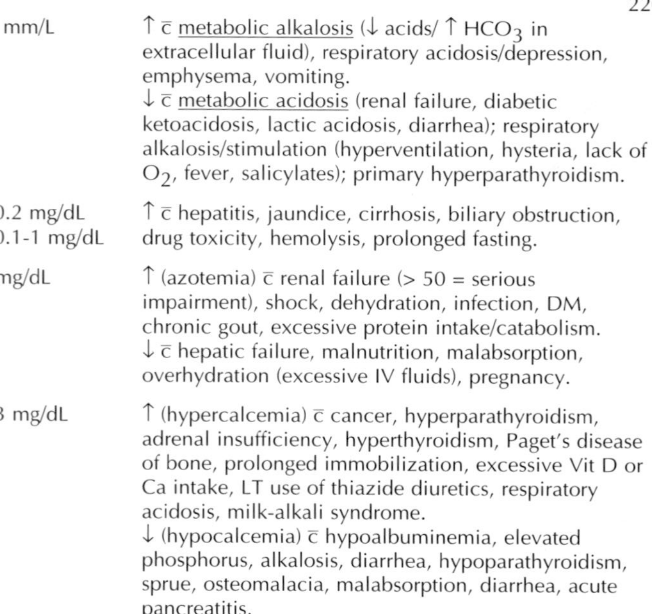

Bicarbonate HCO_3	23-33 mm/L	↑ c̄ <u>metabolic alkalosis</u> (↓ acids/ ↑ HCO_3 in extracellular fluid), respiratory acidosis/depression, emphysema, vomiting. ↓ c̄ <u>metabolic acidosis</u> (renal failure, diabetic ketoacidosis, lactic acidosis, diarrhea); respiratory alkalosis/stimulation (hyperventilation, hysteria, lack of O_2, fever, salicylates); primary hyperparathyroidism.
Bilirubin bil	Direct -< 0.2 mg/dL Total -< 0.1-1 mg/dL	↑ c̄ hepatitis, jaundice, cirrhosis, biliary obstruction, drug toxicity, hemolysis, prolonged fasting.
Blood Urea Nitrogen BUN	8-18 mg/dL	↑ (azotemia) c̄ renal failure (> 50 = serious impairment), shock, dehydration, infection, DM, chronic gout, excessive protein intake/catabolism. ↓ c̄ hepatic failure, malnutrition, malabsorption, overhydration (excessive IV fluids), pregnancy.
Calcium	8.8-10.3 mg/dL	↑ (hypercalcemia) c̄ cancer, hyperparathyroidism, adrenal insufficiency, hyperthyroidism, Paget's disease of bone, prolonged immobilization, excessive Vit D or Ca intake, LT use of thiazide diuretics, respiratory acidosis, milk-alkali syndrome. ↓ (hypocalcemia) c̄ hypoalbuminemia, elevated phosphorus, alkalosis, diarrhea, hypoparathyroidism, sprue, osteomalacia, malabsorption, diarrhea, acute pancreatitis.

Test	Normal values	Interpretation
Carbon Dioxide CO_2	22-28 mEq/L 22-28 mmol/L	Measure of blood alkalinity/acidity: See bicarbonate (HCO_3) above.
Ceruloplasmin (transports copper)	17-34 mg/dL	↑ c̄ Rheumatoid arthritis, biliary cirrhosis, infectious disease, thyrotoxicosis, cancer. ↓ c̄ Wilson's Disease, Menke's steely hair disease, long term hyperalimentation and parenteral nutrition, transient nephrosis, sprue, kwashiorkor.
Chloride Cl	95-105 mEq/L or mmol/L	↑ c̄ dehydration, eclampsia, anemia, hyperventilation, cardiac decompensation, renal insufficiency, aspirin toxicity, Cushing's syndrome, metabolic acidosis. ↓ c̄ diabetic acidosis, fever, acute infections, metabolic alkalosis, protracted vomiting, K deficiency.
*Cholesterol chol	desirable: 120-199 mg/dL borderline: 200-240 high risk: > 240 mg/dL child: 70-175 mg/dL	↑ c̄ hyperlipidemia, obstructive jaundice, DM, hypothroidism, obesity, high fat diet. (strong risk factor for CAD) In public screening a patient c̄ CHOL > 200 mg/dL should be further evaluated by a physician. ↓ c̄ malabsorption, malnutrition, hepatic disease, stress, anemia, sepsis.
Cholesterol-High Density Lipoprotein fraction HDL	F: 35-85 mg/dL M: 35-70 mg/dL child: 30-65 mg/dL	↑ c̄ regular, vigorous exercise, estrogen or insulin therapy, moderate alcohol intake. ↓ c̄ starvation, obesity, liver disease, DM, hyperthyroidism, smoking.

Test	Normal values	Notes
Cholesterol-Low Density Lipoprotein fraction LDL	desirable: < 130 mg/dL borderline: 130-159 mg/dL high risk: > 160 mg/dL	A **calculated value** (Friedwald formula): LDL = total CHOL - HDL CHOL - (TG/5) ↑ c̄ familial type II hyperlipidemia, ↑ fat diet, hypothyroidism, hepatic disease, acute trauma, DM, pregnancy.
*Complete Blood Count (CBC)	Consists of:	WBC, RBC, Hgb, HCT, MCV, MCH, MCHC,
*CBC Differential CBC c̄ diff (see White Blood Cells)		Diff WBC = # of neutrophils, lymphocytes, monocytes, eosinophils, basophils as % of total WBC count. (Many labs include platelets in CBC.)
*Copper Cu	70-150 ug/dL	↑ c̄ anemias, leukemia, infection, biliary cirrhosis, collagen diseases, pregnancy, estrogen use, hypo/hyperthyroidism, hemochromatosis. ↓ c̄ Wilson's disease, severe Cu def, nephrosis, Kwashiorkor.
Creatinine crea	adult: 0.6-1.5 mg/dL	↑ c̄ acute & chronic renal disease; muscle damage, MI, hyperthyroidism, muscle mass, starvation, diabetic acidosis, high meat intake.
Creatine Phosphokinase CPK/CK	F: 96-140 U/L M: 38-174 U/L	Index of muscle/myocardium injury/disease. ↑ c̄ MI or cardiac trauma, acute CVA, ALS, muscular dystrophy, hypothyroidism, vigorous exercise, electric burns/shock, chronic alcoholism, hypokalemia, pulmonary edema.

Ferritin	F: 12-150 ng/mL M: 15-300 ng/mL	↑ c̄ inflammatory diseases, chronic renal disease, malignancy, hepatitis, Fe overload, hemochromatosis. ↓ c̄ Fe def anemia.
*Folic acid Folate	3-17 ng/mL	↓ c̄ megaloblastic & hemolytic anemias, malnutrition, folate antagonist drug (eg anticonvulsant, methotrexate, OC), malabsorption (eg sprue/celiac disease), alcoholic hepatic disease, hyperthyroidism, Vit C def, dialysis, febrile states, pregnancy, cancer.
GGT gamma glutamyl transpeptidase	0-65 U/L	↑ c̄ hepatic disease, hepatoxicity, biliary tract obstruction, pancreatitis.
*Globulin	2.3-3.5 gm/dL (40-48% of TP)	↑ c̄ infection, dehydration, Hodgkin's, Lupus, multiple myeloma, collagen disease, chronic alcoholism, shock, tuberculosis, leukemia. ↓ c̄ malnutrition.
Glucose, fasting Fasting blood sugar FBS	80-115 mg/dL	↑ c̄ DM, Cushing's syndrome, chronic hepatic dysfunction, MI, severe infections, hyperthyroidism, pancreatitis, chronic hepatic disease, prolonged physical inactivity, chronic malnutrition, K def, drugs: eg corticosteroids, high dose antihypertensives. ↓ c̄ insulin overdose, islet-cell carcinoma, bacterial sepsis, hypothyroidism, Addison's disease, extensive liver disease, glycogen storage disease, alcohol abuse, starvation, vigorous exercise.

Test	Normal value	Significance
Glucose-6-Phosphate Dehydrogenase G6PD	8.34 ± 1.59 IU/gm Hgb[49] 8.6-18.6 IU/gm[62]	↑ $\bar{c}$ pernicious anemia, hepatic coma, hyperthyroidism, MI, chronic blood loss, other megaloblastic anemias. ↓ $\bar{c}$ inherited G6PD def (X chromosome linked, ↑ in black males) =increased susceptibility to hemolytic anemia/hemolysis.
Glycosylated hemoglobin thalassemia. GHGB or HGB $A1_C$ Index of LT glucose control (2-3 months)	4.0-7.0% (% of Hgb bound $\bar{c}$ glucose)	↑ $\bar{c}$ poorly controlled/newly diagnosed DM, Good control: < 9.0%, Fair control: 9.0 - 12.0, Poor control: > 12.0% ↓ $\bar{c}$ pregnancy, sickle-cell anemia.
*Hematocrit HCT	F: 33-47% M: 39-54%	↑ $\bar{c}$ dehydration, polycythemia, shock. ↓ $\bar{c}$ anemia (< 30), blood loss, hemolysis, leukemia, hyperthyroidism, cirrhosis, over hydration.
*Hemoglobin Hgb	F: 11.5-15.5 gm/dL M: 14.0-18.0 gm/dL	↑ $\bar{c}$ severe burns, polycythemia, CHF, thalassemia, COPD, dehydration. ↓ $\bar{c}$ anemia, hyperthyroidism, cirrhosis, many systemic diseases (eg leukemia, Lupus, Hodgkin's disease).
International Normalized Ratio (INR) (for PT)	2-3	$INR = \left[\frac{\text{Patient PT}}{\text{Mean Normal PT}}\right]^{ISI}$ Where Patient PT is in secs. Where Mean Normal PT is 11.5 sec Where ISI is the International Sensitivity Index for the thromboplastic product used.

Test	Normal value	Significance
*Iron Fe	F: 60-160 ug/dL M: 80-180 ug/dL	↑ $\bar{c}$ excessive Fe intake, hemolytic anemias, hepatic disease, estrogen use, hemochromatosis. ↓ $\bar{c}$ Fe def anemia, chronic diseases (eg Lupus, rheumatoid arthritis), infections, hepatic disease, surgery, MI.
Ketones, URINE Acetone	0	↑ $\bar{c}$ diabetic ketoacidosis, fever, prolonged vomiting, diarrhea, ↑ fat-pro/ ↓ CHO diet, starvation, anorexia, drug therapy (eg levodopa, insulin).
Lactic Dehydrogenase LDH/LD	50-150 U/L	↑ $\bar{c}$ MI, leukemia, megaloblastic or hemolytic anemias, pulmonary infarction, cancer, renal failure, shock $\bar{c}$ anoxia, mononucleosis, muscular dystrophy. Minor ↑ $\bar{c}$ cirrhosis, hepatitis, jaundice.
Magnesium Mg	1.3-2.1 mEq/L	↑ $\bar{c}$ renal failure, diabetic acidosis, hypothyroidism, Addison's, dehydration, overuse of Mg suppl or antacid. ↓ $\bar{c}$ chronic diarrhea, alcoholism, pancreatitis, renal disease, hepatic cirrhosis, toxemia of pregnancy, hyperthyroidism, malabsorption, ulcerative colitis, K-depleting diuretics.
*Mean Corpuscular Hemoglobin (MCH)	26-34 pg/RBC	↑ $\bar{c}$ macrocytic anemia, false ↑ $\bar{c}$ hyperlipidemia. ↓ $\bar{c}$ microcytic anemia.
*Mean Corpuscular Hemoglobin Concentration MCHC	32-37 gm/dL (gm Hgb/dl RBC)	↑ usually indicates spherocytosis ↓ $\bar{c}$ Fe def, macrocytic anemias, thalassemia, chronic blood loss, Pyr-responsive anemia.

*Mean Corpuscular Volume (MCV)	87-103 um^3/RBC	$\uparrow \bar{c}$ alcohol abuse, macrocytic/megaloblastic pernicious anemias, Vit B_{12} &/or Fol def.
PT (Prothrombin Time)	10-14 secs.	$\uparrow \bar{c}$ prothrombin def, Vit K def, liver disease, anticoagulant therapy, biliary obstruction, salicylate intoxication, hypervitaminosis A, DIC disease.
PTT (Partial Thromboplastin time)	30-45 secs.	Screen for coagulation/clotting disorders & to monitor heparin therapy. $\uparrow \bar{c}$ Vit K def, hemophilia, hepatic disease, DIC disease, antibiotic therapy. $\downarrow \bar{c}$ extensive cancer (except $\bar{c}$ hepatic involvement), acute hemorrhage, early DIC.
pH Arterial Venous	7.35-7.45 7.31-7.41	$\uparrow$ (alkalemia) $\bar{c}$ respiratory or metabolic alkalosis, vomiting, $\downarrow$ K or Cl, high fever, hyperventilation, anoxia, cerebral hemorrhage. $\downarrow$ (acidemia) $\bar{c}$ respiratory or metabolic acidosis, diabetic ketoacidosis, renal failure, diarrhea, respiratory depression, airway obstruction, shock, CHF.
Phosphorus, inorganic P (Phosphate PO_4) (P)	2.5-4.5 mg/dL	$\uparrow \bar{c}$ ESRD & severe nephritis, hypocalcemia, hypervitaminosis D, bone tumors, Addison's, hypoparathyroidism, acromegaly. $\downarrow \bar{c}$ hyperparathyroidism ($\bar{c} \uparrow$ Ca), alcoholism, hypovitaminosis D, rickets or osteomalacia, hyperinsulinism, acute gout, overuse of P binders.

Potassium K	3.5-5.0 mEq/L	↑ (hyperkalemia) c̄ renal failure, tissue damage, acidosis, Addison's, uncontrolled DM, internal hemorrhage, overuse of K suppl. ↓ (hypokalemia) c̄ GI loss, IV fluid s̄ K suppl, alcohol abuse, malabsorption, malnutrition, diarrhea, vomiting, chronic stress or fever, K depleting diuretic, steroid, estrogen use, hepatic disease c̄ ascites, excessive licorice.
Prealbumin better indicator of dietary change than albumin	19-43 mg/dL <11 mg/dL indicates malnutrition significant	Prealbumin is a better indicator of dietary change than albumin. Half-life is 2-3 days. Value not affected by Fe def. ↑ c̄ renal failure. ↓ c̄ acute catabolic states, hepatic disease, stress, infection, surgery, malnutrition, low protein intake.
Protein, Total TP	6.0-8.0 gm/dL	↑ c̄ dehydration, diseases that ↑ globulin. ↓ c̄ protein def, severe hepatic disease, malabsorption, diarrhea, severe burns or infection, edema.
*RBC Red Blood Cell Count erythrocytes	F: 3.5-5.0-5.9 million/mm^3 M: 4.3-5.9	↑ c̄ polycythemia, dehydration, severe diarrhea. ↓ c̄ anemia, hemorrhage, Fe def, systemic disease (eg Hodgkin's, leukemia, Lupus).
Reticulocyte Count	Percent of Total Erythrocytes Men: 0.5%-1.5% Women: 0.5%-2.5% Children: 0.5%-4.0%	↑ Hemolytic anemias, 3-4 days post hemorrhage, therapeutic-diagnostic test, sickle cell disease. ↓ Iron Def anemias, aplastic amenia, untreated pernicious anemia, chronic infection, radiation therapy, endocrine problems, tumor in marrow, myelodysplastic syndromes.

Serum glutamic oxaloacetic transaminase SGOT Aspartate amino transferase (AST)	< 35 U/L[7] F: 6-18 U/L M: 8-20 U/L Child: 25-75 U/L[49]	↑ c̄ cell injury/death: MI (4-10 x normal, ↓ to base by 4th day), acute cirrhosis, hepatitis, pancreatitis or renal disease, cancer, alcoholism, burns, trauma, crushing injury, muscular dystrophy, gangrene. ↓ c̄ uncontrolled DM (c̄ acidosis), beriberi (Thi def.)
Serum glutamic pyruvic transaminase SGPT Alanine amino transferase (ALT)	< 35 U/L[7] F: 7-17 U/L M: 7-24 U/L Child: 5-28 U/L[49]	↑ c̄ hepatitis, jaundice, cirrhosis, hepatic cancer, MI, severe burns, trauma, shock, mononucleosis, pancreatitis.
Sodium Na	135-147mEq/L	↑ (hypernatremia) c̄ dehydration & low fluid intake, diabetes insipidus, Cushing's disease, coma, primary aldosteronism. ↓ (hyponatremia) c̄ edema, severe burns, severe diarrhea/vomiting, diuretics, SIADH, H_2O intoxication, Addison's disease, severe nephritis, starvation, diabetic acidosis, malabsorption.
Specific Gravity URINE SG	1.003-1.035	↑ SG (concentrated urine) c̄ DM, nephrosis, fever, dehydration, vomiting, diarrhea, low fluid intake. ↓ SG (dilute urine) c̄ diabetes insipidus, chronic pyelo- or glomerulo-nephritis, severe renal damage, H_2O intoxication.

Total thyroxine T_4 (by RIA)	4-12 ug/dL	↑ $\bar{c}$ hyperthyroidism, hepatitis (first 4 weeks), estrogen use, pregnancy. ↓ hypothyroidism, nephrosis, cirrhosis, malnutrition, hypoproteinemia.
Total triiodothyronine T_3	75-220 ng/dL	↑ $\bar{c}$ hyperthyroidism, thyroid hormone therapy (daily dosage of T3 > 25 ug or T4 > 300 ug).
Thyroid-stimulating hormone TSH	0.5-6.0 uU/mL	↑ $\bar{c}$ primary hypothyroidism. ↓ $\bar{c}$ hyperthyroidism; secondary hypothyroidism. thyroid hormone therapy.
Total Iron-Binding Capacity TIBC	240-450 ug/dL	↑ $\bar{c}$ Fe def, pregnancy, Fe deficiency anemia. ↓ $\bar{c}$ chronic inflammatory states, Fe overload, hemochromatosis.
Triglycerides TG	F: 35-135 mg/dL M: 40-160 mg/dL	↑ $\bar{c}$ hyperlipidemias, hepatic disease, pancreatitis, poorly controlled DM, hypothyroidism, MI, alcoholism, high sugar &/or fat intake. ↓ $\bar{c}$ malnutrition, malabsorption syndrome, hyperthyroidism, COPD.

Transferrin Transferrin = 0.8 (TIBX) –43	240-480 mg/dL	↑ $\bar{c}$ inadequate Fe stores, Fe def anemia, acute hepatitis, polycythemia, OC use, pregnancy. ↓ $\bar{c}$ pernicious & sickle-cell anemia, chronic infection, cancer, hepatic disease, malnutrition, nephrotic syndrome, thalassemia. Mild ↓ = 150-200; Moderate ↓ = 100-150; Severe ↓ = < 100. (Transferrin = 0.8 (TIBC) - 43).
Uric Acid	F: 2.6-6.0 mg/dL M: 3.5-7.2 mg/dL	↑ $\bar{c}$ renal failure, gout, anorexia, leukemias, acute infectious disease, metastatic cancer, severe eclampsia, shock, diabetic ketosis, metabolic acidosis, lead poisoning, stress, alcoholism, rigorous exercise, polythycemia. ↓ $\bar{c}$ antigout drugs eg allopurinol, probenecid, Wilson's disease, cancer.
Vitamin B_{12} Vit B_{12}	160-1300 pg/mL or 118-959 pmo/L	↑ (> 1100 pg/mL) $\bar{c}$ hepatic disease, some leukemias, cancer (especially $\bar{c}$ hepatic metastasis), pregnancy, OC. ↓ (< 100 pg/mL) $\bar{c}$ pernicious anemia, malabsorption syndromes, primary hypothyroidism, ↓ gastric mucosa (eg gastrectomy or stomach cancer), vegetarian diet, achlorhydria.

Test		Normal values		Interpretation
*White Blood Cells WBC Leukocyte Count		$5\text{-}10^3$/uL		↑ (leukocytosis) c̄ leukemia, bacterial infection, hemorrhage, trauma or tissue injury, cancer. ↓ (leukopenia) c̄ some viral infections, chemotherapy, radiation, bone-marrow depression.
		Absolute		
	Aver %	Value #/uL		
*WBC diff	Neutrophils	56	3000-7000	The relative percentage or number of each type of leukocyte in the blood.
Differential	Eosinophils	2.7	50-400	Formula:[49]
Leukocyte	Basophils	0.3	25-100	Absolute value = Relative value x total WBC ct
Count	Lymphocytes	34	100-4000	WBC/mm^3 = (%) x (cells mm^3)
	Monocytes	2-6	100-600	
Zinc Zn		50-150 ug/dL		↑ c̄ CHD, arteriosclerosis, osteosarcoma. ↓ c̄ malnutrition, dialysis, protein-losing enteropathy, inflammatory bowel disease, nephrotic syndrome, burns or trauma, prolonged TPN, alcoholism, alcoholic cirrhosis or pancreatitis, anorexia, pernicious or sickle cell anemia, cancer c̄ hepatic metastasis, tuberculosis, thalassemia, hypoalbuminemia.

*These tests indicate possible blood dyscrasia (any abnormal or pathological condition of the blood).
References: 7, 11b, 38, 45, 49, 52, 58, 63.

COMPARISON OF HEIGHT-WEIGHT TABLES

Height	Metropolitan 1983 Weights for Ages 25-59		Gerontology Research Center Weight Range for Men and Women by Age (Years)				
	Men	Women	20-29	30-39	40-49	50-59	60-69
ft-in	lb		lb				
4-10		100-131	84-111	92-119	99-127	107-135	115-142
4-11		101-134	87-115	95-123	103-131	111-139	119-147
5-0		103-137	90-119	98-127	106-135	114-143	123-152
5-1	123-145	105-140	93-123	101-131	110-140	118-148	127-157
5-2	125-148	108-144	96-127	105-136	113-144	122-153	131-163
5-3	127-151	111-148	99-131	108-140	117-149	126-158	135-168
5-4	129-155	114-152	102-135	112-145	121-154	130-163	140-173
5-5	131-159	117-156	106-140	115-149	125-159	134-168	144-179
5-6	133-163	120-160	109-144	119-154	129-164	138-174	148-184
5-7	135-167	123-164	112-148	122-159	133-169	143-179	153-190
5-8	137-171	126-167	116-153	126-163	137-174	147-184	158-196
5-9	139-175	129-170	119-157	130-168	141-179	151-190	162-201
5-10	141-179	132-173	122-162	134-173	145-184	156-195	167-207
5-11	144-183	135-176	126-167	137-178	149-190	160-210	172-213
6-0	147-187		129-171	141-183	153-195	165-207	177-219
6-1	150-192		133-176	145-188	157-200	169-213	182-225
6-2	153-197		137-181	149-194	162-206	174-219	187-232
6-3	157-202		141-186	153-199	166-212	179-225	192-238
6-4			144-191	157-205	171-218	184-231	197-244

From: Environmental Nutrition, Vol II, #3, March 1988.

Values in these tables are for height without shoes and weight without clothes.
Weight ranges are the weight for small frame at the lower limit and large frame at the upper limit.

Segmental Weights for Limbs

This information may be used to estimate body weight for patients with amputations.

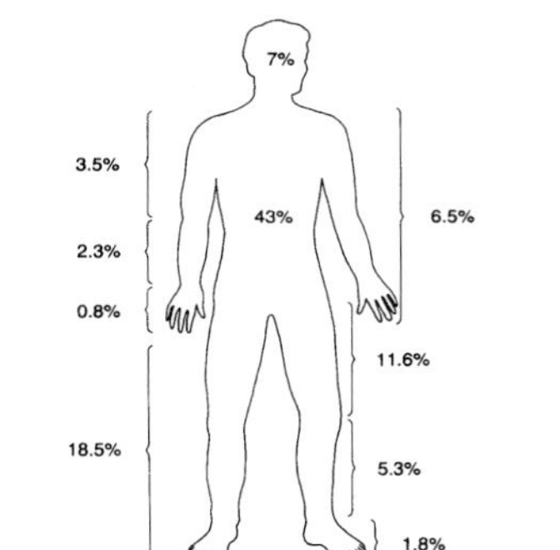

Reference

Reproduced with permission from Braune and Fischer in Brunnstom, S.: Clinical Kinesiology. Philadelphia: F.A. Davis Co., 1972 & adaptation by ASPEN, 1984.

CALCULATION of DESIRABLE BODY WEIGHT

Build	Height	Calculation
Women:		
Medium Frame	1st 5 ft	Allow 100 lbs & add 5 lbs/inch
Large Frame		Add 10%
Small Frame		Subtract 10%
Men:		
Medium Frame	1st 5 ft	Allow 106 lbs & add 6 lbs/inch
Large Frame		Add 10%
Small Frame		Subtract 10%

BODY MASS INDEX (BMI)

Corrects body weight for height, correlated c̄ body fat.

$$\text{BMI} = \frac{\text{weight (kilograms)}}{\text{height}^2\text{ (meters)}}$$

Reference #16

GERIATRIC STANDARDS

FEMALE

Height	Ideal Body Weight	(lbs.) Average	Fluid Minimum (30 cc/kg/day)	(cc)	Protein Minimum (kg x 0.8 gm)
4'9"	89-115	102	5.75 cups	1380	37
4'10"	92-119	106	6 cups	1440	39
4'11"	94-122	108	6 cups	1440	39
5'0"	96-125	111	6.33 cups	1519	40
5'1"	99-128	114	6.5 cups	1560	41
5'2"	102-131	117	6.75 cups	1620	43
5'3"	105-134	120	7 cups	1680	44
5'4"	108-138	123	7 cups	1680	45
5'5"	111-142	127	7.25 cups	1740	46
5'6"	114-146	130	7.5 cups	1800	47
5'7"	118-150	134	7.5 cups	1800	49
5'8"	122-154	138	7.75 cups	1860	50
5'9"	126-158	142	8 cups	1920	52
5'10"	130-163	146	8.33 cups	2000	53
5'11"	134-168	151	8.5 cups	2040	55
6'0"	138-173	158	9 cups	2160	58

Approximate average calories needed to maintain ideal body weight 1564.
Approximate average calories needed to gain body weight 2064.

GERIATRIC STANDARDS

MALE

Height	Ideal Body Weight	(lbs.) Average	Fluid Minimum (30 cc/kg/day)	(cc)	Protein Minimum (kg x 0.8 gm)
5'0"	106-136	121	6.75 cups	1620	44
5'1"	109-138	124	7 cups	1680	45
5'2"	112-141	127	7.25 cups	1740	46
5'3"	115-144	130	7.5 cups	1800	47
5'4"	118-148	133	7.5 cups	1800	48
5'5"	121-152	137	7.75 cups	1860	50
5'6"	124-156	140	8 cups	1920	51
5'7"	128-161	145	8.25 cups	1980	53
5'8"	132-166	149	8.5 cups	2040	54
5'9"	140-174	153	8.75 cups	2100	56
5'10"	140-174	157	8.75 cups	2100	57
5'11"	144-179	162	9.25 cups	2200	59
6'0"	148-184	166	9.5 cups	2280	60
6'1"	152-189	171	9.75 cups	2340	62
6'2"	156-194	177	10 cups	2400	64
6'3"	160-199	180	10.25 cups	2460	65
6'4"	164-204	184	10.5 cups	2520	67

Approximate average calories needed to maintain ideal body weight 2015.
Approximate average calories needed to gain body weight 2154.
Adapted with permission from research by Nancy Powers Siler, M.S., R.D.; Coordinator-Coordinated Program; Department of Nutrition and Medical Dietetics; College of Associated Health Profession; The University of Illinois at Chicago.

NON-NUTRIENTS AND ADDITIVES

Food may contain components with pharmacologic activity that is not manifested under normal circumstances. Bioactive food substances and dyes may augment or antagonize the pharmacologic activity of certain drugs.

Alcohol (ethanol): Excessive alcohol intake results in anorexia by caloric replacement and major organ injury. Ingestion, absorption and/or metabolism of essential nutrients, protein, vitamins and minerals are reduced leading to malnutrition in chronic alcoholics.

One gram of alcohol yields 7.1 kilocalories. (kcal = ozs. of beverage x proof x .8 kcal/proof oz). One pint of 86 proof whiskey daily provides 1/2 the caloric requirement for an average adult.[1] These are "empty calories".

Deficiencies of B-complex vitamins (especially thamin, Vit B_{12}, and folic acid as well as decreased niacin, riboflavin and pyridoxine), protein, magnesium, potassium, and zinc are most prevalent. Vitamin C absorption is affected leading to low tisue levels. Vitamin D metabolism may also be disturbed, contributing to poor utilization of calcium. Diets deficient in both protein and calories may result in muscle wasting and edema. Folic acid depression leads to blood dyscrasias, such as megaloblastic anemia.

Alcohol abuse has an immunity-weakening effect on every component of the immune system. Prolonged episodes of heavy alcohol ingestion lead to general dehydration and mild to severe acidosis. Long term excessive use results in hyperlipidemia and cardiomyopathy. Harmful hepatic effects occur due to alcohol metabolism, including accumulation of fat, alcoholic hepatitis and cirrhosis.

Dietary modifications may be needed to treat complications of cirrhosis, gastritis, pancreatitis and heart disease. A diet rich in protein and vitamins may repair a fat-infiltrated liver.

Alcohol-drug interactions are common. See individual drug listings and the chart on p 239 for additional information. Do not serve patients alcohol-containing beverages or food without a physician's order.

Benzyl Alcohol: Bacteriostatic agent used in parenteral solution. It causes allergic reactions in some people. Benzyl Alcohol has been associated with a fatal "Gasping Syndrome" in premature infants.

Caffeine: Caffeine belongs to a family of chemical compounds called xanthines. Caffeine and its related compounds act as central nervous system and heart muscle stimulants, diuretics, and muscle relaxants. Intake of 100-200 mg caffeine at one time produces significant effects.[6] See caffeine medication entry and Caffeine Content table.

Lactose: Lactose, a natural sweetener in milk, is hydrolyzed in the small intestine by the enzyme lactase to glucose and galactose. Lactase deficiency may cause GI distress when lactose is ingested. In order to avoid possible adverse effects, individuals with lactose intolerance need to be aware that lactose is found as a filler in some medications.

Licorice -- glycyrrhizic acid: Natural extract of glycyrrhiza root used in "natural" licorice candies may antagonize the action of diuretics and complicate antihypertensive therapy. Two or more twists per day (approximately 100 g) of natural (usually imported) licorice enhance sodium reabsorption and potassium excretion along with subsequent water retention. Licorice induced hypokalemia may alter the action of some drugs.

Mannitol: The alcohol form of the sugar mannose. Mannitol is absorbed more slowly, yielding 1/2 as many calories per gram as glucose. Due to slow absorption, mannitol can cause soft stools and diarrhea.[52]

Oxalates (oxalic acid): Oxalate-containing foods need to be avoided during drug treatment of specific disorders. Certain types of kidney stones contain large amounts of oxalates. Low oxalate intake is 40-50 mg per day. See High Oxalate Foods table.

Phenylalanine: Patients with PKU (phenylketonuria) need to be informed that some drugs contain phenylalanine, a component of the synthetic sweetener aspartame. If ingested in significant quantities by the PKU patient, adverse effects may occur.

Phytate (phytic acid): Phosphorus-containing compound found in the outer husks of cereal grains. The amount of phytate increases with the maturity of the seed. Phytate forms non-absorbable complexes with minerals (Ca, Mg, Zn). See High Phytate Foods table.

Sorbitol: The alcohol form of sucrose. Sorbitol is absorbed more slowly than sucrose thus inhibiting a rapid rise in blood glucose. It yields the same calories per gram as glucose. Due to slow absorption, sorbitol can cause soft stools or diarrhea.[52]

Starch (wheat starch): Patients with celiac disease have a permanent intolerance to dietary gluten. Gliadins (grain kernel storage prolamins) are frequently present in pharmaceutical products as part of pharmaceutical starch which is used as filler, binder, or diluent. This can be an unexpected source of gluten for the celiac disease patient who is otherwise on a gluten free diet. If starch is listed under medication it refers to wheat starch. Corn, potato, or rice starches have no deleterious effect on the celiac disease patient and are not noted.

Sulfites: Sulfiting agents are used in foods, beverages and pharmaceuticals as antioxidants. Sulfites may cause severe hypersensitivity reactions in some people, particularly asthmatics. They include sulfur dioxide, sodium sulfite, sodium and potassium metabisulfite. FDA regulations ban the use of sulfites on fresh fruits and vegetables served raw, and require that prescription products list inactive ingredients, including sulfites. Sulfite ingredients, when found in the literature, are noted under each drug listing.

Tartrazine: Tartrazine is Yellow Dye No. 5 color additive, which causes severe allergic reactions in some people (1 in 10,000). The FDA requires the listing of tartrazine when present in foods or drugs.

Tyramine and other pressor agents (dopamine, phenylethylamine, histamine): Tyramine is the decarboxylation product of amino acid tyrosine. It is a vasoconstrictor which, in combination with some drugs [eg monoamine oxidase inhibitors (MAOI)] may cause a hypertensive crisis. Such a crisis includes dangerous increases in blood pressure and possibly increased heart rate, flushing, headache, stroke and death. Large quantities are found in aged, fermented or spoiled foods. See Pressor Agents table.

POSSIBLE ALCOHOL (ETHANOL)-DRUG INTERACTIONS

	Drug Type	Possible Effects
**	amebacidal (metronidazole)	disulfiram-like reaction
*	analgesic (acetaminophen)	↑ hepatoxicity
**	antianxiety (meprobamate)	↑ CNS depression c acute intoxication, ↓ sedation c chronic use
*	anticoagulant (warfarin)	↑ anticoagulant effect c acute intoxication, ↓ c chronic abuse
**	anticonvulsant (phenytoin)	↑ drug effects c acute intoxication, ↓ effect c chronic abuse
**	antidepressant-tricyclic (amitriptyline)	↑ CNS & respiratory depression, ↓ BP, ↑ alcohol effect
**	antidepressant-MAOI (phenelzine)	↑ CNS depression
**	antihistamine (diphenhydramine)	↑ CNS depression
*	antimanic (lithium)	↑ lithium effect
**	antipsychotic (phenothiazine)	↑ CNS & respiratory depression, ↓ BP, impaired motor coordination
*	antitubercular (isoniazid)	↑ hepatoxicity, ↓ drug effect
*	anti-ulcer (cimetidine)	↑ alcohol effect
**	barbiturates (phenobarbital)	↑ CNS depression
**	benzodiazepines (diazepam)	↑ CNS depression impaired motor coordination
*	beta blockers (propranolol)	↑ alcohol effects, ↓ drug effect
***	cephalosporins (cefamandole, cefoperazone, cefotetan, moxalactam)	disulfiram-like reaction
***	disulfiram (Antabuse)	↑ heart rate, chest pains, flushing, N/V, cramps, ↓ BP, confusion
*	diuretics, loop (furosemide)	↓ blood pressure, ↑diuresis
*	insulin	↑ hypoglycemic effect
**	narcotic analgesic (morphine)	↑ CNS & respiratory depression, ↓ BP
*	NSAID (ibuprofen)	↑ gastric mucosal damage, ↑ GI bleeding
*	oral hypoglycemic, sulfonylureas	↑ hypoglycemic effect c acute intoxication, ↓ c chronic abuse
*	oral hypoglycemic (chlorpropamide)	disulfarim-like reaction
*	salicylates (aspirin)	↑ gastric mucosal damage, ↑ GI bleeding
**	sedative, hypnotic (chloral hydrate)	↑ CNS depression, impaired motor coordination, flushing

These suggestions for ethanol intake are meant as general guidelines: Consult the physician.

* Abstinence not required; intake should be limited (1-2 oz c physician's permission.)

** Abstinence recommended. *** Total abstinence required.

From: Vol. 5, *Drug Interactions Newsletter,* November, 1985; Vol. *Medical Letter,* April 1981 and references 1, 4, 6, 7, 9b, and 13.

CAFFEINE CONTENT OF FOODS & BEVERAGES

Item	Caffeine /mg Range
Coffee (5 oz cup)	
Brewed: drip	110-150
percolated	40-70
decaffeinated	2-5
Instant: freeze dried	40-108
decaffeinated	2-3
Tea (bags or loose) (5 oz)	
1 minute brew	9-33
3 minute brew	20-46
5 minute brew	20-50
Tea products	
instant (5 oz cup)	12-29
iced tea (12 oz cup)	22-36

Item	Caffeine /mg Range
Chocolate Products	
cocoa hot (5 oz)	2-15
dry (1 oz)	6
chocolate milk (8 oz)	8
milk chocolate (1 oz)	1-15
dark chocolate, semi-sweet (1 oz)	5-35
Bakers chocolate (1 oz)	25
chocolate-flavored syrup (2 Tbsp)	5
chocolate malted-milk powder (3 hp Tbsp)	8
chocolate chips, semi-sweet (2 oz)	12-15

Soft Drinks

Item	Caffeine /mg Range
Regular (12 oz)	
Mello Yello, Mountain Dew, Kick	52-55
Cola, Dr Pepper, Barqs Root Beer	35-46
Pepsi, RC Cola, Big Red, Aspen	18-38
Mr. PIBB	40
Club soda, seltzer, sparkling water, caffeine-free cola, ginger ale, Sprite, Slice, Fresca, 7-Up, root beer orange/grape/strawberry, PowerAde, tonic water	0

Item	Caffeine /mg Range
Diet (12 oz)	
Tab	46
diet cola, Dr Pepper	36-59
Sugar-free Big Red	38
diet Mr PIBB	40
diet Mello Yello	52
Canada Dry Diet Cola, Fresca	1-4
caffeine-free diet cola	0
Diet Sprite, Diet Slice, Diet Orange Diet Root Beer, Diet 7-Up	0

See also caffeine medication entry, p 38 and caffeine section, p 237.
References: 6, 7, 13, 28, 55, 56, 57.

SALT SUBSTITUTES

BRAND	**K/5 gm**	**Na/5 gm**
Accent	600 mg	0
Adolph's	2340 mg	0
Lawry's Seasoned Salt Substitute	1160 mg	0
NoSalt	2500 mg	0
Morton Seasoned Salt Free	2542 mg	0

BRAND	**K/5 gm**	**Na/5 gm**
Nu-salt	2640 mg	1 mg
Papa Dash (85% Na free)	2000 mg	360 mg
Morton Lite Salt	1214 mg	1036 mg
McCormick's Saltless	0	0
Mrs. Dash (multiple var.)	0	0
(One of many Na- and K free herbal mixtures)		

HIGH OXALATE (OXALIC ACID) FOOD SOURCES

(All > 15 mg oxalate per 100 gm serving)

Fruits
*rhubarb
*gooseberries
*citrus peel
raspberries, black
grapes, Concord
currants, red
blueberries
blackberries
raspberries, red
strawberries

Vegetables
*swiss chard
*cassava root
*amaranth
*spinach, raw
*collards
*pursalane
*parsley, raw
*okra
*beet leaves/root
*leeks
sweet potatoes

Beverages (5 - 10 oz)
beer: Lager draft, Pilsner
juices (containing berries)
Ovaltine and other mixes
tea (oxalate content ↑ $\overline{c}$ ↑ brewing time)
Coffee powder (Nescafe)
colas

Miscellaneous
nuts: *almonds
*peanuts
*pecans
*wheat germ
*poppy seeds
*peanut butter
*chocolate, cocoa
*soybean crackers
*pepper (> 1 tsp/day)
grits (white corn)

Foods are listed in decreasing oxalate content. 40-50 mg/day = low-oxalate intake. Reference 40.
* = > 70 mg/100 gm.

HIGH PHYTATE (PHYTIC ACID) FOOD SOURCES

FOOD ITEM	PHYTIC ACID (mg)
Grain/Grain Products	
wheat bran, crude - 1 oz (28 gm)	843
wheat germ - 1 T (6 gm)	244
barley, whole grain - 3.5 oz (100 gm)	970
barley, pearl, raw - 3.5 oz (100 gm)	491
oats, raw - 3.5 oz (100 gm)	943
corn chips - 1 oz (28 gm)	178
Cereals - 1 oz: All Bran	679
Shredded Wheat	415
wheat flakes	411
oatmeal (cooked) .5 cup	113
Bread, rye 1 slice	235
Nuts, Nut products and Seeds	
nuts: 3.5 oz (100 gm)	
almonds	1280
brazil nuts	1799
coconut, raw	270
hazelnuts	604
peanuts	748
walnuts	760
peanut butter - 1T (16 gm)	200
sesame seeds, raw - 1 oz (28 gm)	1319

FOOD ITEM	PHYTIC ACID (mg)
Vegetables 3.5 oz (100 gm)	
rice, wild, raw	2200
rice, brown, raw	890
rice, white, long-grain, raw	340
rice, white, short-grain, raw	140
kidney beans, raw	1200-2060
garbanzo beans, raw	280
navy beans, raw	280
peas, dried, raw	851
pinto beans, raw	620-1950
white beans, raw	1030
Miscellaneous 3.5 oz (100 gm)	
cocoa, dry pwd 1 T (5 gm)	94
soybean meal	1400-1600
soybean protein concentrate	1240-2170
soybean protein isolate	430-1170

The phytic acid content varies according to plant part and state of maturity at harvest.[55] References: 13, 52, 55 (14th edition).

PRESSOR AGENTS IN FOODS AND BEVERAGES

(Tyramine, Dopamine, Phenylethylamine)

FOODS THAT MUST BE AVOIDED

aged cheeses and meats
salami or mortadella
air-dried sausage
fermented bean curd
soya bean, soya bean paste
MSG
Miso Soup
fava (Italian green beans), snowpea or broad bean pods (contain dopamine)
sauerkraut, kim chee
pickled herring brine
hydrolyzed protein extracts (soup/gravy bases)
concentrated yeast extracts (Marmite)
Brewer's yeast (vitamin supplements)
malt beverages, Chianti wine
alcohol-free beer (also 'home brew')

FOODS THAT MAY BE USED WITH CAUTION* (Limit total intake to 1/4-1/2 cup or 2-4 ozs per day.)

bologna, pepperoni
fresh liver, liverwurst
aged kielbasa sausage
pate, lumpfish roe
smoked meats and fish
Schmaltz herring in oil
soy sauce
avocado, figs, banana, raspberries
peanuts
chocolate, coffee, cola*
pickled herring (avoid brine)

FOODS NOT LIMITED (Based on current analyses)

unfermented cheeses (cream, cottage, ricotta, processed)
smoked white fish, salmon, carp, smoked anchovies
canned figs, raisins
fresh pineapple
beetroot, cucumber
sweet corn, mushrooms
salad dressings, tomato sauce
baked raised products, English cookies
boiled egg, yogurt, junket
Worcestershire sauce,
curry powder
other beers, wines, vodka, gin

HISTAMINE: Content is highest in fish (tuna, sardines, skipjack) that is beyond optimal freshness.

*Caffeine, a weak pressor agent, in quantities > 500 mg per day may exacerbate reactions.
See also Tyramine p 238. References: 9, 10, 21, 52, 59

HERBAL TEAS AND REMEDIES: CAUTIONS

Burdock, juniper, jimson weed, paniculata hydrangea: Can induce bizarre anticholinergic effects.
Chamomile, yarrow: Allergic reactions in people allergic to ragweed, asters, marigold, golden rod, or chrysanthemums.
Chaparral: Acute toxic hepatitis reported.
Coltsfoot: Contains senkirkine and hepatotoxic, carcinogenic pyrrolizidine alkaloid.
Comfrey: Contains hepatotoxic pyrrolizidine alkaloids. Deadly nightshade contamination may cause atropine poisoning.
Foxglove, dogbane, lily-of-the-valley, oleander: Have digitalis-like activity and can cause digitalis toxicity.
Gurana: Commonly found in herbal remedies, contains more caffeine than any other plant (3-5x).
Ginseng: Contains triterpenoid saponins, ↓ serum glucose; LT use mimics corticosteroid poisoning (↑ or ↓ BP, CNS effects).
Horse chestnut, buckeye (aesculus): Contains a toxic coumarin glycoside.
Jin bu huan: contains natural morphine-like compounds, and levotetrahydropalmatine which is believed to cause acute hepatitis even when the remedy is taken according to package directions.
Licorice root: ↑ amounts may cause Na & H_2O retention, K loss, diarrhea, ↑ BP, & c̄ LT use- cardiac arrest.
Ma Huang (Ephedra): Contains ephedrine, a cardiac stimulant.
Mandrake (may be packaged for sale as ginseng): Contains a strong hallucinogen.
Mistletoe (viscum) all varieties: Contains pressor amines B-phenylethylamine and tyramine.
Sassafras: Contains safrole a potent carcinogen (FDA banned for food use but sold in health food stores).
Seeds, pits, bark or leaves of apple, apricot, bitter almond, cassava bean, cherry, peach: Contain compounds that liberate hydrogen cyanide. Large intake may cause cyanide poisoning.
Senna, aloe, buckthorn bark, dock roots: Strong irritant cathartic laxatives, can cause diarrhea.
Shave grass, wormwood: Can cause acute neurotoxicity, diarrhea.
Symphytum (Comfrey): Contains hepatotoxic pyrrolizidine alkaloids; highest levels occur in roots.
Indian Tobacco: Contains lobeline, a CNS stimulant - large doses can cause coma and death.
Tonka beans, melilot, woodruff: Contain natural coumarins and can cause coagulation defects, liver damage.
Vinca (greater and lesser periwinkle): senecio longilobus (thread-leafed groundsel): Contain toxic alkaloids vinblastine and vincristine that cause cytotoxic and neurological actions, hepatotoxicity.

References: 15, 34, 60, 73

OSMOLALITIES OF SELECTED BEVERAGES AND FOODS

Osmolality refers to the number and size of particles per kilogram of water. Expressed in osmoles or milliosmoles per kg water. Extracellular fluid is 280 to 300 mOsms/kg water. Normal serum is 275 to 325.

Patients with limited gastrointestinal tolerance should receive hyposmolar or mildly hyperosmolar liquids (< 400 mOsm). Because of high osmolality some food/liquids may need to be diluted initially.

Beverage	Dilution	mOsm/kg
Juices		
prune	1:3	1,076
cranberry	1:3	836
pineapple	-	772
apple	-	705
tomato, grapefruit	-	619
orange	-	601
V-8	-	578
low-calorie cranberry	-	287
Coffee/tea (1 cup)		
coffee with 1 tsp sugar	-	128
tea with 1 tsp sugar	-	106
coffee	-	83
tea	-	8
Enteral Formulas		
isotonic (Isocal, Jevity, Osmolite, Ultracal)	-	300-310
1.0 cal/mL (Ensure, Resource, Sustacal)	-	430-650
1.5 cal/mL (Ensure Plus, Sustacal HC, Resource Plus)	-	600-690

Beverage	Dilution	mOsm/kg
Broth		
↓ Na, low-fat chicken	-	452
regular chicken	-	389
Jello		
cherry, ($\bar{c}$ sugar)	1:4	735
sugar-free	-	57
Milk/Milk Products		
human milk	-	277-303
ice cream	-	1,150
Carnation Instant Breakfast		
made $\bar{c}$ skim milk	-	617
made $\bar{c}$ whole milk	-	653
eggnog	-	695
skim milk $\bar{c}$ Lactaid	-	375
whole milk $\bar{c}$ Lactaid		413
skim milk		280
whole milk	-	277
Soft Drinks		
cola	-	714
ginger ale	-	565
diet ginger ale/cola	-	43-50
Water Ice, cherry	1:3	1,064

References: 16, 32, 52, 61 & manufacturer's information

pH and ACID CONTENT OF BEVERAGES

Active peptic ulcer or GERD: Some juices and most carbonated beverages have a pH low enough (< 3.5) to activate pepsin. Acid content is comparable to or exceeds the basal gastric secretion. Avoidance of extrinsic sources of acid may decrease patient discomfort.

Fruit or vegetable products	**pH**	**mEq acid/cc**
vinegar (cider)	3.1-3.2	0.60-.64
grapefruit, pineapple, orange	3.4-3.8	0.12-.17
cranberry	2.6-2.8	0.080-.081
grape, apple, apricot nectar	3.3-3.8	0.055-.096
orange drink	2.6	0.055
tomato	4.3	0.049-.059
peach nectar	3.6	0.038-.039
prune	4.1-4.2	0.031-.036
pear nectar	3.7	0.021-.022
Milk		
skim	6.5-6.7	0.007-.009
half & half cream	6.6-6.7	0.005-.007
whole	6.6-6.7	0.005-.006

Carbonated beverages	**pH**	**mEq acid/cc**
orange soda	2.8	0.056-.058
cola (average)	2.4	0.037-.057
diet cola (can)	2.9	0.042
(soda open 1 hour)	2.9-3.1	0.057-.082
7-Up	3.0-3.1	0.048-.055
ginger ale (can)	2.7-2.9	0.041-0.054
club soda	3.7	0.046
Other beverages		
coffee (whole)	4.9-5.1	0.004-.006
Sanka (instant)	5.1-5.4	0.004-.006
cocoa (instant)	6.7-6.9	0.001-.002
tea (instant)	6.8-6.9	0.001-.002
tap water	7.6-8.2	————

References: #64; Manufacturer's information; New England Journal of Medicine; 11/21/85, p. 1351

MAGNESIUM (Mg) SIGNIFICANT DIETARY SOURCES*

Fruits and Vegetables

Avocado, banana, adzuki beans, blackeye peas (cowpeas), cassava (raw), chickpeas (garbanzo beans), great northern beans, kidney beans, lentils, lima beans, lupins, navy beans, pigeonpeas, pink beans, pinto beans, potato with skin (baked or microwaved), raisins, seaweed, soybeans, spinach, Swiss chard, white beans, yellow beans.

Grains and Grain Products

(More than 80% of the Mg is lost by removal of the germ and outer layers of cereal grains.)[47]
Amaranth, barley, buckwheat, buckwheat flour, granola, oats (whole grain), oat bran, rice (brown), rice (wild), rice bran, rye flour, triticale flour, wheat bran, wheat germ, whole wheat flour. Whole wheat pasta. High bran cereals (eg All Bran, 100% Bran, Bran Buds, bran flakes, raisin bran).

Nuts and Seeds

(Dried nuts or seeds provide more Mg than roasted.)
Pumpkin seeds, sunflower seeds, sesame seeds, almonds, cashews, sunflower seeds, hazel nuts, brazil nuts, peanuts, black walnuts, pistachios, English walnuts, macadamia nuts, pecans.

Other

Molasses, hummus, soybean products: flour, natto, miso, tempeh, raw tofu.

* 30 mg or more Magnesium/100 g See also **magnesium p 122.** References: 16, 34, 47, 52, 55

POTASSIUM (K) SIGNIFICANT DIETARY SOURCES

Vegetables and Fruits

Standard servings provide approximately 150-600 mg potassium

asparagus	cauliflower	pumpkin, cooked
artichoke	celery, Pascal type raw 2 stalks	seaweed
bamboo shoots, raw	kale	spinach, turnip greens
beets, cooked drained	mushrooms, raw boiled	squash, winter
broccoli	okra pods, cooked	sweet potato
Brussels sprouts, raw, cooked	potato	tomato, tomato juice
carrots, carrot juice	potato chips	tomato paste
beans: adzuki, black, kidney, lentil, lima, pinto, red, soy, white		vegetable juice 6 oz

Standard servings provide approximately 300-500 mg potassium

apricots, raw	cantaloupe	kiwifruit	prune juice 5 oz
avocado 1/3 whole	grapefruit juice	orange juice	strawberries
banana 1 small	honeydew	orange, 1	tangerine juice
dried fruit: apple, apricots, dates, pear, peach, prune, raisins,			

Cereal and Breads

Serving sizes average approximately 230 mg K

All Bran	Bran Flakes	Mueslix	Raisin Bran
Bread pumpernickel, 2 slices			

Miscellaneous 100-200 mg K

almonds, 12-15	coffee, 10 oz	pecans	tea, 14 oz
Brazil nuts, 5 medium	filberts, hazelnuts	peanuts	tofu
cashews	fruitcake	peanut butter	sunflower seeds
chestnuts, 4 large	molasses	pumpkin seeds	walnuts

Table prepared by Joanna Steinman, RD, LD; Polybytes & Zaneta Pronsky, MS, RD.

VITAMIN K SIGNIFICANT DIETARY SOURCES*

Fats and Oils

(Exposure to fluorescent and sunlight rapidly destroys vitamin K in oils.)

Canola (rapeseed) oil, soybean oil

Vegetables

(Higher concentrations of Vitamin K are found in the outer leaves and peels of vegetables.) Broccoli, brussel sprouts, cabbage (green raw), cauliflower, chayote leaf, chickpeas (garbanzo beans), chive (raw), coriander leaf, cucumber peel, endive, kale, lettuce, lentils, mint, mung beans, mustard greens, nettle leaves, purslane, scallions (green onions), seaweed (extremely high levels), soybeans, spinach, Swiss chard, turnip greens, watercress.

Other

Beef liver, chicken liver, pork liver, egg yolk, green tea leaves, algae (purple laver and hijiki).

* 50 mg or more Vit K/100 g See also **Vitamin K p 212** References: 47, 52, 55, 81

DRUGS NOT COMPATIBLE WITH TUBE FEEDING

The following drugs, when combined with enteral products*, cause thickening or clumping as detected by visual inspection. This may clog the feeding tube. This occurs most frequently with highly acidic syrups (pH > 4.0) & bulk-forming agents. Liquid forms of drugs should be used whenever possible.

Many drugs have not been tested. Lack of inclusion in this list does not guarantee compatibility.

aluminum hydroxide (Amphogel)
al-mg hydroxide, double strength (Mylanta II)
(regular strength was compatible)
calcium glubionate (Neo-Calglucon Syrup)
chlorpromazine (Thorazine Concentrate)
cimetidine HCl (Tagamet Liquid)
dicyclomine (Bentyl Liquid)
Dimetane/Dimetapp Elixir
ferrous sulfate (Feosol Elixir)
Fleet Phospho-soda (Na biphosphate + Na phosphate)
guaifenesin (Robitussin Syrup)

lithium carbonate (Cibalith-S syrup)
magaldrate (Riopan)**
mandelamine suspension (see below)
metoclopromide (Reglan Syrup)
Paregoric Elixir (opium, 45% alcohol)
potassium chloride (some liquid forms)
(KCl Liquid 10 & 20%, Klorvess Syrup)
pseudoephedrine (Sudafed Syrup)
thioridazine (Mellaril Solution)[70]
(concentrate was compatible)[71]
zinc sulfate (capsules)

Administer separately from tube feedings due to possible effects on bioavailability:
phenytoin (Dilantin) tetracycline theophylline

* Ensure, Ensure HN, Ensure Plus, Ensure Plus HN, Enrich, Osmolite, Osmolite HN, Two-Cal HN. Elemental products, Vital and Vivonex TEN were also tested. No incompatibility was found with these products, except c̄ mandelamine suspension (incompatible c̄ Vital)

** Compatible c̄ Osmolite HN, but not Osmolite.

References: 8, 11a, 32, 69, 70, 71, 72

REFERENCES

1. **AMA Drug Evaluations**, 1995 Annual, American Medical Assoc. (Chicago, IL, Amer Med Assoc., 1995)
2. **Handbook of Nonprescription Drugs**, 9th Edition, American Pharmaceutical Assoc. (Washington, DC, American Pharmaceutical Assoc., 1990)
3. **Drug Interaction Facts**, Tatro, D.S., Editor (St Louis, MO, Facts and Comparisons, thru July, 1995)
4. Gilman, A.G.; Rall, T.W.; Nies, A.S. & Taylor, P., **The Pharmacological Basis of Therapeutics**, 8th Edition (New York City, NY, McGraw Hill, 1990)
5. Hansten, P.D., **Drug Interactions**, 5th Edition (Philadelphia, PA, Lea & Febiger, 1985)
6. **AHFS Drug Information 95**, McEvoy, G.K., Editor (Bethesda, MD, American Society of Health Pharmacists, 1995)
7. **Facts and Comparisons**, Olin, B.R., Editor-in-Chief (St. Louis, MO, Facts & Comparisons, thru July, 1995)
8. **Nutrition and Drug Therapy: Clinical Pharmacology, Drug Compatibility and Stability** (Silver Spring, MD, A.S.P.E.N., 1992)

9 a. "The Medical Letter on Drugs and Therapeutics" (New Rochelle, NY, The Medical Letter, Inc.) thru Vol. 37 (952), July, 1995

b. **The Medical Letter Handbook of Adverse Drug Interactions**, 1995

10 a. **Physicians Desk Reference**, 49th Edition (Montvale, NJ, Medical Economics Co., 1995)

b. **PDR for Nonprescription Drugs**, 16th Edition

c. **PDR Guide to Drug Interactions, Side Effects, Indications,** 49th Edition

11. Roe, D.A.:

a. **Diet and Drug Interactions** (New York, NY, Van Nostrand Reinhold, 1989)

b. **Geriatric Nutrition**, 3rd Edition (Englewood Cliffs, NJ, Prentice-Hall Inc., 1992)

c. **Handbook on Drug & Nutrient Interactions**, 4th Edition
(Chicago, IL, American Dietetic Assoc., 1989)
d. **Drugs & Nutrition in the Geriatric Patient,** Editor (New York City, NY, Churchill-Livingston, 1984)
e. "Therapeutic Effects of Drug-Nutrient Interactions in the Elderly", 1985 JADA 85(2):174

12. Schneider, H.A.; Anderson, C.E. & Coursin, D.B. **Nutritional Support of Medical Practice** (Hagerstown, MD, Medical Dept., Harper & Row, 1977)
13. **United States Pharmacopeia Dispensing Information**, 15th Edition (Rockville, MD, U.S. Pharmacopeial Convention, 1995)
    Vol. I, **Drug Information for the Care Professional**; Vol. II, **Advice for the Patient** & Updates
14. Smith, C.H., Editor, "Dietary Concerns Associated with the Use of Medications, 1984 JADA 84(8):901
    "Drug-Food/Food-Drug Interactions" Chapter 30, **Geriatric Nutrition** (New York, NY, Raven Press, 1995)
15. Tyler, V.E., **The Honest Herbal** (Binghamton, NY, Haworth Press, 1993)
16. **Manual of Clinical Dietetics**, 4th Edition, American Dietetic Assoc, Chicago, IL, 1992
17. **Psychotropic Drugs**, Keltner, N.L. & Folks, D.G.; (St Louis, MO, Mosby Year Book, 1993)
18. Pandit, M.K., et al "Drug-induced Disorders of Glucose Tolerance", 1993 Ann Intern Med 118:529-539
19. Bezchlidnyk, K.Z., "Should Psychiatric Patients Drink Coffee?", 1981 Can Med Assoc J, 124:4, Feb 15, 1981
20. Smith, C.H. & Bidlack, W.R.:
    "Food and Drug Interactions", Food Technology, Oct. 1982, 99-103
    "Effect of Nutritional Factors on Hepatic Drug & Toxicant Metabolism", 1984 JADA 84(8):892
21. Gelenberg, A.J.; *Biological Therapies in Psychiatry Newsletter* (St. Louis, MO, Mosby-Year Book) thru July, 1995

22. Fairweather-Tait, S., et al "Orange Juice enhances Aluminum Absorption from Antacid Preparation", 1994 Eur Jour Clin Nutr 48: 71
23. **Remington: The Science and Practice of Pharmacy**, Gennaro, A.R., Editor, 19th Edition (Easton, Pa, Mack Publishing, 1995)
24. Strain, E.C. et al, "Caffeine Dependence Syndrome" 1994 JAMA 272: 1043-1048
25. **Psychotropic Drug Handbook**, 6th Edition, Perry, A.J., Editor (Cincinnati, OH, Harvey Whitney, 1991)
26. Gahart, B.L., **Intravenous Medications**, 11th Edition (St. Louis, MO., Mosby Year Book, 1995)
27. Murray, J.J. & Healy, M.D.; "Drug-Mineral Interactions: a New Responsibility for The Hospital Dietitian", 1991 JADA; 91: 66-73
28. *FDA Consumer*, US Dept. of Health Services, Rockville, MD, 1983-1990.
29. Miletic, I.D. et al, "Identification of Gliadin Presence in Pharmaceutical Products", 1994 Jour Ped Gastro Nutr 19: 27-33
30. Lamy, P.P.:
    a. "How Your Patient's Diet Can Affect Drug Response", 1980 Drug Therapy, 10(8): 82-90
    b. "Effects of Diet & Nutrition on Drug Therapy", 1982 J Am Geriatr Soc, supplement Vol. 30:(11): 99
    c. "A Consideration of NSAID Use in the Elderly", 1988 Geriatric Medicine Today, 7(4)
31. National Research Council **Health Effects of Ingested Fluoride** (Washington, DC, National Academy Press, 1993)
32. **Nutrition Support Handbook**, Teasley-Strausburg, K.M., Editor (Cincinnati, OH, Harvey-Whitney Books, 1992)
33. Richter, W.O. et al, "Interaction between Fibre and Lovastatin", 1994 The Lancet 338: 706
34. Merritt, R.J., editor *Nutrition & the MD*, San Diego, CA, Quest Publishing, thru Vol. 21, #6, 1995

35. "Protein Distribution Diets in the Management of Fluctuations in Levodopa Response" Special Report 1994 Drugs & Nutrients in Neurology, NMIN
36. Karstaedt, P.J. & Pincus, J.H., "Protein Redistribution Diet Remains Effective in Patients with Fluctuating Parkinsonism", 1992 Arch Neurol 49(2): 149-151.
37. Haas, E., & Lemmons, A., "Drug-induced Taste Disorders", Current Concepts in Hosp Phar Management, 1988, p 16
38. Grant, A. & DeHoog, S. **Nutritional Assessment and Support**, 4th Edition (Seattle, WA, Grant & DeHoog, 1991)
39. Wodarski, L.A., et al, "Hypercholesterolemia and Developmental Disabilities", 1993 Topics in Clin Nutr 8(4): 66-74
40. Ney, D.M.; Hofmann, A.F.; Fischer, C. & Stubblefield, H. **Low Oxalate Diet Book** (San Diego, U Calif Med Ctr, 1981)
41. Pinto J.T & Rivlin R.S., "Drugs That Promote Renal Excretion of Riboflavin", 1987 Drug Nutrient Interactions 5:143-151
42. The Psychiatric Times Vol. V (6), June, 1988
43. Emerson, A.P., "Foods High in Fiber and Phytobezoar Formation", 1987 JADA, 87:1675
44. Garabedian-Ruffalo, S.M. & Ruffalo, R.L., "Drug and Nutrient Interactions", 1986 Am Fam Physician 33(2):165-174
45. Petersdor, R.G. et al **Harrison's Principles of Internal Medicine**, 11th Ed (NYC, NY, McGraw-Hill Book Co., 1987)
46. Houts, S.S., "Lactose Intolerance", Food Technology, March, 1988, p. 110
47. National Academy of Sciences (NRC), **1989 Recommended Dietary Allowances**, 10th Edition, Washington, DC, 1989

48. Pinto, J.T., "The Pharmacokinetic and Pharmacodynamic Interactions of Food and Drugs", 1991 Top Clin Nutr, 6(3):14
49. Fischbach, F.T., **A Manual of Laboratory & Diagnostic Tests**; 4th Edition (Philadelphia, PA, J.B. Lippincott Co., 1992)
50. Bailey, D.G. et al, "Grapefruit Juice and Drugs: How Significant is the Interaction?" 1994 Clin Pharm 26(2): 91-98
51. Menon, I.S, et al, "Effect of Onions on Blood Fibrinolytic Activity", 1968 Br Med J, 3:351
52. Mahan, L.K. & Arlin, M.T.; **Krause's Food, Nutrition, & Diet Therapy**, 8th Edition (Phila, PA, W.B. Saunders, 1992)
53. Long, P., "The Vitamin Wars", Health, May/June 1993, p. 45.
54. **Vitamin Preparations as Dietary Supplements and as Therapeutic Agents**, Council on Scientific Affairs, AMA, 1987 JAMA, 257:1929
55. Pennington, J.A.T., **Bowes & Church's Food Values of Portions Commonly Used**, 15th Ed (NYC, NY, Harper & Row, 1989)
56. **Evaluation of Caffeine Safety. A Scientific Status Summary**. Institute of Food Technologist's Expert Panel, June, 1987
57. Consumer Information, Coca-Cola Co., Consumer Information Center, (PO Box 1734, Atlanta, GA 30301), 1993
58. Tilkian, S.M., Conover, M.B. & Tilkian, A.G.; **Clinical Implications of Laboratory Tests**, 3rd Edition (St. Louis, MO, Mosby Year-Book, 1983)

59. McCabe, B.J.:
& Tsuang, M.T., "Dietary Considerations in MAO Inhibitor Regimens", J Clin Psychiatry Vol. 43:5, May, 1982.
"The MAOI Diet", Massachusetts General Hospital Newsletter, Biological Therapies in Psychiatry 1987 10(2)
"Dietary Tyramine and Other Pressor Amines in MAOI Regimes: A Review", 1986 JADA, Perspectives in Practice 86:1059
60. Siler, N.P., "Problems with Ingestion of Herbs or Plant Products", Nutrition Faddism, TDA Diet Manual, Texas Diet Assoc., 1988
61. Robinson, C.H.; Lawler, M.R.; Chenoweth, W.L. & Garwick, A.E.; **Normal and Therapeutic Nutrition**, 17th Edition (NYC, NY, Macmillan Publishing Co., 1986)
62. National Soft Drink Assoc., "What's in Soft Drinks?" pamphlet, Washington, DC, September, 1982
63. Wallach, J. **Interpretation of Diagnostic Tests**, 4th Edition (Boston/Toronto, Little, Brown and Company", 1986)
64. Flick, A.L., "Acid Content of Common Beverages" 1970 Digestive Diseases, 15:317-320, University Hospital, San Diego, CA.
65. Trovato, A., et al, "Drug-Nutrient Interactions", 1991 Am Fam Physician 44(5): 1651-1658
66. Simonsen, L. L., "Top 200 Drugs" April 1995 Pharmacy Times p 17- 24
67. Huxtable, R.J., "The Myth of Beneficent Nature: The Risks of Herbal Preparations", 1992 Ann Int Med 117(2): 165-166
68. Charuhas, P.M. & Aker, S.N., "Nutritional Implications of Antineoplastic Chemotherapeutic Agents", 1992 Clin Applied Nutr 2(2): 20-33
69. Holtz, L et al Compatibility of Medications with Enteral Feedings", 1987 JPEN 11(2); 183-186

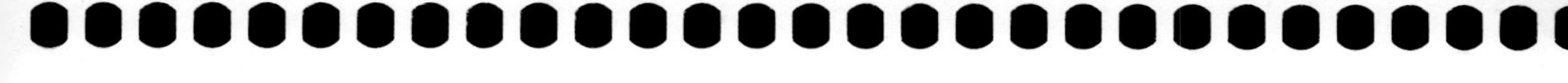

70. Cutie, A.J et al "Compatibility of Enteral Products with Commonly Employed Drug Additives," 1983 JPEN 7(2):186-191
71. Burns, P.E et al "Physical Compatibility of Enteral Formulas with Various Common Medications." 1988 JADA 88(9): 1094-6
72. Rombeau, J.L. & Caldwell, M.D. **Enteral and Tube Feeding**, 2nd Edition (W.B. Saunders, 1990, Philadelphia, PA)
73. *Environmental Nutrition,* New York City, NY, Environmental Nutrition, Inc. thru Vol. 18, #7, 1995
74. Hartshorn, E.A. "Effect of Histamine H2-Receptor Antagonists on Vitamin B12 Absorption", 1992 Ann Pharmacother 26: 1283-6
75. Buchman, A.L. et al, "Selenium Renal Homeostasis is Impaired in Patients Receiving Long-Term Total Parenteral Nutrition", 1994 JPEN 18:231-233
76. Love, R.R. et al, "Effects of Tamoxifen on Cardiovascular Risk Factors in Postmenopausal Women" 1991 Ann Intern Med 115:860-864
77. Shils, M.E., Olson, J.A., Shike, M., **Modern Nutrition in Health and Disease**, 8th Ed (Phila, PA, Lea & Febiger, 1994)
78. *Tufts University Diet & Nutrition Letter,* New York City, NY, thru Vol. 13, #4, June, 1995
79. Harris, J.E., "Interaction of Dietary Factors with Oral Anticoagulants: Review and Applications" 1995 JADA 95(5):580-584
80. Giraud, D.W. et al, "Plasma and Dietary Vitamin C and E Levels of Tobacco Chewers, Smokers and Nonusers" 1995 JADA 95(7) 798-799

NOTES

NOTES

NOTES

WINDOWS SOFTWARE ORDER FORM

SEND SOFTWARE TO:

NAME: ____________________

ADDRESS: ____________________

____

CITY: ____________ STATE: ________ ZIP: ________

PHONE: (   ) ____________ QUANTITY: ________ @ ________ $ ________

SOFTWARE REQUIREMENTS:

IBM PC OR COMPATIBLE
4 MB RAM
6 MB FREE HARD DISK
80386 CPU OR HIGHER
WINDOWS VER 3.1 OR LATER

☐ **SEND 3 1/2" (1.44MB) DISKETTES OR**
☐ **SEND 5 1/4" (1.2MB) DISKETTES**

PRICE: (INCLUDES ONE COPY NINTH EDITION BOOK)

$189.95

NETWORK COMPATIBLE
CALL FOR MULTI-USER PRICING

SHIPPING AND HANDLING:
$8.00 PER PROGRAM
$25.00 PER PROGRAM ORDER-CANADA
$40.00 PER PROGRAM ORDER-INTERNATIONAL

☐ VISA ☐ MasterCard

CREDIT CARD NUMBER ____________________

EXP DATE ____________________

SIGNATURE ____________________

PENNSYLVANIA RESIDENTS
ADD 6% SALES TAX $ ________

SHIPPING & HANDLING $ ________

TOTAL ENCLOSED $ ________

PREPAYMENT REQUIRED.

CHECKS MUST BE IN US FUNDS DRAWN ON A US BANK.

ALLOW 4-6 WEEKS FOR DELIVERY.

ENCLOSE THIS ORDER FORM WITH YOUR CHECK, MONEY ORDER OR CREDIT CARD INFORMATION TO:

FOOD-MEDICATION INTERACTIONS
PO BOX 659
POTTSTOWN, PA 19464
PHONE: 610-970-7143 FAX 610-970-5470

SEE OTHER SIDE FOR NINTH EDITION BOOK ORDER FORM